TRANSFERRIN BIOLOGY

Papers by
Stuart Kornfeld, Roberta M. Palmour, A. Stratil, J. Williams, Rainer Hans Zschocke, Andrew Ferguson, Shou-Hsian Mao, R.L. Spooner, Robert H. Tamarin, Leona Caroline. T.A. Douglas, Jeffrey A. Frelinger, H. McFarlane, E.H. Morgan, et al.

MSS Information Corporation
655 Madison Avenue, New York, N.Y. 10021

Library of Congress Cataloging in Publication Data
Main entry under title:

Transferrin biology.

1. Transferrin--Addresses, essays, lectures.
I. Kornfeld, Stuart. [DNLM: 1. Transferrin--
Collected works. WH 400 T772 1973]
QP551.T724 599'.01'13 72-13431
ISBN 0-8422-7088-4

TABLE OF CONTENTS

CREDITS AND ACKNOWLEDGEMENTS

Caroline, Leona; Fred Rosner; and Philip J. Kozinn, "Elevated Serum Iron, Low Unbound Transferrin and Candidiasis in Acute Leukemia," *Blood*, 1969, 34:441-451.

Douglas, T.A.; J.P. Renton; and C. Watts, "Placental Transfer of Iron in the Rabbit," *British Journal of Haematology*, 1971, 20:185-194.

Ferguson, Andrew, "Geographic and Species Variation in Transferrin and Ovotransferrin Polymorphism in the Columbidae," *Comparative Biochemistry and Physiology*, 1971, 38B:477-486.

Frelinger, Jeffrey A., "Maternally Derived Transferrin in Pigeon Squabs," *Science*, 1971, 171:1259-1261.

Kornfeld, Stuart, "The Effect of Metal Attachment to Human Apotransferrin on Its Binding to Reticulocytes," *Biochimica et Biophysica Acta*, 1969, 194:25-33.

Mao, Shou-Hsian; and Herbert C. Dessauer, "Selectively Neutral Mutations: Transferrins and the Evolution of Natricine Snakes,"*Comparative Biochemistry and Physiology*, 1971, 40A:669-680.

McFarlane, H.; S. Reddy;K.J. Adcock; H. Adeshina; and A.R. Cooke, "Immunity, Transferrin, and Survival in Kwashiorkor," *British Medical Journal*, 1970, 4:268-270.

Morgan, E.H., "A Study of Iron Transfer from Rabbit Transferrin to Reticulocytes Using Synthetic Chelating Agents," *Biochimica et Biophysica Acta*, 1971, 103:116.

Morgan, E.H., "Factors Affecting the Synthesis of Transferrin by Rat Tissue Slices," *The Journal of Biological Chemistry*, 1969, 244: 4193-4199.

Morgan, E.H., "Transferrin and Albumin Distribution and Turnover in the Rabbit," *Australian Journal of Experimental Biology and Medical Science*, 1969, 47:361-366.

Morgan, E.H.; and Erica Baker, "The Effect of Metabolic Inhibitors on Transferrin and Iron Uptake and Transferrin Release from Reticulocytes," *Biochimica et Biophysica Acta*, 1969, 184:442-454.

Palmour, Roberta M.; and H. Eldon Sutton, "Vertebrate Transferrins: Molecular Weights, Chemical Compositions, and Iron-Binding Studies," *Biochemistry*, 1971, 10:4026-4032.

Spooner, R.L.; and G. Baxter, "Abnormal Expression of Normal Transferrin Alleles in Cattle," *Biochemical Genetics*, 1969, 2:371-382.

Spooner, R.L.; R.B. Land; R.A. Oliver; and A. Stratil, "Foetal and Neonatal Transferrins in Cattle," *Animal Blood Groups and Biochemical Genetics*, 1970, 1:241-246.

Stratil, A.; and R.L. Spooner, "Isolation and Properties of Individual Components of Cattle Transferrin: The Role of Sialic Acid," *Biochemical Genetics*, 1971, 5:347-365.

Tamarin, Robert H.; and Charles J. Krebs, "*Microtus* Population Biology. II. Genetic Changes at the Transferrin Locus in Fluctuating Populations of Two Vole Species," *Evolution*, 1969, 23:183-211.

Williams, J.; C.F. Phelps; and J.M. Lowe, "Ovotransferrin with One Iron Atom," *Nature*, 1970, 226:858-859.

Zschocke, Rainer Hans; and Anatoly Bezkorovainy, "Some Immunochemical Properties of Succinylated Human Transferrin and Related Proteins," *Biochimica et Biophysica Acta*, 1970, 200:241-246.

PREFACE

Transferrins are a group of non-heme iron binding proteins. Since their initial description in 1952, they have been the subject of research from a biochemical, physiological and genetic point of view. Biochemists have centered on the primary structure and ligand binding of the protein. The physiologists have been interested in its role in the regulation of erythropoeisis and in iron metabolism in general. The geneticists have been intrigued with its widespread polymorphism, and have studied it with the hope that it will lead to a better understanding of the evolutionary process.

The basic role of transferrin in iron transport is well established. Current work in physiology focuses on the interaction of transferrin and reticulocytes. Considerable progress has been made in the area, and evidence suggests that this will develop into a model system for the study of protein-membrane interactions. Genetics has turned its attention to the problem of maintaining polymorphism in populations with some success, while biochemistry is still struggling with the structure of the molecule.

These readings were selected to present an overview of this exciting research. Although the articles chosen are not meant to be all inclusive, they will provide one with a basic understanding of transferrin genetics — from populations to molecules.

Jeffrey A. Frelinger, Ph.D.
Ronald T. Acton, Ph.D.
January, 1973

The Biochemistry of Transferrins

THE EFFECT OF METAL ATTACHMENT TO HUMAN APOTRANSFERRIN ON ITS BINDING TO RETICULOCYTES

STUART KORNFELD

INTRODUCTION

The plasma glycoprotein transferrin functions primarily in the transport of Fe^{3+} from sites of Fe^{3+} absorption and storage to immature red blood cells[1-3]. The molecule has a molecular weight of approx. 90 000 and binds 2 moles of Fe^{3+} per mole of protein. The two metal binding sites are independent of each other and have approximately equal stability constants[4,5]. Several investigators have shown that when Fe^{3+} binds to apotransferrin a number of changes occur in the physical and chemical properties of the molecule[6-9]. However, considerably less is known about the consequences of metal binding to apotransferrin on the biological properties of the molecule. There are conflicting reports concerning the effect that bound Fe^{3+} exerts on the binding of transferrin to reticulocyte receptor sites[10,11]. Further, while Cu^{2+} and Cr^{3+} can occupy the Fe^{3+} binding sites of transferrin, the biological results of this binding have not been examined. The present experiments were designed to test the effect of Fe^{3+}, Cr^{3+} and Cu^{2+} binding to apotransferrin on its ability to bind to transferrin receptor sites on the reticulocyte cell surface.

Materials

Purified human Fe^{3+}-free transferrin (Behringwerke) was purchased from Hoechst Pharmaceutical Co., Cincinnati, Ohio. Sephadex G-150 was obtained from Pharmacia Fine Chemicals, Piscataway, New Jersey.

Methods

Rabbit reticulocytes. Reticulocytes were obtained from bled rabbits as previously described[12].

Iodination of transferrin. Fe^{3+}-free transferrin was iodinated by the method of AWAI AND BROWN[13].

Determination of the dissociation constant for transferrin binding to reticulocytes. A. Direct determination using iodinated transferrin. To aliquots of iodinated apotransferrin (2.0 mg/ml dissolved in 0.9% NaCl–0.01 M $NaHCO_3$, pH 7.4) were added various amounts of either $FeSO_4$, $CrCl_3$ or $CuSO_4$. The amount of metal added to achieve a certain saturation of the metal binding capacity was calculated on the basis that one mole of transferrin binds two moles of metal. When 100% metal saturation of the protein was desired, 10% more metal was added than the calculated maximum to insure complete saturation. Measurements of the maximal absorption of Fe^{3+}–transferrin at 465 mμ and Cu^{2+}–transferrin at 440 mμ following repeated addition confirmed that the transferrins were really saturated. The solutions were incubated at 37° for at least 1 h prior to use. When 100% Fe^{3+}–saturated transferrin was prepared, the solutions were incubated for an additional 20 h at 4° prior to use. The standard reaction mixtures contained 0.25 ml of reticulocytes and 0.75 ml of 0.9% NaCl–0.01 M $NaHCO_3$ containing various concentrations of iodinated transferrin ranging from 0.02 to 0.4 mg. After incubation at 37° for 30 min, the reticulocytes were washed 3 times with 5 vol. of cold saline and then transferred to counting tubes; the amounts of bound radioactive transferrin were determined in a Packard Autogamma well counter. Duplicate determinations in the same experiment gave a maximum difference of only 5%. These data were plotted as described by STECK AND WALLACH[14] for a reversible bimolecular reaction according to the equation:

$$\frac{1}{r} = \frac{1}{Kn} \cdot \frac{1}{[T]} + \frac{1}{n}$$

where $1/r = [C]/[TS]$ and $[C]$ = reticulocytes/ml, $[TS]$ = µg/ml of transferrin bound to cell receptor sites, $[T]$ = µg/ml free transferrin, n = number of receptor sites per reticulocyte, and K is the association constant. The values for the dissociation constant, $1/K$, were calculated and used to compare the different transferrins. *B. Indirect determination using* $^{59}Fe^{3+}$*–transferrin.* These assays were performed as described above except that $^{59}FeSO_4$ was substituted for $^{56}FeSO_4$ and the uptake of $^{59}Fe^{3+}$ by the reticulocytes was determined. The Fe^{3+}-binding capacity of the transferrin was one-third saturated except where noted. The rationale for plotting these data by the method of LINEWEAVER AND BURK[15] to obtain the apparent dissociation constants has been previously discussed[12].

Gel filtration. Sephadex G-150 was mixed with 0.9% NaCl–0.01 M $NaHCO_3$–0.01 M Tris, pH 7.4 for 48 h prior to use. The column (2.5 cm × 80 cm) was fitted for upward flow and equilibrated with the same buffer. The sample (1 ml) containing the various transferrins was introduced through a three-way valve and then the flow rate was maintained at 10 ml/h with a peristaltic pump.

RESULTS

Effect of Fe^{3+} *on transferrin binding to reticulocytes*

AISEN *et al.*[5] have shown that transferrin can exist in three states: apotransferrin, mono-Fe^{3+}–transferrin and di-Fe^{3+}–transferrin. When apo[^{131}I]transferrin was completely saturated with Fe^{3+} to form di-Fe^{3+}–transferrin, its binding affinity to reticulocytes was enhanced about 5-fold, as shown in Fig. 1. In this experiment the apparent dissociation constant (K_a) for transferrin binding to its cell surface receptor sites

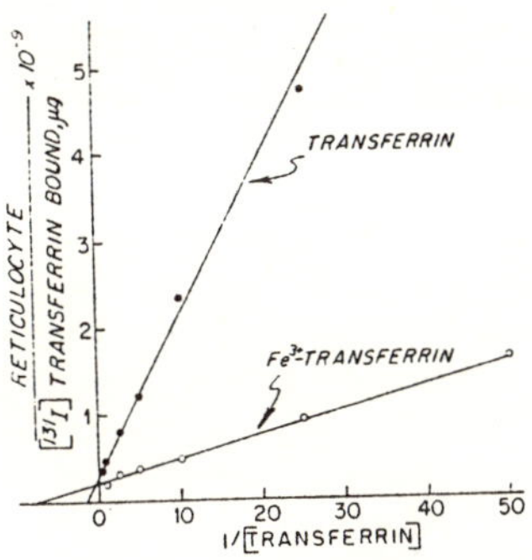

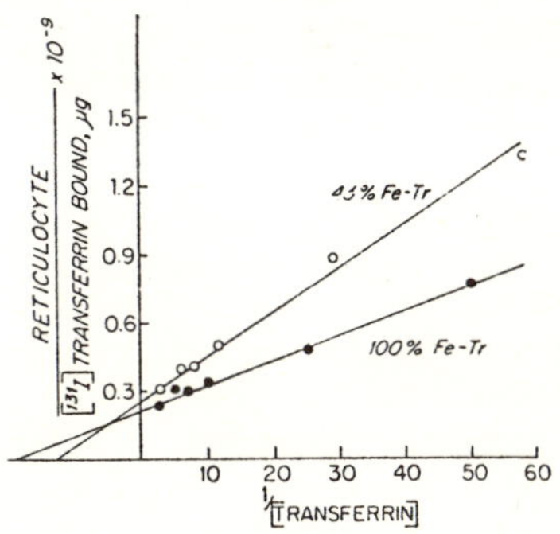

Fig. 1. Effect of Fe^{3+} attachment to transferrin on transferrin binding to reticulocytes. Standard assay conditions were used with varying concentrations (mg/ml) of apo[^{131}I]transferrin (●—●) and 100% Fe^{3+}–[^{131}I]transferrin (○—○).

Fig. 2. Binding of 43% (○—○) and 100% (●—●) Fe^{3+}–[^{131}I]transferrin to reticulocytes. Standard assay conditions were used.

was 0.66 mg/ml for apotransferrin and 0.13 mg/ml for 100% Fe^{3+}–transferrin*. Fig. 2 compares the binding affinity of 43% and 100% Fe^{3+}-saturated transferrin to reticulocytes. These species of transferrin presumably represent predominantly mono-Fe^{3+}–transferrin and di-Fe^{3+}–transferrin respectively. The apparent dissociation constants derived from these data are 0.077 mg/ml for 43% Fe^{3+}–transferrin and 0.053 mg/ml for 100% Fe^{3+}–transferrin, demonstrating that the addition of the first Fe^{3+} to transferrin has a much greater effect on the binding affinity than does the addition of the second Fe^{3+}.

Effect of Cr^{3+} and Cu^{2+} on transferrin binding to reticulocytes

Several metals, including Cr^{3+} and Cu^{2+} also bind to the Fe^{3+} binding sites of transferrin. Cr^{3+} binds as the trivalent metal while Cu^{2+} binds as the divalent metal. The effect of these metals on the binding of transferrin to reticulocytes is shown in Fig. 3. Cu^{2+}–transferrin has the same apparent dissociation constant as apotransferrin (0.5 mg/ml) while Cr^{3+}–transferrin has a significantly lower dissociation constant (0.28 mg/ml). The dissociation constant of Fe^{3+}–transferrin was the lowest of all (0.13 mg/ml).

Inhibition of normal transferrin function by various transferrins

Another way to determine the binding affinities of the various transferrins for the cell receptor sites is by competition experiments. When the rate of $^{59}Fe^{3+}$ uptake is determined as a function of transferrin concentration and the data are plotted by the method of LINEWEAVER AND BURK[15], it is possible to calculate a dissociation constant for transferrin binding to reticulocytes[12]. This method is particularly useful since it only determines transferrin binding to functional receptor sites; that is, those sites capable of transferring Fe^{3+} into the cell. Non-specific binding of transferrin to the cell surface is excluded. If one then determines the ability of unlabeled metal

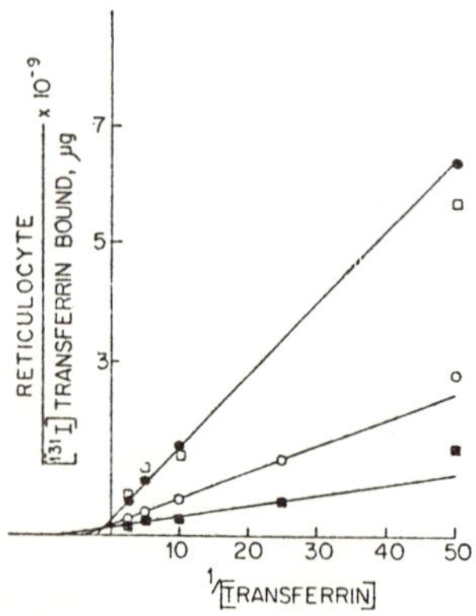

Fig. 3. Effect of 100% Cu^{2+}, Cr^{3+} and Fe^{3+} saturation of [^{131}I]transferrin on its binding to reticulocytes. The standard assay conditions were used. ■—■, Fe^{3+}–transferrin; ○—○, Cr^{3+}–transferrin; □—□, Cu^{2+}–transferrin; ●—●, apotransferrin.

* Since the absolute values for the apparent affinity constants for 100% Fe^{3+}–transferrin varied between 0.03 mg/ml and 0.15 mg/ml depending on the individual batch of reticulocytes, each set of experiments was performed with a single preparation of reticulocytes.

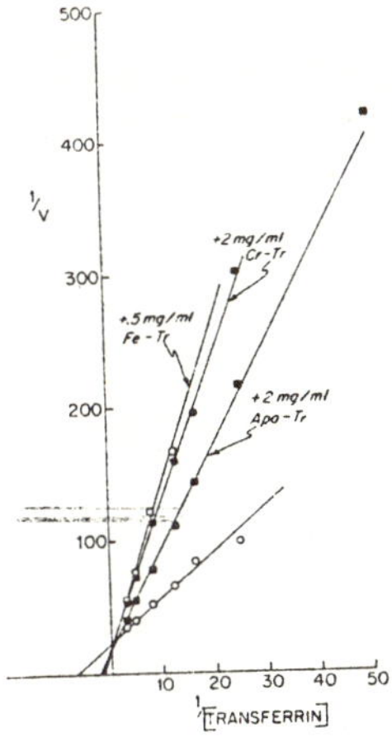

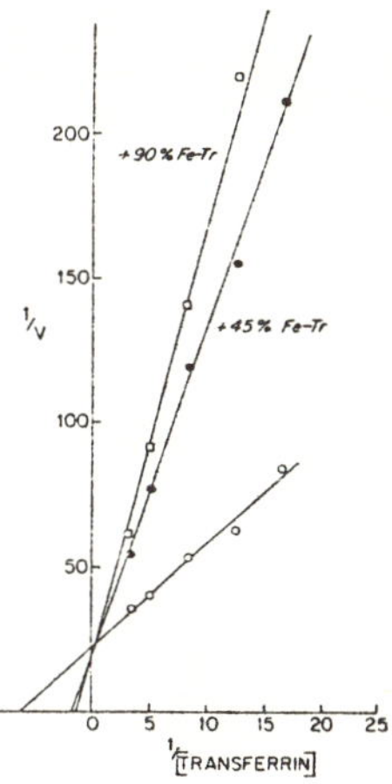

Fig. 4. Inhibition of $^{59}Fe^{3+}$ uptake by reticulocytes from $^{59}Fe^{3+}$–transferrin by the presence of various transferrins. The assay conditions are described in the text. The concentration (mg/ml) of $^{59}Fe^{3+}$–transferrin was varied as noted. The velocity, v, is expressed as μg $^{59}Fe^{3+}$ uptake in 25 min. ○—○, $^{59}Fe^{3+}$–transferrin alone; ■—■, +2 mg/ml apotransferrin; ●—●, +2 mg/ml Cr^{3+}–transferrin; □—□, +0.5 mg/ml Fe^{3+}–transferrin.

Fig. 5. Inhibition of $^{59}Fe^{3+}$ uptake by reticulocytes from $^{59}Fe^{3+}$–transferrin by the presence of 45% (●—●) and 90% (□—□) $^{56}Fe^{3+}$–transferrin. The concentration of the inhibitor transferrins was 0.5 mg/ml. The experimental details were the same as those described in the legend of Fig. 4.

transferrins to inhibit the intracellular uptake of $^{59}Fe^{3+}$ from $^{59}Fe^{3+}$–transferrin, it is possible to calculate the affinity with which these unlabeled transferrins bind to the physiologic receptor sites. The results of such an experiment are shown in Fig. 4. In this experiment the effect of unlabeled apotransferrin, 100% Cr^{3+}–transferrin and 100% $^{56}Fe^{3+}$–transferrin on the ability of $^{59}Fe^{3+}$–transferrin to donate Fe^{3+} to reticulocytes was determined. The results again show that Fe^{3+}–transferrin binds better to reticulocyte receptor sites than Cr^{3+}–transferrin which in turn binds better than apotransferrin. The calculated K_i's from these data are 1.06 mg/ml for apotransferrin, 0.65 mg/ml for Cr^{3+}–transferrin and 0.15 mg/ml for Fe^{3+}–transferrin. The inhibitory capacity of 90% and 45% $^{56}Fe^{3+}$–transferrin was compared as shown in Fig. 5. Based on these data, 90% $^{56}Fe^{3+}$–transferrin has a K_i of 0.14 mg/ml while 45% $^{56}Fe^{3+}$–transferrin has a K_i of 0.19 mg/ml. Again, these data suggest that the attachment of the first Fe^{3+} to transferrin has a greater effect on its binding to reticulocytes than does the attachment of the second Fe^{3+}.

Effect of Fe^{3+} saturation of transferrin on its capacity to donate Fe^{3+} to reticulocytes

The ability of 50% and 100% $^{59}Fe^{3+}$–transferrins to bind to reticulocytes and to transfer Fe^{3+} were compared as shown in Fig. 6. This double reciprocal plot shows that 50% Fe^{3+}–transferrin has a maximal rate of Fe^{3+} transfer that is 75% that of 100% Fe^{3+}–transferrin. The dissociation constant for binding to the cell surface is slightly lower with 100% than with 50% saturated transferrin. Similar results were obtained when bone marrow erythroid precursors were used as the receptors.

Gel filtration of various transferrins

The previous data have demonstrated that the binding of metals to apotransferrin greatly affects the binding of the protein to reticulocyte receptor sites. One explanation for this phenomenon is that metal attachment to the apoprotein results in a conformation change in the protein which enhances its binding to the receptor site. HABEEB[16] has pointed out the usefulness of gel filtration as a means of detecting various conformational states of proteins that result in changes in the Stokes radius of the molecule. In Fig. 7 are shown the results of typical gel filtration patterns of

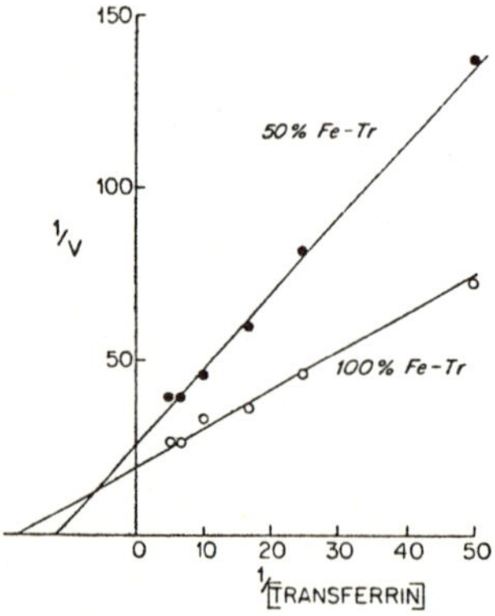

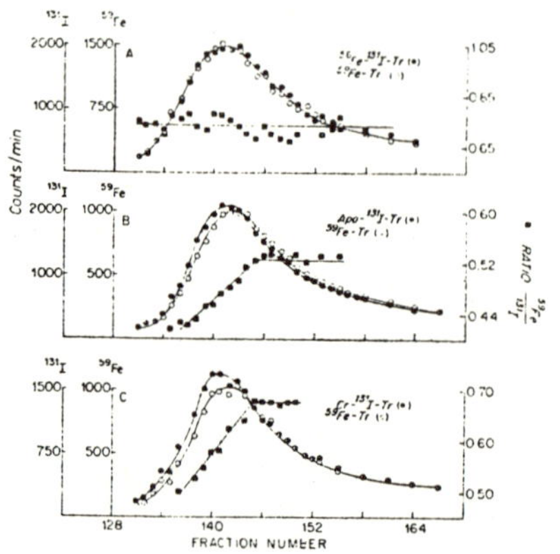

Fig. 6. Double reciprocal plot of $^{59}Fe^{3+}$ uptake *versus* transferrin concentration of 50% (●—●) and 100% (○—○) $^{59}Fe^{3+}$–transferrins. Standard assay conditions were used. The transferrin concentration (mg/ml) was varied as noted. The velocity, v, is expressed as μg $^{59}Fe^{3+}$ uptake in 20 min.

Fig. 7. The elution patterns of various transferrins on Sephadex G-150 (2.5 cm × 80 cm) with a buffer containing 0.9% NaCl–0.01 M $NaHCO_3$–0.01 M Tris, pH 7.4. The Fe^{3+}– and Cr^{3+}–transferrins were 100% saturated. The flow rate was 10 ml/h and fractions were collected every 6 min. ○—○, $^{59}Fe^{3+}$–transferrin; ●—●, (A) $^{56}Fe^{3+}$–[^{131}I]transferrin, (B) apo[^{131}I]transferrin, (C) Cr^{3+}–[^{131}I]transferrin; ■—■, ratio $^{59}Fe^{3+}/^{131}I$.

apotransferrin, 100% Fe^{3+}–transferrin and 100% Cr^{3+}–transferrin. Iodinated transferrin has an identical elution pattern as untreated transferrin (Panel A). The elution patterns obtained when either metal-free or $^{52}Cr^{3+}$–saturated [^{131}I]transferrin was mixed with $^{59}Fe^{3+}$–transferrin and then subjected to gel filtration are shown in Panels B and C. In these experiments Fe^{3+}–transferrin was slightly more retarded than both apotransferrin and Cr^{3+}–transferrin. Since the separation of the two transferrins was not very great, the ratios of the two isotopes present in each fraction are also plotted. These ratios show a progressive enrichment for Fe^{3+}–transferrin compared to either apotransferrin or Cr^{3+}–transferrin, confirming that Fe^{3+}–transferrin is eluted later from the column. Each experiment shown in Fig. 7 was repeated 3 times, always with the same results. These data suggest that the Stokes radius of Fe^{3+}–transferrin is somewhat less than that of the other molecules. In another experiment a mixture of apo[^{131}I]transferrin and $^{51}Cr^{3+}$–transferrin were eluted as a single superimposable peak.

DISCUSSION

Binding of metals to apotransferrin results in several changes in the physical and chemical properties of the molecule. KOECHLIN[6] found that Fe^{3+}–transferrin is 10 times more soluble in 50% ethanol at pH 7.0 than apotransferrin; other metals, including Cu^{2+}, did not enhance the solubility of the apoprotein. AZARI AND FEENEY[7] have demonstrated that apotransferrin is more susceptible to proteolysis with chymotrypsin and to thermal denaturation than Fe^{3+}–transferrin. BUTTKUS *et al.*[8] showed that with acetylation apotransferrin lost its metal binding capacity sooner then Fe^{3+}–transferrin. KOURILSKY AND BURTIN[9] have found that binding of Fe^{3+} to apotransferrin resulted in the loss of an antigenic determinant which could be recovered by removing the metal from the protein with a chelating agent. Several of these investigators have postulated that the alterations in the properties of transferrin are related to the effect of metal binding on the conformation of the protein.

There is considerably less information about the effect of metal binding on the biologic properties of transferrin. JANDL AND KATZ[10] showed that Fe^{3+}–transferrin has a greater affinity for reticulocyte receptor sites than apotransferrin, but there was some ambiguity in quantitating the difference. Contrary to these findings, MORGAN *et al.*[11] suggested that both apotransferrin and Fe^{3+}–transferrin compete equally well for transferrin receptor sites. Their experiments, however, were concerned with the release from reticulocytes of bound transferrin while JANDL AND KATZ[10] measured directly the binding of transferrin to reticulocytes. FLETCHER AND HUEHNS[17] have presented data which indicate that Fe^{3+} transfer to reticulocytes may occur preferentially from one metal binding site than the other. This phenomenon may relate to differences in structure around the two metal binding sites of the transferrin molecule.

The data presented in this paper demonstrate by both direct binding studies and competition experiments that the binding of metals to apotransferrin affects the binding of the protein to its receptor site on the surface of reticulocytes. The extent of the effect is primarily related to the particular metal that is bound and is less dependent on whether 1 or 2 molecules of metal are bound per molecule of protein. Thus, at saturation of the metal binding sites, Fe^{3+}–transferrin binds better to reticulocytes than Cr^{3+}–transferrin which in turn binds better than Cu^{2+}–transferrin. However, di-Fe^{3+}–transferrin binds to receptor sites only slightly better than mono-Fe^{3+}–transferrin. While it is known that Fe^{3+} binding to the two transferrin metal binding sites is a random process[5], our results show that binding of the first Fe^{3+} to transferrin results in a significantly greater effect on the biologic properties of the molecule than does the addition of the second Fe^{3+}.

From the data shown in Figs. 1–3, it can be calculated that the number of cellular receptor sites for the various transferrins is approximately the same, indicating that they all bind to the same sites on the cell surface. Direct evidence for this postulate comes from the competition experiments (Figs. 4 and 5). The actual number of receptor sites per reticulocyte is a function of the age of the reticulocyte, with young reticulocytes having more transferrin receptor sites than old reticulocytes[10,18]. The reticulocytes used in these experiments had between 26 000 and 45 000 sites per cell.

The effect that metal binding to transferrin exerts on the binding of the protein to its reticulocyte receptor sites could come about in two ways: First, the metal itself could be involved in the binding to the receptor site and/or, second, binding of the metal to the apoprotein could result in a conformational change in the protein which enhances its binding to the receptor site. That different conformational states of the various transferrins do occur is demonstrated by the gel filtration studies which show that Fe^{3+}–transferrin has a smaller Stokes radius than either Cr^{3+}– or apotransferrin. These results provide the first direct evidence that Fe^{3+} attachment to apotransferrin results in a conformational change in the molecule. Still it is not possible as yet to attribute the change in binding to the receptor site to this effect. Experiments performed with $^{51}Cr^{3+}$–transferrin have shown that reticulocytes do not take up this metal even though the transferrin binds to the proper cell receptor sites. Therefore, since the identity of the metal itself must be recognized at some stage in the process of Fe^{3+} uptake by reticulocytes, the possibility that Fe^{3+} itself participates in the binding of transferrin to its receptor site must be considered.

The enhanced binding affinity to reticulocyte receptor sites of Fe^{3+}–transferrin compared to apotransferrin is teleologically appropriate for efficient Fe^{3+} uptake by reticulocytes. Thus, both mono- and di-Fe^{3+}–transferrins would compete successfully with apotransferrin for cellular receptor sites* and bound transferrin that had transferred its Fe^{3+} would be displaced by an incoming Fe^{3+}–transferrin molecule. That the maximal rate of Fe^{3+} transfer from mono-Fe^{3+}–transferrin is about 75% that of di-Fe^{3+}–transferrin suggests either that both Fe^{3+} atoms are not transferred simultaneously when a di-Fe^{3+}–transferrin molecule binds to its cellular receptor site or that the rate of Fe^{3+} uptake from the two metal binding sites is unequal. The latter possibility is consistent with the data of FLETCHER AND HUEHNS[17].

The assumption is made in this work that the isotopically labeled transferrin behaves in a manner very similar to the native protein. The evidence in favor of this assumption comes primarily from the studies of AWAI AND BROWN[13], whose iodination procedure was followed in this work. These authors showed that the electrophoretic mobility on paper and starch gel, the immunoelectrophoretic and ultracentrifugation patterns and the rate and extent of Fe^{3+} uptake was identical between native and iodinated transferrin. They further showed in double-label experiments with human volunteers that the rate of Fe^{3+} clearance from iodinated transferrin was the same as that of the patients' own plasma transferrin. The data in Fig. 7 shows that native and iodinated transferrin behave identically on gel filtration. These data strongly suggest that the iodinated transferrin at least closely approximates the native molecule.

ADDENDUM

After this manuscript was submitted for publication, BAKER AND MORGAN[19] reported studies on the binding of iodinated rabbit transferrin to rabbit reticulocytes. The average association constant for transferrin binding was 207 000 $l \cdot mole^{-1}$ with a range from 49 000 to 590 000. These values are in fairly good agreement with the dissociation constants for human transferrin reported in this paper and previously[12]. The mean number of transferrin binding sites per reticulocyte was determined to be 334 000, a value considerably higher than that reported here. The reason for this discrepancy is not apparent.

---

* Since plasma transferrin is normally about one-third saturated, both apo- and Fe^{3+}–transferrin molecules would be present.

ACKNOWLEDGMENTS

This investigation was supported by grants from the U.S. Public Health Service, CA-08759-01 and HE 00022-22, the American Cancer Society, PRA-31, and gifts in memory of Bill Burns, Mark Edison, and Russell Kelce.

REFERENCES

1 J. H. JANDL, J. K. INMAN, R. L. SIMMONS AND D. W. ALLEN, *J. Clin. Invest.*, 38 (1959) 161.
2 E. H. MORGAN AND C. B. LAURELL, *Brit. J. Haematol.*, 9 (1963) 471.
3 A. L. SCHADE, *Farmaco*, 19 (1964) 185.
4 R. AASA, B. G. MALMSTROM, P. SALTMAN AND T. VANNGARD, *Biochim. Biophys. Acta*, 75 (1963) 203.
5 P. AISEN, A. LEIBMAN AND H. A. REICH, *J. Biol. Chem.*, 241 (1966) 1666.
6 B. A. KOECHLIN, *J. Am. Chem. Soc.*, 74 (1952) 2649.
7 P. R. AZARI AND R. E. FEENEY, *J. Biol. Chem.*, 232 (1958) 293.
8 H. BUTTKUS, J. R. CLARK AND R. F. FEENEY, *Biochemistry*, 4 (1965) 998.
9 F. M. KOURILSKY AND P. BURTIN, *Nature*, 218 (1968) 375.
10 J. H. JANDL AND J. H. KATZ, *J. Clin. Invest.*, 42 (1963) 314.
11 E. H. MORGAN, E. R. HUEHNS AND C. A. FINCH, *Am. J. Physiol.*, 210 (1966) 579.
12 S. KORNFELD, *Biochemistry*, 7 (1968) 945.
13 M. AWAI AND E. B. BROWN, *J. Lab. Clin. Med.*, 61 (1963) 363.
14 T. L. STECK AND D. F. H. WALLACH, *Biochim. Biophys. Acta*, 97 (1965) 510.
15 H. LINEWEAVER AND D. BURK, *J. Am. Chem. Soc.*, 56 (1934) 658.
16 A. F. S. A. HABEEB, *Biochim. Biophys. Acta*, 121 (1966) 21.
17 J. FLETCHER AND E. R. HUEHNS, *Nature*, 218 (1968) 1211.
18 S. KORNFELD, *Abstr. 12th Congr. Intern. Soc. Hematol., New York, 1968*, p. 86.
19 E. BAKER AND E. H. MORGAN, *Biochemistry*, 8 (1969) 1133.

Vertebrate Transferrins. Molecular Weights, Chemical Compositions, and Iron-Binding Studies

Roberta M. Palmour and H. Eldon Sutton

The structure of human transferrin (Tf)[1] has been investigated in several laboratories. Two identical carbohydrate chains (Jamieson, 1966) and two iron-binding sites (Surgenor *et al.*, 1949) suggest that a gene duplication may have occurred at some time during the evolution of the molecule (Greene and Feeney, 1968). Early reports gave a molecular weight for human Tf of 88,000–90,000, but more recent analyses of sedimentation and diffusion, sedimentation equilibrium, osmotic pressure, iron content, and gel filtration yield values of 68,000–78,000 for human Tf (Charlwood, 1963; Roberts *et al.*, 1966). Intensive studies of the sedimentation velocities of RCM Tf in 8 M urea and 6 M Gdn·HCl (Greene and Feeney, 1968) and of the sedimentation equilibrium values for RCM Tf in 8 M urea and 6 M Gdn·HCl (Mann *et al.*, 1970) have failed to demonstrate the presence of disulfide-linked subunit chains. However, the possibility of a complete or partial duplication of amino acid sequence within a single polypeptide chain exists. We have surveyed iron-binding proteins in lower vertebrates and invertebrates in the search for forms of transferrin that would correspond to a primordial gene prior to duplication.

Boffa *et al.* (1966) reported an iron-binding protein in lampreys with a sedimentation value of $s_{20,w}$ = 4.8–5.1 S, corresponding to a molecular weight of 70,000–80,000. Manwell (1963) reported iron-binding proteins in both marine

[1] Abbreviations used are: Tf, transferrin; SDS, sodium dodecyl sulfate; RCM, reduced carboxymethylated; BSA, bovine serum albumin; IgG, immunoglobulin G; Gdn·HCl, guanidine hydrochloride.

lampreys and hagfish but did not determine the molecular weight of hagfish Tf. As lampreys and hagfish are members of the most primitive vertebrate class, Cyclostomata, we examined the serum of the California hagfish, *Eptatretus stoutii*, for iron-binding proteins. The Tf's from the New Zealand white rabbit, the bullfrog (*Rana catesbiana*), and the red-eared slider turtle (*Pseudemys scripta*) were studied for comparative evolutionary purposes.

Materials

Human Tf was purchased from Behringwerke Co. (Certified Blood Donor Service) and further purified by starch block electrophoresis in pH 8.6 barbital buffer (Sutton and Karp, 1965). Frogs and turtles were purchased from Carolina Biological Supply and were bled by heart puncture. Hagfish serum was obtained from Pacific Bio-Marine Co. BSA, ovalbumin, cytochrome *c*, and iodoacetamide were purchased from Sigma Chemical Co., and pepsin and trypsin from Worthington Biochemical Corp. β-Mercaptoethanol was obtained from Eastman Organic Chemicals and $^{59}FeCl_3$ from International Nuclear Corp. Urea (Baker analyzed reagent) was deionized before use.

Methods

Identification of Tf's. Serum samples containing 0.236 μg of ^{59}Fe/ml of serum (a final concentration of 6–7 μCi of ^{59}Fe/ml) were subjected to polyacrylamide gel electrophoresis (0.1 M Tris–0.05 M glycine buffer, pH 8.8) or to horizontal starch gel electrophoresis (0.3 M LiOH, pH 8.2). The gel was sliced longitudinally, one-half was stained with Amido-Schwarz 10B, and autoradiography was performed with the second slice (Giblett *et al.*, 1959).

Purification of Tf's. Rabbit Tf was purified by a combination of rivanol (2-ethoxy-6,9-diaminoacridine lactate) precipitation and starch block electrophoresis (Sutton and Karp, 1965). Frog and turtle Tf's were purified by rivanol precipitation, followed by preparative acrylamide slab electrophoresis (pH 8.9 Tris·HCl buffer) and subsequent electrophoretic elution of the Tf band (Chen, 1968). Alternatively, the rivanol precipitates from frog or turtle serum were chromatographed on Bio-Gel A-5 m agarose columns (2.5 × 70 cm) equilibrated with 0.05 M Tris–0.1 M KCl buffer (pH 7.6). Hagfish serum was fractionated by gel filtration on Bio-Gel A-5 m agarose columns, followed by ion-exchange chromatography on a 1.5 × 30 cm DEAE-Cellex (Bio-Rad) column equilibrated with 0.01 M Tris·HCl (pH 7.8). Proteins were eluted by a linear concentration gradient from 0.01 to 0.45 M Tris·HCl (pH 7.8). All Tf's were saturated with iron (ferric ammonium citrate) prior to purification.

Protein Concentration. The protein concentration of most samples was determined by weighing the dried samples or by reading optical density at 280 nm, assuming $E_{1\,cm}^{1\%} = 13.8$ for Fe-Tf or 11.2 for apoTf (Laurell, 1960). For quantitative iron-binding determinations and sialic acid assays, protein concentration was determined by the method of Lowry *et al.* (1951).

Ultracentrifugal Studies. Sedimentation velocities of human, rabbit, turtle, frog, and hagfish Tf's were determined in the Spinco Model E analytical ultracentrifuge at protein concentrations of 1.0, 0.6, 0.4, and 0.2% in 0.1 M sodium phosphate buffer (pH 7.5). Sedimentation coefficients for all Tf's were calculated from the slopes of plots of log $\bar{x}$ *vs.* t (Svedberg and Pedersen, 1940).

The molecular weights of the purified Tf's were determined at a protein concentration of 0.15% in 0.1 M sodium phosphate (pH 7.5) buffer by sedimentation equilibrium at 20° and 10,589 rpm. Samples were dialyzed against the solvent for at least 24 hr prior to analysis. The molecular weight was calculated from the slope of plots of ln $j(r)$ *vs.* r^2 (where j, the fringe number, is proportional to c, the concentration) according to the equation $d \ln c/dr = w^2M(1 - \bar{v}\rho)r/2RT$ (Svedberg and Pedersen, 1940). The partial specific volumes ($\bar{v}$) of native Tf's were calculated from the amino acid composition, after the example of Schachman (1967). For human and rabbit Tf's, $\bar{v} = 0.725$; for turtle Tf, $\bar{v} = 0.726$; for frog Tf, $\bar{v} = 0.733$; and for hagfish Tf, $\bar{v} = 0.721$.

Gel Filtration Studies. The molecular weights of purified Tf's were studied by gel filtration on a 1.5 × 60 cm Sephadex G-100 column (Andrews, 1966) using 0.05 M Tris–0.1 M KCl buffer (pH 7.7). The elution volumes for appropriate protein standards were measured and plotted against the log of the molecular weight of each standard; the elution volume of each Tf was then located on the standard curve.

SDS Electrophoresis. Acrylamide gel electrophoresis using SDS was performed according to the technique of Weber and Osborne (1969). Purified proteins (3 mg/ml) were dissolved in 0.01 M sodium phosphate buffer (pH 7.0) containing 1% SDS and 1% β-mercaptoethanol and incubated at 37° for 3 hr. After electrophoresis of 75-μg samples on 10% acrylamide gels, the migration distance of each protein was measured in millimeters and divided by the migration distance of a standard (cytochrome c) to yield a relative mobility which was plotted against the log of the molecular weight of the protein being studied. A standard curve for similarly treated proteins of known molecular weights was prepared, and unknown proteins were located on that curve.

RCM Tf's. Purified Tf's were reduced and alkylated following the procedure of Crestfield *et al.* (1963), as modified by Greene and Feeney (1968). Tf in 8 M urea–0.3 M Tris·HCl (pH 8.6) was reduced with a 100-fold molar excess of β-mercaptoethanol (based on the potentially available sulfhydryl groups in each protein) for 16 hr at 50°, then alkylated with a 10% excess of iodoacetamide (based on the amount of β-mercaptoethanol used). These solutions were then dialyzed for 96 hr against several changes of 8 M urea–0.1 M Tris·HCl buffer (pH 8.6) to remove the reagents. BSA and pepsin were prepared in this fashion for use as standards. Sedimentation coefficients for RCM proteins were determined in a synthetic boundary cell, using 8 M urea–0.1 M Tris·HCl buffer in the reference side. Samples were centrifuged at 42,040 rpm and 20° using a protein concentration of 0.2%. The solvent density value for the 8 M urea system was taken as 1.116 g/cm^3 (Greene and Feeney, 1968), and the values used for $\bar{v}$ were 0.723 for human and rabbit Tf's, 0.725 for turtle Tf, 0.730 for frog Tf, 0.721 for hagfish Tf, 0.725 for pepsin, and 0.729 for BSA (after Greene and Feeney, 1968).

Amino Acid Analysis. Total amino acid content of each purified Tf was determined on a Spinco Model 120B automatic amino acid analyzer (modified to the sensitivity of a Model 120C), using duplicate samples of 18-, 36-, and 72-hr 6 N HCl hydrolysates of both performic acid oxidized (Hirs, 1956) and untreated Tf's. Tryptophan was determined in triplicate by the thioglycolic acid method of Matsubara and Sasaki (1969).

Sialic Acid Content. Sialic acid was assayed by the thiobarbituric acid method (Warren, 1959). A known standard containing 0.15 μmole of sialic acid/ml was included for calibration.

Absorption spectra in the visible region were determined for 1% solutions of both apoTf's and iron-saturated Tf's using a Cary Model 15 recording spectrophotometer with a 1-cm light path. Samples were dissolved in 0.1 M Tris·HCl (pH 7.5), containing 0.015 M $NaHCO_3$, then dialyzed extensively against several changes of the same buffer to remove any excess iron. An aliquot of the final dialysis fluid was used as a blank. Extinction coefficients were determined at the wavelengths of maximum absorbance.

Quantitative Iron-Binding Analysis. Quantitative iron-binding determinations were carried out on each purified Tf (Schade and Reinhart, 1966; Masson and Heremans, 1968;

Spik, 1968). The Tf's were deprived of iron by dialysis against 1.0 M citric acid, followed by extensive dialysis against deionized water. The protein was lyophilized and dissolved in 0.1 M Tris·HCl–0.015 M $NaHCO_3$ (pH 7.5). An aliquot was removed for protein determination, and the absorbance of the apoTf solution was read at 465 nm to provide a reference point. Stepwise 2-μl aliquots of a standard iron solution (0.00179 M ferric ammonium sulfate, 0.00179 M citric acid, 8.5×10^{-5} M ascorbic acid) containing 0.1 μg of Fe/μl were added to 1-ml portions of the apoTf solutions. These preparations were incubated at 25° for 1 hr, then optical densities at wavelengths of 465 and 410 nm were read in a Gilford Model 240 spectrophotometer. When absorbance was plotted as a function of microliters of Fe solution added, a plateau was reached at which further addition of iron caused no significant increase in optical density. The inflection point

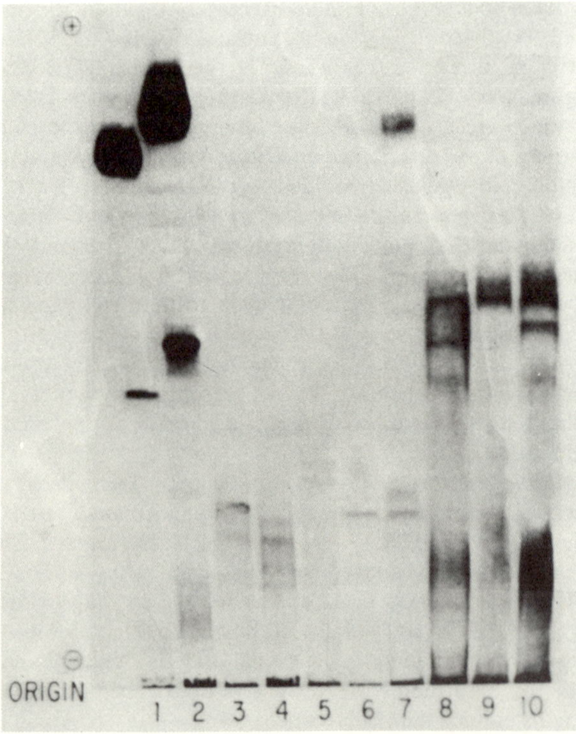

FIGURE 1: Polyacrylamide gel electrophoresis of $^{59}FeCl_3$ labeled human serum (1), rabbit serum (2), turtle sera (3–5), frog sera (6–7), and hagfish sera (8–10).

of the curve was located in terms of microliters of Fe solution added, and this value was converted to micrograms of Fe bound per milligram of protein.

Results

Iron-binding proteins were identified by acrylamide electrophoresis in all vertebrate species examined, as seen in Figure 1. The sera or body fluids from several invertebrate animals (*Amphioxus;* three moth species, *Anatherea polyphemus, Hyalophora cecropia*, and *Actias luna;* the horseshoe crab,

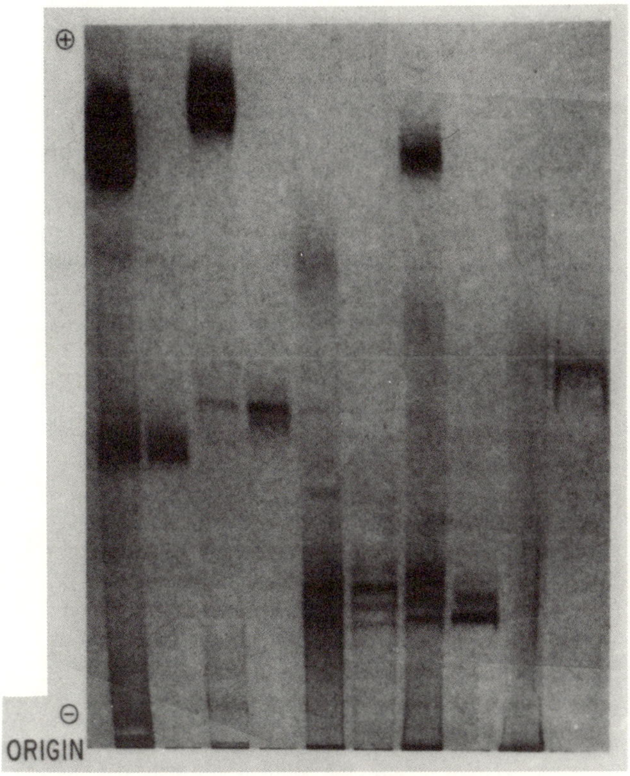

FIGURE 2: Polyacrylamide gel electrophoresis from left to right of human serum, human Tf, rabbit serum, rabbit Tf, turtle serum, turtle Tf, frog serum, frog Tf, hagfish serum, and hagfish Tf.

TABLE I: Comparative Sedimentation Coefficients of Tf's in 0.1 M Na_2HPO_4 (pH 7.5).

Tf	$s^0_{20,w}$ (S)	Comparative s^a
Human	5.32 ± 0.19	1.00000
Rabbit	5.29 ± 0.10	0.99436
Turtle	5.63 ± 0.26	1.05827
Frog	5.16 ± 0.12	0.96992
Hagfish	3.45 ± 0.14	0.64850

[a] Ratio of $s^0_{20,w}$ of each Tf to $s^0_{20,w}$ of human Tf.

Limulus; Daphnia, the water flea; the crab, *Cambarus;* the sea cucumbers, *Cucumaria* and *Malpodia;* the snail, *Helix;* the clam, *Arca;* the limpet, *Megathuria;* the leech, *Haemopis;* two earthworms, *Lumbricus* and *Tubifex;* two marine worms, *Glycera* and *Amphitrite;* a nematode, *Cephalobus;* two sipunculoids, *Dendrostrom* and *Golfingia;* and *Dugesia*, the brown planaria) were screened for the presence of iron-binding proteins. Positive results were obtained from the hemolymph of the moth species only.

Transferrins from human, rabbit, turtle, frog, and hagfish sera were purified for further study. A comparison of the purified Tfs with the serum from which each Tf was derived is shown in Figure 2; the purified Tf's all retained their ability to bind radioactive iron. In addition, each preparation showed a single, symmetrical peak during analytical ultracentrifugation and gel filtration. The human Tf preparations contain less than 5% hemopexin, as estimated from immunoelectrophoresis and immunodiffusion against antihemopexin.

Each purified Tf was examined by several different physical methods in order to determine its molecular weight. The sedimentation coefficient of each Tf was determined at three different protein concentrations and then extrapolated to standard conditions and infinite dilution by the usual methods (Table I). Molecular weight values were determined by sedimentation equilibrium studies. Values for human and rabbit Tf's were determined in duplicate; three independently isolated samples of each of the other Tf's (turtle, frog, and hagfish) were analyzed. An average of the values obtained for each protein yields the following molecular weights: human Tf, 76,200; rabbit Tf, 74,500; turtle Tf, 93,790; frog Tf, 79,370; and hagfish Tf, 44,340. Gel filtration properties of each protein were examined as a further indication of molecular size (Figure 3). This approach indicated molecular weights of 78,000, 76,000, and 72,000, respectively, for human, rabbit, and frog Tf's. Turtle Tf was located at a molecular weight of 96,000, while hagfish Tf appeared to have a molecular weight of 45,500. Finally, electrophoretic migration after treatment with SDS and a reducing agent was studied. Table II summarizes the migration distances of a series of molecular weight standards and of each Tf being studied, while Figure 4 relates the relative mobility to the log of the molecular weight. By this method, human and frog Tf's showed molecular weights of 81,000, rabbit Tf yielded a value of 79,500, and turtle Tf had a molecular weight of 85,000. The main protein band for hagfish Tf indicated a molecular weight of 41,500; however, a faint band corresponding to a molecular weight of 85,000 was observed. The molecular weight values determined by the foregoing methods are summarized for each Tf in Table III. For pur

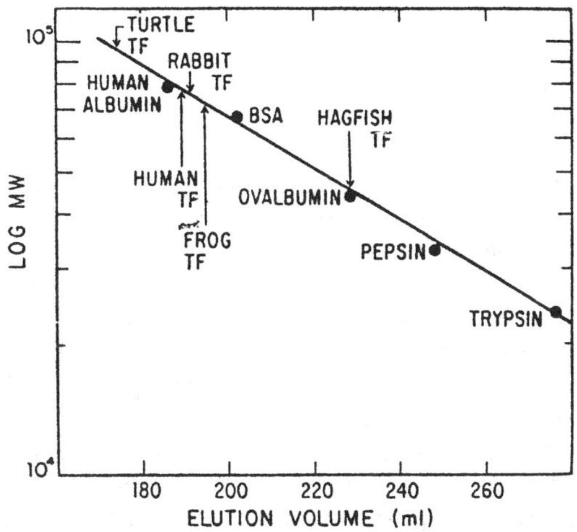

FIGURE 3: Gel filtration analysis of vertebrate Tf's on Sephadex G-100, pH 7.7, Tris–KCl buffer, with the log of the molecular weight of selected standards plotted against their elution volumes.

poses of calculations, the molecular weight of human, rabbit, and frog Tf's was taken as 76,000; turtle Tf was considered to have a molecular weight of 92,000; while the molecular weight of hagfish Tf was estimated as 44,000.

Each Tf was examined for the presence of disulfide-linked subunit chains. Following the approach of Greene and Feeney (1968), the sedimentation velocity of each RCM Tf was

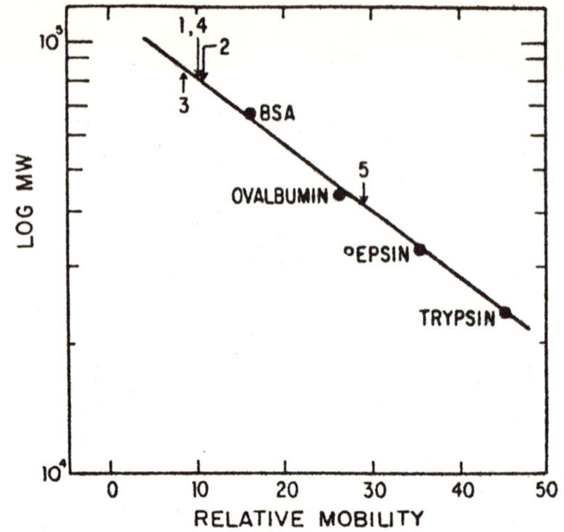

FIGURE 4: The relative electrophoretic mobilities of SDS-treated human Tf (1), rabbit Tf (2), turtle Tf (3), frog Tf (4), and hagfish Tf (5), located on a curve standardized with SDS-treated reference proteins.

determined in 8 M urea and compared to the sedimentation velocity of RCM BSA and RCM pepsin (Table IV). Amino acid analysis of an aliquot of each RCM protein indicated that conversion of cystine to carboxymethylcysteine was complete. Assuming that RCM proteins assume a random coil form (Tanford *et al.*, 1967), their sedimentation behavior should be solely a function of chain length or particle weight. The sedimentation coefficients of RCM human, rabbit, and frog Tf's are all higher than the sedimentation coefficient for RCM BSA, with a known chain weight of 67,800. The sedimentation coefficient for RCM hagfish Tf is lower than that for RCM BSA, but higher than that of RCM pepsin, with a particle weight of 33,000. RCM turtle Tf has two components, one of which sediments faster than RCM BSA, while the second component sediments slightly slower than RCM BSA.

Tanford *et al.* (1967), in a study of the sedimentation properties of a variety of RCM proteins, found that for proteins the relationship of s_{obsd} to chain length is $\log s/(1 - \bar{v}\rho) \propto 0.5 \log M$. Thus a plot of $\log s/(1 - \bar{v}\rho)$ *vs.* $\log M$ should yield a line with a slope of approximately 0.5. Figure 5 graphically demonstrates that human, rabbit, frog, and hagfish Tf's are single polypeptide chains; turtle Tf may be composed of two polypeptide chains.

TABLE II: Electrophoretic Migration of Proteins on SDS Acrylamide Gels.

	Absolute Migration (mm)	Rel Migration (mm)	Mol Wt
Reference Proteins			
IgG half-molecule	8	6.45	90,000
BSA	20	16.12	67,000
Ovalbumin	33	26.60	44,000
Pepsin	44	35.46	33,000
Trypsin	56	45.15	23,500
Purified Tfs[a]			
Human	12.5	10.08	81,000
Rabbit	13.0	10.48	79,000
Turtle	11.0	8.87	85,000
Frog	12.5	10.08	81,000
Hagfish	36.0	29.02	41,500

[a] Molecular weight as determined by this technique.

Total amino acid content was determined for each isolated Tf after 18-, 36-, and 72-hr hydrolysis. Very few differences were observed in the amino acid yields for different hydrolysis periods. However, some valylvaline, identified by elution on a Beckman automatic amino acid analyzer (J. R. Brown, personal communication), remained in the hydrolysates of hagfish Tf even after 72 hr. Duplicate samples of this protein were hydrolyzed for 102 hr to assure complete cleavage of valine residues; the valine value for these hydrolysates was used in computing molar ratios of amino acids for hagfish Tf. Amino acid content in grams of protein is given for each Tf in Table V. All values are the average of at least three determinations and are corrected to include tryptophan as determined following thioglycolic acid hydrolysis and half-cystine as determined after performic acid oxidation. By analogy to human Tf, 5.8% carbohydrate was allowed for

TABLE III: Molecular Weight Values for Tf's.

Tf's	Method of Determination		
	Sedimentation Equil	Gel Filtration	Migration on SDS Gels
Human	76,200	78,000	81,000
Rabbit	74,590	76,000	79,500
Turtle	93,700	96,000	85,000
Frog	79,370	72,000	81,000
Hagfish	44,340	45,500	41,500

each Tf; this allowance was taken into account when calculating the number of residues of each amino acid per molecule of protein.

In addition, amino acid analysis indicated the presence of glucosamine in all samples studied; galactosamine peaks were seen for turtle and hagfish Tf's only. Both amino sugars elute from the basic column immediately following the neutral and acidic amino acid peak. Quantitative assay for the amino sugars was not performed.

The sialic acid content of each protein was determined;

TABLE IV: Sedimentation Behavior of RCM Proteins in 8 M Urea.

RCM Proteins	Particle Wt[a]	$s_{20,\mathrm{obsd}}$	$\bar{v}^b$
Human Tf	77,900	0.75	0.723
Rabbit Tf	77,900	0.76	0.723
Turtle Tf	92,900[c]	0.83	0.725
	46,450[d]	0.59	0.725
Frog Tf	77,300	0.73	0.731
Hagfish Tf	44,400	0.53	0.719
BSA	67,800	0.68	0.729
Pepsin	33,000	0.45	0.725

[a] Particle weight of RCM proteins using molecular weights calculated from this study. [b] Calculated from amino acid composition and corrected for CM-cysteine content, after Greene and Feeney (1968). [c] Particle weight for a single-chain structure. [d] Particle weight for a double-chain structure.

the results are summarized in Table VI. Based on determined molecular weights, human and turtle Tf's contain an average of four residues of sialic acid per molecule, while rabbit, frog, and hagfish Tf's each contain an average of two residues per molecule. The sialic acid content of turtle Tf may well account for the multiple bands seen on acrylamide electrophoresis, in a fashion analogous to that described by Chen and Sutton (1967) for bovine Tf.

The visible absorption curve for each of the Fe–Tf complexes is shown in Figure 6. Both human and rabbit Tf's show

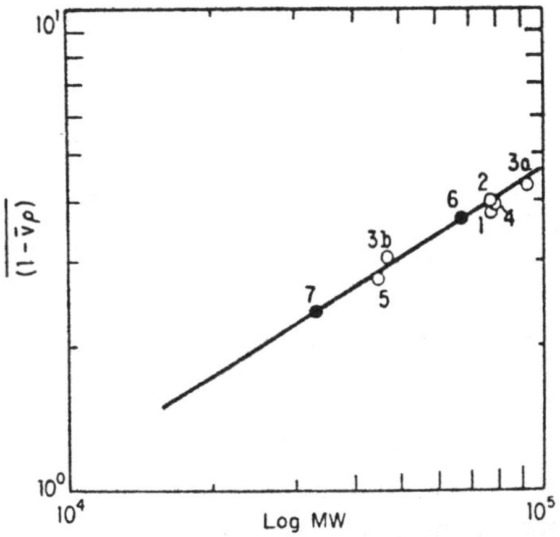

FIGURE 5: The relationship between sedimentation behavior of RCM proteins in 8 M urea and chain length or particle weight. The calculated values for $s/(1 - v\rho)$ are plotted against particle weights of RCM human Tf (1), RCM rabbit Tf (2), RCM turtle Tf (3), RCM frog Tf (4), RCM hagfish Tf (5), RCM BSA (6), and RCM pepsin (7) on a log–log scale.

maximum absorbance at 465 nm. Although all three other vertebrate Tf's have a shoulder on the absorption curve at 465 nm, maximum absorbance is seen at 405 nm for turtle Tf, 407 nm for frog Tf, and 415 nm for hagfish Tf. Extinction coefficients for all Tf's were calculated at wavelengths of 465, 410, and 280 nm; they are summarized in Table VII. Although this region corresponds to that of heme absorption, we have ruled out contamination by a non-Tf component.

TABLE V: Amino Acid Content of Tfs (g of AA/100 g of Protein).

Amino Acid	Human[a]	Rabbit	Turtle	Frog	Hagfish
Lysine	9.60	8.95	8.40	12.12	7.37
Histidine	3.11	3.10	2.34	2.80	3.48
Arginine	5.29	5.16	4.82	4.15	4.62
Aspartic acid	11.11	11.07	10.10	10.23	10.57
Threonine	3.92	2.81	5.93	4.89	5.52
Serine	3.99	4.03	6.34	4.47	5.30
Glutamic acid	10.24	10.68	11.46	11.11	11.22
Proline	4.30	4.32	3.61	4.68	3.97
Glycine	3.65	3.54	4.13	3.70	3.75
Alanine	5.19	5.06	4.71	5.16	5.09
Half-cystine	4.31	4.40	1.95	3.30	2.61
Valine	5.30	5.73	6.16	4.85	4.85
Methionine	1.25	1.09	1.15	1.30	2.52
Isoleucine	2.08	2.34	3.81	3.41	4.51
Leucine	8.51	9.03	7.61	7.49	7.87
Tyrosine	5.28	5.19	4.30	4.40	3.25
Phenylalanine	5.26	4.96	4.99	5.23	5.42
Tryptophan	1.81	2.23	1.91	1.10	2.28
Total[b]	94.20	93.66	94.20	94.29	94.20

[a] Wang (1966). [b] Calculations are corrected to include 5.8% carbohydrate, by analogy to human Tf.

The absorbance peak at 410 nm disappears when the Tf is deprived of bound iron and returns when the iron content is restored stoichiometrically to that same sample.

The iron-binding capacity of each Tf was quantitatively determined; the values for each experiment were read at wavelengths of 465 and 410 nm. Each experiment was continued until several successive tubes showed no change in optical density. The increase in optical density was plotted

TABLE VI: Sialic Acid Assay of Tf's.

Tf	Protein Concn (mg/ml)[a]	Sialic Acid (μmole/ml)	Sialic Acid (μmole/mg)	Av No. of Residues/ Molecule[b]
Human	3.00	0.1503	0.0501	3.81 (76,000)
Rabbit	3.00	0.0822	0.0274	2.08 (76,000)
Turtle	3.08	0.1445	0.0469	4.31 (92,000)
Frog	2.96	0.0687	0.0232	1.76 (76,000)
Hagfish	2.52	0.1230	0.0488	2.15 (44,000)

[a] Protein concentration determined by the Folin reaction.
[b] Based on the molecule weight in parentheses.

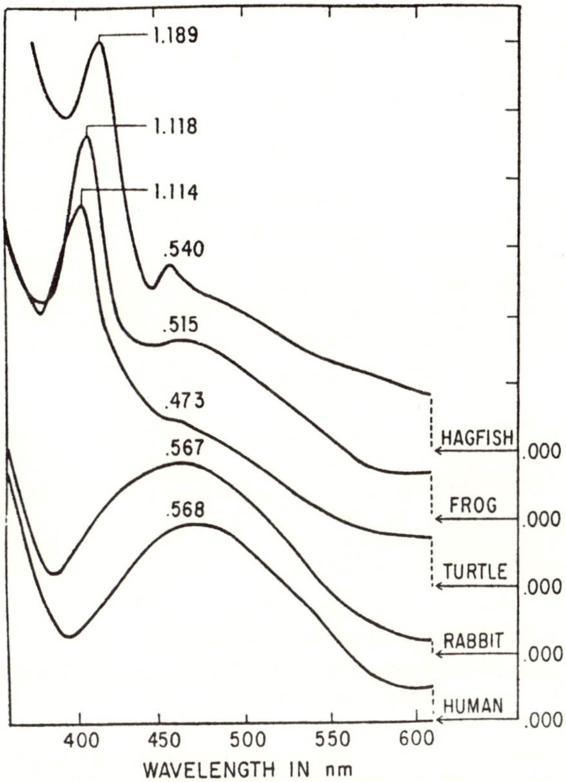

FIGURE 6: Spectral absorbance curves for 1% solutions of purified Tf's, with zero points and extinction coefficients for each curve.

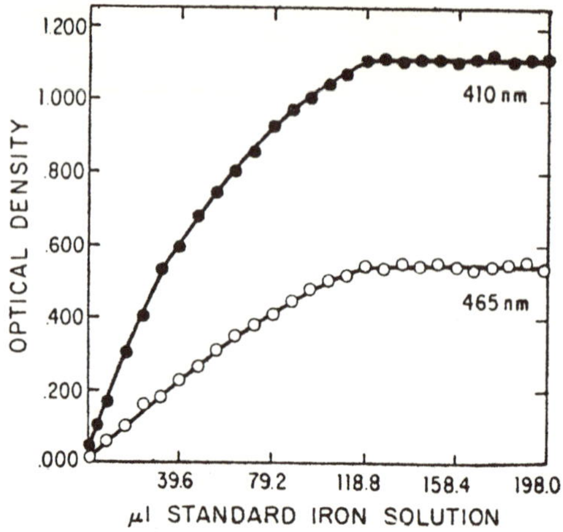

FIGURE 7: Quantitative determination of the iron-binding capacity of hagfish Tf, with the protein concentration corrected to a 1% solution. The optical density at 410 and 465 nm was plotted as a function of the amount of a standard iron solution required to achieve the absorbance indicated.

against the increments of iron solution for each protein (Figure 7). The iron-binding capacity of each protein was calculated in micrograms per milliliter and in atoms per molecule based on the determined molecular weights; these data are compared in Table VIII. Hagfish Tf bound 1.19 μg of Fe/mg of protein, corresponding to one atom per molecule, while the other Tf's being studied bound from 1.23 to 1.43 μg of Fe per mg of protein (two atoms of Fe per molecule).

Discussion

This study examines a series of animal proteins which show the physiologically important capacity for binding iron. Many electrophoretic variants of human Tf have been reported in the literature (Sutton and Jamieson, 1971), and two electrophoretic forms of rabbit Tf have been seen (Jordan *et al.*, 1967). The turtle sera examined in this study each contained multiple iron-binding bands; the variability between samples may be due to subspecies differences. Two electrophoretic variants of frog Tf were found, and several variants of hagfish

TABLE VII: Extinction Coefficients of Iron-Saturated Tf's in 0.1 M Tris–0.015 M $NaHCO_3$ (pH 7.8).

Tf	$E^{1\%}_{1\,cm}$ 280 nm	$E^{1\%}_{1\,cm}$ 410 nm	$E^{1\%}_{1\,cm}$ 465 nm
Human	14.06	0.315	0.568
Rabbit	13.74	0.308	0.567
Turtle	13.33	1.012	0.473
Frog	11.91	1.082	0.515
Hagfish	10.78	1.166	0.499

Tf were observed. An examination of the primary amino acid sequence of each molecule, together with the determination of the functional ability to donate iron to reticulocytes, would be necessary before absolute homology could be established.

The fact that iron-binding proteins are present in moth hemolymph argues that precursors to vertebrate Tf may have existed in some other invertebrate animals. Other arthropods were examined, but iron-binding proteins were not found in the species studied. An analogy between moth iron-binding proteins and vertebrate Tf's may be expected on the basis of their iron-binding capacities; until sequence studies are completed, however, no homology can be assumed.

For many years, the structure of human Tf has been an enigma to investigators; the circumstantial evidences for a gene duplication (two iron-binding sites, two identical carbohydrate side chains) are quite strong, but the most diligent methods have failed to identify any subunit structure. The initial purpose of this study was to locate either a primordial low molecular weight Tf or to locate a Tf which had maintained its subunit structure. From the available evidence, hagfish Tf, with a molecular weight of 44,000 and a binding capacity of one atom of Fe per molecule, fulfills the immediate requirements. Although a comparison of the amino acid content of human and hagfish Tf's clearly indicates that human Tf is not an exact duplicate of hagfish Tf, the theory of a partial gene duplication, followed by multiple point mutations in both human and hagfish Tf's, is plausible.

Furthermore, the data accumulated by Boffa's laboratory on lamprey Tf's indicate that the hagfish may be the only vertebrate now living which has a Tf of low molecular weight. If the hagfish is a degenerate, rather than a primitive, organism, its Tf may be the result of massive gene deletions rather than the precursor for subsequent gene duplication. In most well-studied genetic systems, massive gene deletions tend to be

TABLE VIII: Iron-Binding Capacities of Tf's.

Tf	Protein Content[a] (mg/ml)	μl of Fe Soln Added	μg of Fe Bound/ mg of Protein	Atoms of Fe Bound/Molecule[b]
Human	3.00	42	1.40	1.91 (76,000)
Rabbit	3.00	43	1.43	1.95 (76,000)
Turtle	3.08	38	1.23	2.04 (92,000)
Frog	2.96	40	1.35	1.85 (76,000)
Hagfish	2.52	30	1.19	0.94 (44,000)

[a] Protein concentration determined by the Folin method.
[b] Based on the molecular weights indicated in the parentheses.

lethal, whereas gene duplication can be advantageous. In addition, preliminary reports (Ohno *et al.*, 1968) indicate that lamprey erythrocytes contain twice as many chromosomes as hagfish erythrocytes do, suggesting that the whole genome may have duplicated early in vertebrate evolution.

The subunit structures of the Tf's from *Pseudemys scripta* and several fish species are under investigation in this laboratory. A recent study suggests that chicken ovoTf may have maintained a duplicate structure, as Phillips and Azari (1971) have found that 2 moles of each of the cyanogen bromide fragments are recovered from each mole of ovoTf. However, Elleman and Williams (1970) find no evidence of duplicate structure in their sequences of 34 unique cysteic acid containing peptides from chicken ovoTf.

In order to establish unequivocally that a gene duplication is responsible for the differences in molecular size and chemical composition of the Tf's studied here, sequence data on the primary amino acid structure of the proteins will be required. Sequence studies on human Tf are well under way at the present time, while sequencing of the hagfish molecule has been initiated.

Acknowledgments

The authors thank Dr. Charles R. Shaw, Department of Biology, The University of Texas M. D. Anderson Hospital and Tumor Institute, Houston, Texas, for the hospitality extended to one of the authors (R. M. P.) during a part of this study.

References

Andrews, P. (1966), *Protides Biol. Fluids Proc. Colloq. 14*, 573.

Boffa, G. A., Faure, A., Got, R., Drilhon, A., and Fine, J. M. (1966), *Protides Biol. Fluids Proc. Colloq. 14*, 97.

Charlwood, P. A. (1963), *Biochem. J. 88*, 394.

Chen, S.-H. (1968), Ph.D. Dissertation, Austin, Texas, The University of Texas at Austin.

Chen, S.-H., and Sutton, H. E. (1967), *Genetics 56*, 425.

Crestfield, A. M., Moore, S., and Stein, W. H. (1963), *J. Biol. Chem. 238*, 522.

Elleman, T. C., and Williams, J. (1970), *Biochem. J. 116*, 515.

Giblett, E. R., Hickman, C. G., and Smithies, O. (1959), *Nature (London) 183*, 1589.

Greene, F. C., and Feeney, R. E. (1968), *Biochemistry 7*, 1366.

Hirs, C. H. W. (1956), *J. Biol. Chem. 219*, 611.

Jamieson, G. A. (1966), *Protides Biol. Fluids Proc. Colloq. 14*, 71.

Jordan, S. M., Kaldor, I., and Morgan, E. H. (1967), *Nature (London) 215*, 76.

Laurell, C.-B. (1960), *Plasma Proteins 1*, 349.

Lowry, O. H., Rosebrough, H. J., Farr, A. L., and Rand, R. S. (1951), *J. Biol. Chem. 193*, 265.

Mann, K. G., Fish, W. W., Cox, A. C., and Tanford, C. (1970), *Biochemistry 9*, 1348.

Manwell, C. (1963), *in* The Biology of Myxine, Brodal, A., and Fange, R., Ed., Oslo, Norway, Scandanavian University Books, p 372.

Masson, P. L., and Heremans, J. F. (1968), *Eur. J. Biochem. 6*, 579.

Matsubara, H., and Sasaki, R. M. (1969), *Biochem. Biophys. Res. Commun. 35*, 175.

Ohno, S., Wolf, U., and Atkin, N. B. (1968), *Hereditas 59*, 169.

Phillips, J. L., and Azari, P. (1971), *Biochemistry 10*, 1160.

Roberts, R. C., Makey, D. G., and Seal, U. S. (1966), *J. Biol. Chem. 241*, 4907.

Schachman, H. A. (1967), *Methods Enzymol. 4*, 32.

Schade, A. L., and Reinhart, R. W. (1966), *Protides Biol. Fluids Proc. Colloq. 14*, 75.

Spik, G. (1968), Ph.D. Dissertation, Lille, France, Université de Lille.

Surgenor, D. M., Koechlin, B. A., and Strong, L. E. (1949), *J. Clin. Invest. 28*, 73.

Sutton, H. E., and Jamieson, G. A. (1971), *in* The Glycoproteins, 2nd ed, Gottschalk, A., Ed., Amsterdam, The Netherlands, Elsevier (in press).

Sutton, H. E., and Karp, G. W. (1965), *Biochim. Biophys.*

Acta 107, 153.
Svedberg, T., and Pedersen, K. O. (1940), The Ultracentrifuge, London, England, Oxford University Press, p 51.
Tanford, C., Kawahara, K., Lapanje, S., Hooker, T. M., Zarlengo, M. H., Salahudoin, A., Aune, K. C., and Takagi, T. (1967), *J. Amer. Chem. Soc. 89*, 5023.
Wang, A.-C. (1966), Ph.D. Dissertation, Austin, Texas, The University of Texas at Austin.
Warren, L. (1959), *J. Biol. Chem. 234*, 1971.
Weber, K., and Osborne, M. (1969), *J. Biol. Chem. 244*, 4406.

Isolation and Properties of Individual Components of Cattle Transferrin: The Role of Sialic Acid

A. Stratil **R. L. Spooner**

INTRODUCTION

The study of the electrophoretic patterns of bovine serum transferrin on starch gel electrophoresis has shown that although the majority of animals fit a set pattern with two main and one weak pair of protein bands for each variant (Makarechian and Howell, 1966), a few animals show a variant pattern with fewer bands (Sartore and Bernoco, 1966; Spooner and Baxter, 1969).

The variation observed by Spooner and Baxter (1969) indicated the presence of a locus separate from the *Tf* locus which controlled the attachment of sialic acid to the polypeptide chain.

More recently, Spooner *et al.* (1970) studied the ontogeny of bovine transferrins and found that, instead of three pairs, there were only three single bands in fetal transferrin and that the formation of pairs did not occur until around term.

Previous studies on the treatment of bovine transferrin with neuraminidase suggested the presence of only two residues of sialic acid available to the enzyme (Parker and Bearn, 1962*b*). More recently, Chen and Sutton (1967), using partially purified transferrin, concluded that all of the heterogeneity was caused by increasing numbers of sialic acid residues for each band seen in gel electrophoresis. Neither of these reports referred to the presence of pairs of bands in adult transferrrin, and their findings did not explain the results of Spooner and Baxter (1969), where it appeared that neuraminidase treatment reduced the mobility of bands in pairs and not singly. Moreover, neither Parker and Bearn (1962*b*) nor Chen and Sutton (1967) were using electrophoretic techniques of sufficient discrimination to visualize all of the bands present in homozygous cattle transferrin. It was therefore decided to attempt to isolate the individual transferrin bands and use these isolated bands to examine the causes of the complex heterogeneity found in this protein. Preliminary results of this work were described by Stratil and Spooner (1970).

MATERIALS AND METHODS

Serum

Serum from cattle with known transferrin genotype was used. No pooled sera were used, though in some cases more than one example of the same phenotype was purified.

Isolation of Transferrins and Individual Transferrin Bands

For separation of transferrins, the method of Rivanol–ammonium sulfate precipitation was used (see Schultze and Heremans, 1966). Further purification of transferrins and separation of individual bands were accomplished by ion exchange chromatography on DEAE-Sephadex A-50 and gel filtration on Sephadex G-200, if needed. The isolation procedure is shown in Fig. 1.

Starch Gel Electrophoresis

Transferrin types and the process of fractionation were checked by starch gel electrophoresis with tris–cacodylic acid buffer (Spooner and Baxter, 1969). For the study of apotransferrins, tris–citric acid, *p*H 7.6, was also used (Spooner *et al.*, 1970).

Immunoelectrophoresis

Rabbit antisera to whole serum and to crude transferrin were used to check the purity of the preparations by immunoelectrophoresis (Scheidegger, 1955) by the use of 1.5% agar in 0.04 M sodium barbitone–HCl buffer, *p*H 8.2, and a voltage gradient of 5 v/cm.

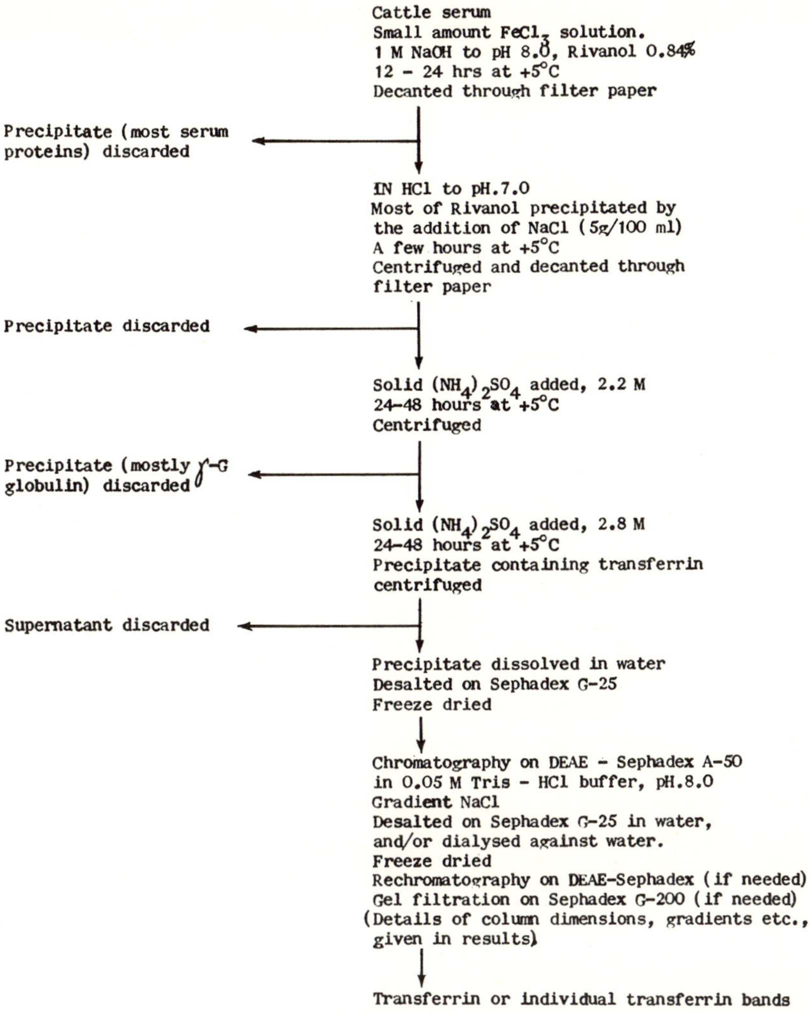

Fig. 1. Scheme for the isolation of bovine transferrin and its individual components.

Homogeneity

Homogeneity of transferrin preparations was studied in an MSE analytical ultracentrifuge; 0.5% transferrin solution in phosphate buffer, *p*H 7.2, was centrifuged at 55,000 rpm for 120 min at 20 C. Photographs were taken at intervals of 8 min.

Estimation of Molecular Weight

Estimation of molecular weight (Andrews, 1964, 1965) was performed by gel filtration on Sephadex G-200. Sephadex was packed into a 4.5 cm^2 by 62 cm column, and 0.1 M tris–HCl buffer + 0.5 M NaCl + 0.02% sodium azide was used as eluant; 10–15 mg samples were dissolved in 2 ml buffer and applied to the top of the Sephadex bed, after excess buffer had drained away. Flow rate of 7.8 ml/cm^2/hr was used, and 3 ml fractions were collected. For calibration of the column and for comparison, the following proteins were used:

Ovalbumin (hen egg)—(Sigma Chemical Co., grade II), further purified on Sephadex G-200 before use; molecular weight 45,000 (Warner, 1954).

Albumin (bovine)—(Sigma Chemical Co., 2× crystallized); molecular weight 67,000 (Putnam, 1965).

IgG (bovine)—isolated from the Rivanol supernatant by precipitation with 2.2 M ammonium sulfate and purified on Sephadex G-200; the purity was confirmed by immunoelectrophoresis; molecular weight 160,000.

Transferrin (pig), conalbumin (hen egg), and conalbumin (duck egg) were generous gifts from Dr. J. Williams (University of Bristol).

Transferrin (human) and IgG (human) were isolated by Rivanol precipitation of most of the serum proteins and further fractionation of the supernatant on Sephadex G-200.

Isoelectric Focusing

Isoelectric focusing was performed as described by Wenn and Williams (1968). Ampholytes of *p*H range 3–6 and 4–6 were used for the separation of approximately 25 mg of Tf A preparation, or artificial mixtures of isolated bands.

Preparation of Apotransferrins and the Method of Reconstitution

Transferrin solution was dialyzed against four changes of 0.25 M sodium citrate–citric acid buffer, *p*H 3.8, and then against water. Finally, the solution was freeze-dried. For starch gel electrophoresis, the apotransferrin preparation was dissolved in the gel buffer. Iron was added to apotransferrin as 0.002 M $FeCl_3$. 6 H_2O in 0.1 M $NaHCO_3$ + 0.1 M sodium citrate. Samples were incubated 1 hr at room temperature, after addition of iron.

Autoradiography

Autoradiography was performed as previously described using Fe^{59}-citrate (Spooner *et al.*, 1970).

Neuraminidase Treatment

Samples (0.5–1.0 mg) of freeze-dried protein were dissolved in 60–70 μl 0.2 M acetate buffer, *p*H 5.25, + 0.04 M $CaCl_2$, and 30–40 μl neuraminidase ex *Vibrio cholerae*

(BDH; activity 500 units/ml) was added. Samples were incubated at 37 C for 2, 6, 24, and 48 hr respectively.

Sialic Acid

Sialic acid was determined by the thiobarbituric acid assay (Aminoff, 1961) after 25 min hydrolysis of the protein at 80 C in 0.1 N sulfuric acid. *N*-acetylneuraminic acid was used as standard.

RESULTS

Starch Gel Electrophoretic Patterns of Cattle Transferrins

With a suitable buffer system, homozygous cattle serum transferrins give three pairs of bands in starch gel electrophoresis, the most anodic pair being the weakest. Figure 2 shows the most common genetic variants (Tf A_1, Tf D_1, Tf D_2, and Tf E) after isolation by Rivanol–ammonium sulfate precipitation. In Fig. 3, three different types are shown—normal adult Tf A, fetal Tf A, and abnormal adult TF A (Spooner and Baxter, 1969). All of these three types are apparently the products of a single allele.

Isolation of Individual Transferrin Bands

To study the nature of the heterogeneity of transferrin variants, it was necesary to isolate individual bands in a pure state. The preparations after Rivanol–ammonium

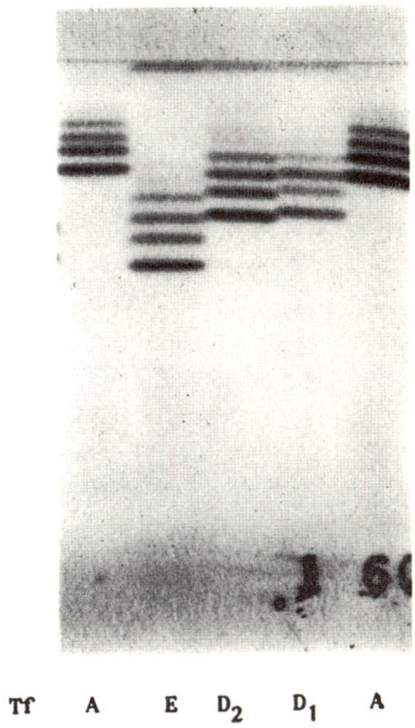

Fig. 2. Starch gel electrophoresis of the four genetic variants of cattle transferrins after Rivanol–ammonium sulfate precipitation.

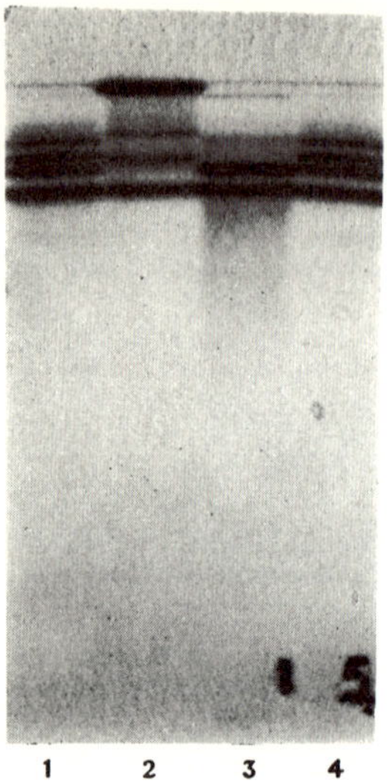

Fig. 3. Starch gel electrophoretic separation of normal adult Tf A (samples 1 and 4), fetal Tf A (sample 2), and abnormal adult Tf A (sample 3). Samples were obtained by DEAE-Sephadex chromatography, except sample 2, which was obtained from Rivanol supernatant.

sulfate precipitation served as a starting material. Initially, following the studies of Wenn and Williams (1968), isoelectric focusing was used to attempt to isolate individual bands, but it did not give satisfactory results. The reason for this failure will be dealt with later in this paper. It was found, however, that in chromatography of transferrin on DEAE-Sephadex A-50 with a linear gradient of NaCl the transferrin formed a nonsymmetrical peak. This experiment indicated that DEAE-Sephadex had the potential to separate proteins as similar as the bands of a single genetic variant. It was found in the course of the study that the use of long columns and shallow gradients was necessary for a satisfactory separation.

Although with this method there was some overlapping of individual bands, it was found possible to separate the major individual components from unfractionated transferrin with a shallow gradient using conditions as given in Fig. 5A. To obtain bands free of visible contaminants, rechromatography on DEAE-Sephadex was, however, found necessary.

During fractionation other bands were detected, some with an electrophoretic mobility slower than the slowest band normally detectable in starch gel electrophoresis of sera and some with a mobility faster than the fastest bands. These slower and faster bands were present in all of the variants studied and both bound Fe^{59}, indicating that they were transferrins (Fig. 4A and Fig. 4B).

Twelve bands found in homozygous Tf A are schematically illustrated in Fig. 5B, and starch gel electrophoresis of all isolated bands is shown in Fig. 5C. It was observed that these always behaved as pairs of bands, hence giving six pairs in the normal homozygous type. When the *p*H of the gel buffer was dropped from 7.45 to 7.25, the distance between pairs of bands was increased, while the distance between the bands within a single pair was decreased. The designation of numbers 0–5 for the pairs of bands is related to their sialic acid content and will be dealt with later in this paper.

In starch gel electrophoresis of sera, only pairs 2 and 3 and a weaker pair 4 are detectable. Pairs 0, 1, and 5 can be detected only after fractionation and concentration. The intensity of bands within a pair is not identical, but generally the slower band, a, is more intense than band b; this is true for all of the pairs. The order of pairs according to decreasing intensity is as follows:

$$2 > 3 > 4 > 1 > 0 > 5$$

The situation in abnormal Tf A is slightly different in that the intensities of pairs 3 and 4 are comparable to the intensities of pairs 4 and 5 in the normal Tf A and pair 2 is more intense in the abnormal Tf A than in the normal. The bands of pair 5 were not detected in abnormal Tf A.

Isoelectric Focusing

Isoelectric focusing of a transferrin preparation (Tf A), when using ampholyte *p*H range 3–6, gave a complicated picture. Six to eight peaks were detected; the most clearly defined peak had a *p*H of 5.2 and contained bands 2a and 2b. Most of the other zones had a lower *p*H (ranging from 4.75 to 4.25). Starch gel electrophoresis of

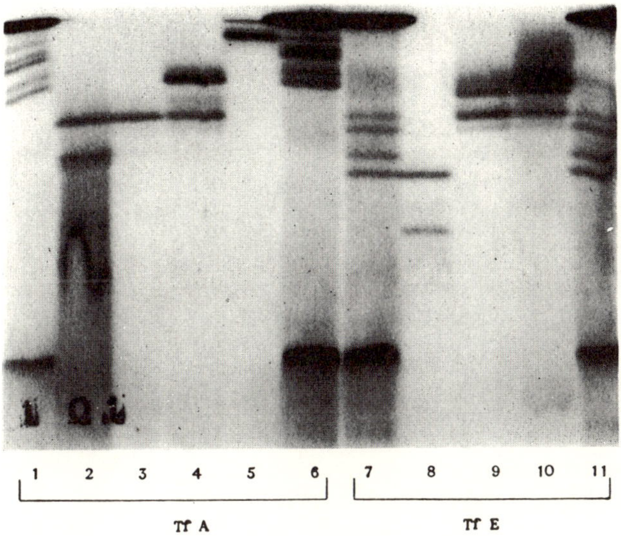

Fig. 4A. Starch gel electrophoresis of transferrin bands, which are slower (samples 2, 3, 4, and 8) and faster (samples 5, 9, and 10) than the bands normally detected in serum. In sample 5 the weak band just near the borate line is not transferrin. Samples 1, 6, 7, and 11—serum. Fe^{59}-citrate was added to the samples before electrophoresis.

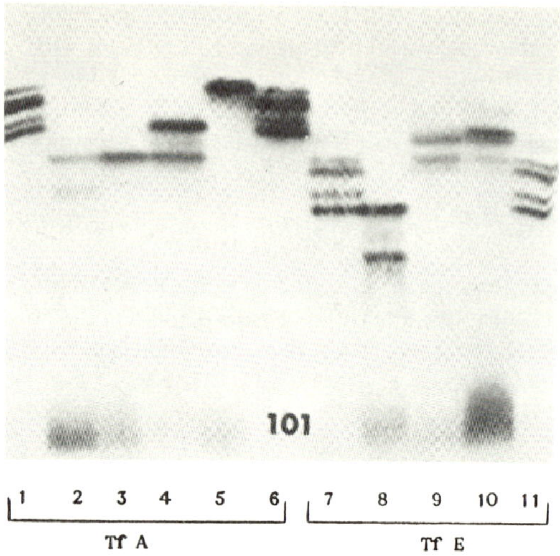

Fig. 4B. Autoradiograph of the gel shown in Fig 4A. The fastest transferrin bands are best seen in sample 10 from Tf E.

the fractions always showed the presence of both bands of a pair, the relative intensity of bands a and b being the same in all cases. In some fractions, two pairs of bands were detected.

In isoelectric focusing of a preparation containing bands 2a and 2b (when using ampholyte *p*H range 4–6), three peaks of about equal intensity were detected, the *p*H

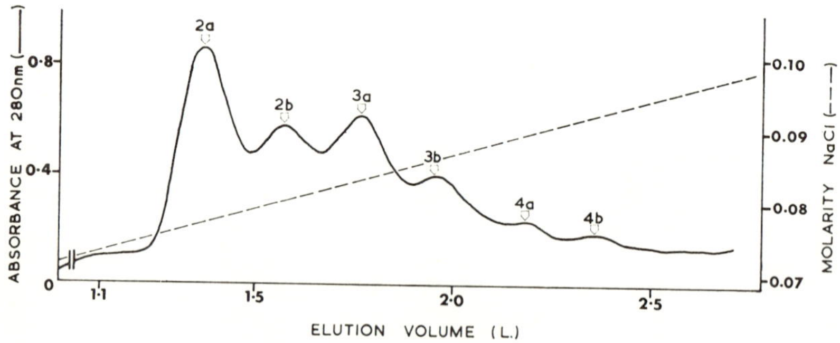

Fig. 5A. Separation of cattle transferrin on DEAE-Sephadex in 0.05 M tris–HCl buffer, *p*H 8.0. A sample (480 mg) was fractionated on the column 8.0 cm^2 by 57 cm. Gradient elution from 0.06 to 0.10 M NaCl; flow rate 50 ml/hr; 12 ml fractions were collected. Numbers 2a, 2b, 3a, 3b, 4a, and 4b refer to the transferrin bands as shown in Fig. 5B.

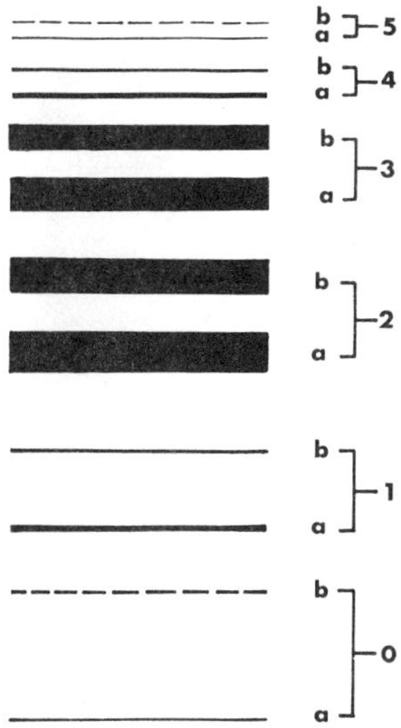

Fig. 5B. Schematic diagram of all transferrin bands isolated from Tf A.

of these peaks being 4.9, 5.2, and 5.7, respectively. However, bands 2a and 2b were present in all peaks in the same ratio.

It is known that iron dissociates from transferrin in isoelectric focusing (Wenn and Williams, 1968), and hence this splitting of pair 2 into three fractions each containing both bands of pair 2 is apparently due to this dissociation and suggests that the three pairs represent transferrin with differing numbers of iron atoms per mole of protein. It can also be seen how this reduplication of pairs produced by differing amounts of iron can produce the complex picture seen when unfractionated bovine transferrin is subjected to isoelectric focusing.

Apotransferrins and the Effect of Iron

As was shown in Figs. 4A and 4B, all detected bands bound Fe^{59}. The addition of further Fe^{3+} had no effect on the transferrin pattern, indicating that all detected bands represented transferrin saturated with iron. Removal of iron from transferrin dramatically changed the electrophoretic pattern when tris–citrate buffer was used for starch gel electrophoresis (Fig. 6). In apotransferrins, two additional regions were detected, each of which contained two or three bands. The region nearest to the origin was more diffuse than that just anodic to it. Moreover, weak bands were present in the position where transferrin bands were normally found. Binding of Fe^{59} was shown to take place in the intermediate and normal transferrin regions after addition of Fe^{59} to apotransferrin, but not in the region nearest to the origin. The position of individual regions varied according to the particular genetic variant. After addition of

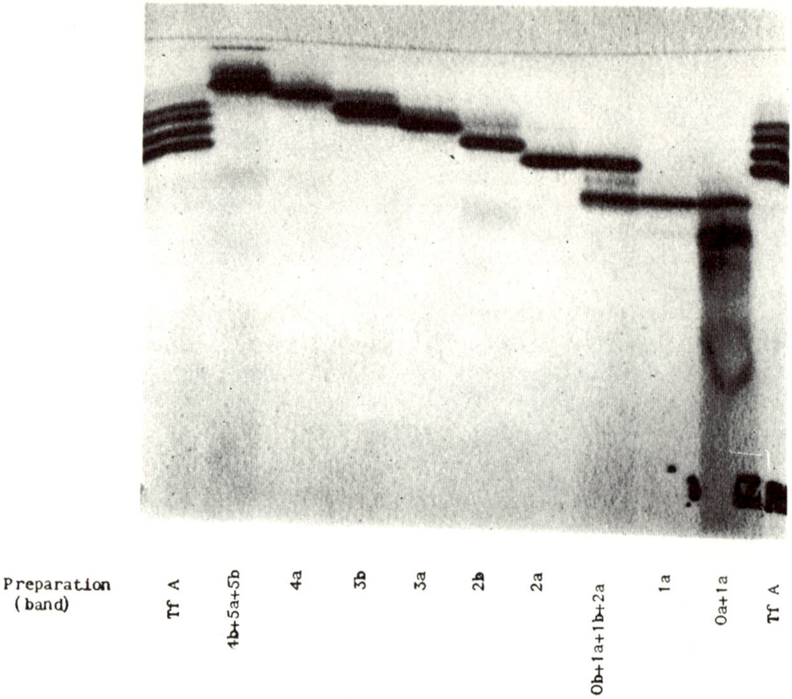

Fig. 5C. Starch gel electrophoretic pattern of all isolated bands from Tf A. Band 5b is very weak in this picture but it can be clearly demonstrated when a higher concentration of the sample is used. Trailing from the origin in sample 10 and the very fast band in sample 2 are not transferrins. Samples 1 and 11—isolated unfractionated Tf A.

buffer with $FeCl_3$, both slower regions disappeared, leaving only the bands migrating in the normal transferrin position, i.e., representing transferrin saturated with iron.

In tris-cacodylic acid buffer, only two regions were detected in apotransferrin preparations, one representing transferrin with iron and the other transferrin without iron.

Degree of Purity of Individual Fractions

In starch gel electrophoresis, most of the preparations are homogeneous, except preparations containing the bands 0 and 1, where diffuse trailing from the origin is present, and preparations of bands 4a and 4b, where another faster migrating band was usually present. Bands 5a and 5b were difficult to isolate in sufficient quantity and purity because of their low concentration.

In immunoelectrophoresis, most preparations of transferrin of 0.5% or above contained, in addition to the main transferrin arc, another faster weak arc. This was

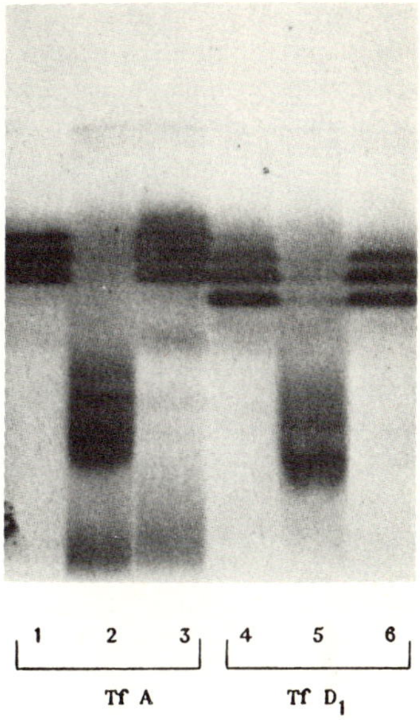

Fig. 6. Starch gel electrophoresis of apo- and Fe-transferrins. Samples 1 and 6—crude transferrin preparations; samples 2 and 5—apotransferrin preparations; samples 3 and 4—apotransferrin + $FeCl_3$ (30 μl of 0.002 M $FeCl_3$ was added to 70 μl of 2.5% protein solution). Samples after Rivanol–ammonium sulfate precipitation, except sample 1, which was chromatographed on DEAE-Sephadex.

not detected when the sample was diluted to 0.1%. The fast component did not bind Fe^{59} and was therefore not transferrin. It is interesting, however, that the relationship of this faster arc to the main transferrin arc is invariant; e.g., the contaminant for Tf E is slower than that for Tf A, suggesting that although it does not bind Fe^{59} this protein may be closely related to or bound to transferrin. This contaminating component is difficult to remove from transferrin preparations. It was neither possible to remove it by chromatography on CM-Sephadex or by gel filtration on Sephadex G-200. Preparations free of this component could only be obtained after rechromatography on DEAE-Sephadex (Fig. 7).

In analytical ultracentrifugation, both band 2a and a mixture of bands 2a and 2b form a single symmetrical peak, giving an S°_{20w} of 5.18.

Estimation of Molecular Weight

Both unfractionated transferrin and mixtures of a few bands or individual bands form a symmetrical peak in gel filtration on Sephadex G-200. To investigate whether or not individual bands differ in their molecular weights, mixtures of bands 2a and 2b were analyzed. The first and last transferrin fractions eluted from the column were tested in starch gel electrophoresis. In both cases, the relative intensity of the two bands was exactly the same, without any sign of them being separated. No difference was found in the elution volumes of bands 2a + 2b, and 3b.

Comparisons of elution volumes of cattle transferrins with other iron-binding proteins and with proteins of known molecular weights are shown in Table I.

Preliminary studies with meniscus depletion sedimentation equilibrium (Yphantis, 1964) in aqueous buffer gave a molecular weight of 77,500 for a mixture of bands 2a and 2b of native Tf A, and results after reduction in 6 M guanidine hydrochloride gave a value of 62,200. Although there is no explanation for this lower value at present, it nevertheless confirms the single-chain nature of bovine transferrin. These studies will be given in detail elsewhere (Feinstein *et al.*, in preparation).

Neuraminidase Treatment and Sialic Acid Determination

Individual bands 2a and 2b were incubated with neuraminidase for 3, 6, 24 (Fig. 8), and 48 hr. Sialic acid splitting was fast during the first 6 hr after which the reaction slowed down. The resulting pattern after 48 hr incubation was little different from that after 24 hr treatment, although in some cases it was not apparently complete even then.

Unfractionated Tf A after incubation with neuraminidase formed two bands, the slow one having the mobility of the band 0a and the fast one that of band 0b. The band 0a was not changed by neuraminidase treatment. However, bands 1a, 2a, 3a,

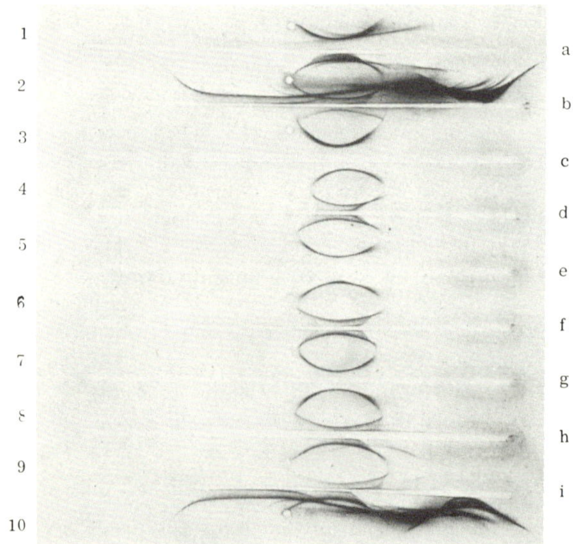

Fig. 7. Immunoelectrophoresis of several transferrin preparations (0.5% solution) and their comparison with cattle serum. Samples 1, 2, and 10—serum; samples 3–7—transferrin preparations after rechromatography on DEAE-Sephadex; samples 8 and 9—transferrin preparations after one chromatography on DEAE-Sephadex. Antiserum against crude transferrin preparation (troughs a, c, e, and g) and cattle serum (troughs b, d, f, h, and i).

Table I. Elution Volumes and Corresponding Molecular Weights for Proteins Studied

Protein	Elution volume (ml)	Molecular weight
Ovalbumin (hen egg)	200.0	45,000[a]
Albumin (bovine)	182.0	67,000[a]
γG-globulin (bovine)	143.0	160,000[a]
Transferrin (bovine)	178.0	74,000
Transferrin (pig)	178.0	74,000
Transferrin (human)	173.0	82,000
Conalbumin (hen egg)	178.0	74,000
Conalbumin (duck egg)	188.0	60,000
γ-Globulin (human)	138.0	180,000

[a] References are given in *Materials and Methods*.

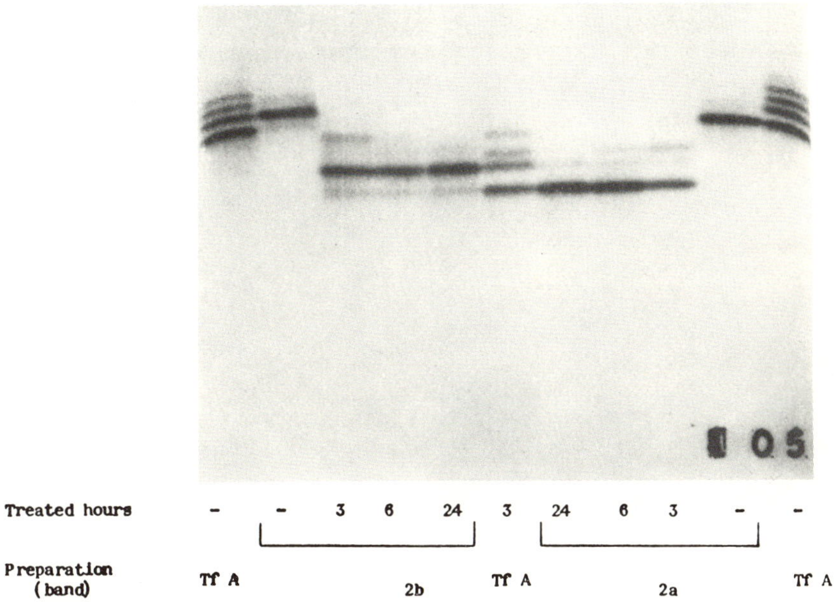

Fig. 8. An example of the effect of neuraminidase treatment on isolated bands to show the stepwise slowing of the bands with increased duration of treatment.

and 4a migrated with the mobility of the band 0a after treatment, and bands 2b, 3b, and 4b with the mobility of the band 0b. Bands 0b, 1b, 5a, and 5b were not studied because of lack of sufficient material.

After neuraminidase treatment of abnormal transferrin, the result was indistinguishable from that of the normal Tf A. However, after treatment of fetal Tf A,

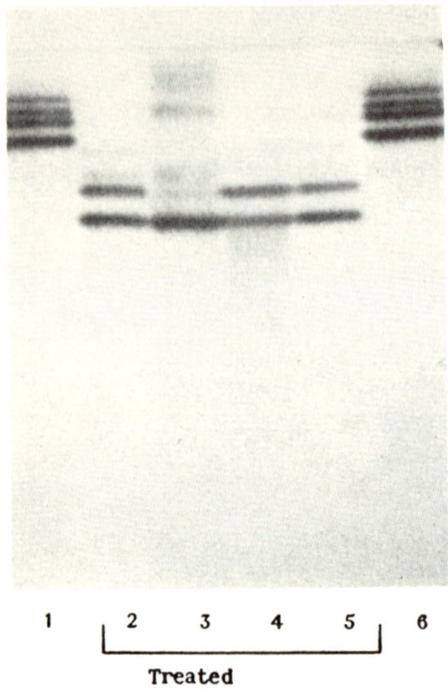

Fig. 9. Comparison of adult normal Tf A (samples 2 and 5), fetal Tf A (sample 3), and adult abnormal Tf A (sample 4) after treatment with neuraminidase. Sample treated 24 hr, except sample 2, which was treated 6 hr. Sample 3 contained in addition to transferrin some faster bands (see Fig. 3), their electrophoretic mobility being also decreased after neuraminidase treatment. Samples 1 and 6—untreated normal Tf A.

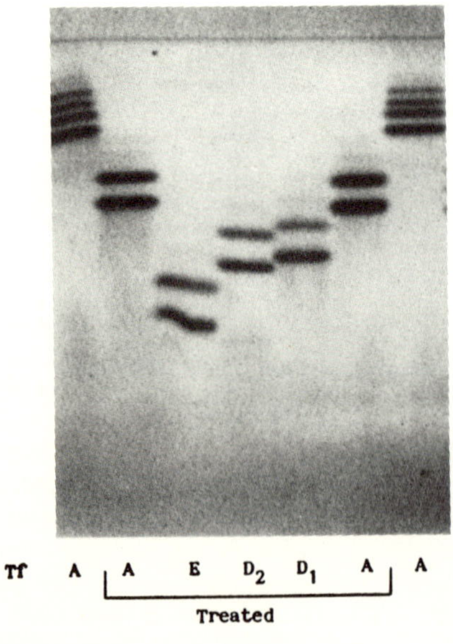

Fig. 10. Starch gel electrophoresis of genetic variants of transferrins (Tf A, Tf D_1, Tf D_2, and Tf E) after 24 hr neuraminidase treatment.

Table II. Sialic Acid Content of Some Transferrin Components

Transferrin variant	Band	μM sialic acid/ mg protein	M sialic acid/ 77,500 g protein	Nearest integer
Normal Tf A	2a	0.0256	1.98	2
	2b	0.0227	1.76	2
	3a	0.0390	3.02	3
	3b	0.0391	3.03	3
	4a+4b	0.0549	4.25	4
	4b	0.0525	4.07	4
Abnormal Tf A	2a	0.0259	2.01	2
	2b	0.0246	1.91	2
	3a+3b	0.0331	2.57	3
	3b	0.0341	2.64	3

only one band was detected having the position of band 0a (Fig. 9). This result fits with the observation that in fetal transferrins only the slower band of each pair is present (Spooner *et al.*, 1970).

Neuraminidase treatment of isolated unfractionated preparations of Tf D_1, Tf D_2, and Tf E showed exactly the same final results of one pair of bands, and the difference in the mobility between individual variants remained (Fig. 10).

Analyses of the sialic acid content of individual bands, which complement the result of neuraminidase treatment, are given in Table II. It seems that all sialic acid present in transferrin is accessible to neuraminidase as the results of neuraminidase treatment are in good agreement with the sialic acid determination. These results show that pair 2 contains two residues of sialic acid, pair 3 three residues, and pair 4 four residues of sialic acid per molecule of protein. It is reasonable to expect that the 0 pair of bands does not contain sialic acid, pair 1 contains one residue, and pair 5 contains five residues of sialic acid per molecule of protein.

DISCUSSION

Properties of Transferrin

The fact that bands a and b of a single pair could neither be separated by isoelectric focusing or by gel filtration on Sephadex G-200 showed that they have the same isoelectric point and very similar molecular weights. However, the finding that they could be separated on DEAE-Sephadex indicates that although they have the same isoelectric point they have different charges at the *p*H of the buffer used (8.0). DEAE-Sephadex has the advantage over starch block electrophoresis and isoelectric focusing that it is also possible to concentrate trace components (0a, 0b, 1a, 1b, 5a, 5b) of transferrins and handle much larger quantities of material.

The weaker bands described above (0a, 0b, 1a, 1b, 5a, and 5b) have been shown to be transferrin. They bind Fe^{59}, they behave like other detectable transferrin bands after neuraminidase treatment, they occur in all transferrin variants, and they are immunologically identical with the faster, stronger bands. There is no reason to think that they might be denaturation products formed during the isolation procedure.

Earlier studies on neuraminidase treatment of cattle transferrins suggested that there were two residues of sialic acid for each protein band (Parker and Bearn, 1962*b*). More recently, using polyacrylamide gel electrophoresis, Chen and Sutton (1967) detected two strong, one weak, and one trace band in homozygous Tf A. They purified the three strongest bands and treated them with neuraminidase and concluded that the heterogeneity was entirely caused by differing numbers of sialic acid residues, with the slowest band having two residues of sialic acid.

In studies on normal and abnormal transferrins, it was found that neuraminidase treatment produced four bands and all of these were slower than the untreated transferrin variant (Spooner and Baxter, 1969). Similar results were obtained on treatment of purified normal bovine transferrins (Dostal and Hunter, 1970*b*). From the results presented in this paper, it can be seen that in the earlier studies sialic acid was not completely removed. Moreover, in the studies by Chen and Sutton (1967), the separation technique was not sufficiently sensitive to discriminate between all transferrin bands within a single variant.

Studies on the iron-binding proteins of other animal species, including man, have shown that these too are heterogeneous. Sialic acid is responsible for most of this heterogeneity, which, depending on the number of residues per protein molecule, produces mostly two or three bands (e.g., chicken serum and seminal plasma transferrins—Williams, 1962 and Stratil, 1970; rabbit serum and milk transferrin—Baker *et al.*, 1968), but up to five bands in human cord transferrins (Parker *et al.*, 1963). Human cerebrospinal transferrin has also been shown to have two to four bands, again produced by differing numbers of sialic acid residues (Parker and Bearn, 1962*b*, and others).

Heterogeneity of iron-binding proteins which is unrelated to sialic acid has also been described (e.g., bird conalbumins—Clark *et al.*, 1963; human transferrins—Parker and Bearn, 1962*a*; see also Schultze and Heremans, 1966). Chicken conalbumin which has no sialic acid has two components. These components were shown to be identical in amino acid composition (Wenn and Williams, 1968) and their peptide maps were very similar (Williams and Wenn, 1970), suggesting that the difference does not lie in the polypeptide chain. However, unlike cattle transferrin, the two components of conalbumin can be separated by isoelectric focusing (Wenn and Williams, 1968). Further studies are in progress to determine the difference between these two basic components of bovine transferrin.

All of the 12 transferrin bands in a single genetic variant represent transferrin saturated with iron. The effect of iron on the electrophoretic mobility of transferrin has theoretical significance, because it makes possible the investigation of the independence of iron-binding sites in iron-binding proteins. Three zones, representing human transferrin or hen egg conalbumin without iron, and with one or two iron atoms per molecule of protein, were demonstrated by free-boundary electrophoresis (Warner and Weber, 1953; Aisen *et al.*, 1966), by isoelectric focusing (Wenn and Williams, 1968), and, with conalbumin, by starch gel electrophoresis (Stratil, 1967). The apotransferrin preparations described in this paper gave comparable results to those with hen egg conalbumins. It is probable, therefore, that the region nearest to the origin represents transferrin without iron, the intermediate region being transferrin with one atom of Fe and the fastest region transferrin with two atoms of iron per molecule of protein.

It is evident that the separation of apotransferrins is dependent on the buffer system used, because only two regions were detected with tris–cacodylic acid. The concentration of protein in the sample used for starch gel electrophoresis is also of great importance; if the concentration is too low, apotransferrin can become saturated with iron with which it comes into contact during electrophoresis, and the resulting pattern is then the same as the pattern of Fe-transferrin.

It is clear from the results of a number of authors (see Feeney and Allison, 1969) that the molecular weights of iron-binding proteins range from 70,000 to 90,000. The molecular weights determined in this study are in accordance with those published. Although the molecular weights estimated by gel filtration on Sephadex are not absolutely accurate (Andrews, 1964, 1965), it is evident that the molecular weight of cattle transferrin is similar to the molecular weight of hen egg conalbumin and pig transferrin and that it is lower than human transferrin and higher than bovine albumin. The value 74,000 found as the molecular weight for cattle transferrin on Sephadex G-200 and the value 77,500 by meniscus depletion sedimentation equilibrium seem to be more exact than the values of 103,000 (Hines, 1965) and 62,000 (Dostal and Hunter, 1970*a*).

Although the problem of subunits in cattle transferrins was not studied adequately it seems from the preliminary results with the meniscus depletion method (Feinstein *et al.*, in preparation), and from comparison with the studies on transferrins of other species (Greene and Feeney, 1968; Elleman and Williams, 1970) and man (Bezkorovainy and Grohlich, 1967; Mann *et al.*, 1970), that cattle transferrins are represented by a single polypeptide chain.

Genetic Consideration

On the basis of the detailed studies presented in this paper and the previous studies of abnormal transferrins (Spooner and Baxter, 1969), and fetal transferrins (Spooner *et al.*, 1970), it appears possible that at least three different loci control the biosynthesis of cattle transferrins.

First, there is the locus responsible for the synthesis of the polypeptide chain (Tf_P). The commonest genetic variants controlled by this locus are Tf A, Tf D_1, Tf D_2, and Tf E. It is to be expected that the nature of the differences between individual variants lies in single amino acid substitutions and that these variants are in fact sequential primary allomers, comparable to the genetic variants of human hemoglobins, human transferrins, and many other polymorphic proteins which have been studied extensively. Codominant inheritance of these variants has been proved convincingly by Ashton (1958), Smithies and Hickman (1958), Kristjansson and Hickman (1965), and others.

Second is a locus controlling the attachment of sialic acid to the polypeptide chain (Tf_{SA}). In abnormal transferrins (Spooner and Baxter, 1969), most of the trans-

D

ferrin has two residues of sialic acid, but that with three and four residues is comparable in intensity to that with four and five residues in the normal transferrin. Evidence presented by Spooner and Baxter (1969) indicated that this attachment of sialic acid was probably controlled by a locus separate from Tf_P. Further family material collected since their paper was written serves to confirm this conclusion. It appears that the normal distribution of sialic acid (0–5) is controlled by a dominant gene, $Tf_{SA}S$, and the abnormal pattern 0–4 by a recessive gene $Tf_{SA}s$ (Spooner and Baxter, unpublished).

It is likely that there are other control mechanisms responsible for variations in the relative proportions of individual transferrin pairs, but there is no experimental evidence available at the moment.

Third, a locus controlling the formation of band b in a single pair of bands (Tf_X) can be postulated. The cause of the difference between bands a and b has not yet been found, but it is quite clear that there must be another type of genetic determination, because the b bands are not present in early fetal life. They appear gradually only a short period before birth, which indicates that locus Tf_X is activated later than loci Tf_P and Tf_{SA}, which are active at least as early as 12 weeks of fetal life (Spooner *et al.*, 1970).

It seems that the locus Tf_X controls the attachment of a component to the polypeptide chain which causes an increase in the negative charge of some transferrin molecules at alkaline *p*H. These then appear as the b bands in each pair. One possible explanation is that this component may be some carbohydrate attached to the transferrin molecule.

ACKNOWLEDGMENTS

We would like to thank Mr. R. A. Oliver for technical assistance and Mr. G. Baxter for the graphs and photographs. We are also most grateful to Dr. A. H. Maddy for the sialic acid assays and Dr. A. E. Stuart for the ultracentrifuge studies.

REFERENCES

Aisen, P., Leibman, A., and Reich, H. A. (1966). Studies on the binding of iron to transferrin and conalbumin. *J. Biol. Chem.* **241**: 1666.

Aminoff, D. (1961). Methods for the quantitative estimation of *N*-acetylneuraminic acid and their application to hydrolysates of sialo mucoids. *Biochem. J.* **81**: 384.

Andrews, P. (1964). Estimation of the molecular weights of proteins by Sephadex gel-filtration. *Biochem. J.* **91**: 222.

Andrews, P. (1965). The gel-filtration behaviour of proteins related to their molecular weights over a wide range. *Biochem. J.* **96**: 595.

Ashton, G. C. (1958). Genetics of *β*-globulin polymorphism in British cattle. *Nature* **182**: 370.

Baker, E., Shaw, D. C., and Morgan, E. H. (1968). Isolation and characterization of rabbit serum and milk transferrins. Evidence for difference in sialic acid content only. *Biochemistry* **7**: 1371.

Bezkorovainy, A., and Grohlich D. (1967). The behaviour of native and reduced–alkylated human transferrin in urea and Guanidine–HCl solutions. *Biochem. Biophys. Acta* **147**: 497.

Chen, S., and Sutton, H. E. (1967). Bovine transferrins: Sialic acid and the complex phenotype. *Genetics* **56**: 425.

Clark, J. R., Osuga, D. T., and Feeney, R. E. (1963). Comparison of avian egg white conalbumins. *J. Biol. Chem.* **238**: 3621.

Dostal, J., and Hunter, A. G. (1970*a*). Isolation of genetic variants of bovine serum transferrin. *J. Dairy Sci.* **53**: 651.

Dostal, J., and Hunter, A. G. (1970*b*). The role of polymorphic proteins in production of cattle. Presented at 12th Conference on Blood Groups and Protein Polymorphism in Animals, Budapest, July 1970 (in press).

Elleman, T. C., and Williams, J. (1970). The amino acid sequences of cysteic acid–containing peptides from performic acid–oxidized ovotransferrin. *Biochem. J.* **116**: 515.

Feeney, R. E., and Allison, R. G. (1969). *Evolutionary Biochemistry of Proteins: Homologous and Analogous Proteins from Avian Egg Whites, Blood Sera, Milk and Other Substances*, Wiley, New York, p. 290.

Green, F. C., and Feeney, R. E. (1968). Physical evidence for transferrins as single polypeptide chains. *Biochemistry* **7**: 1366.

Hines, H. C. (1965). Some biochemical and immunological properties of bovine transferrins and the implication of these properties in genetic control mechanisms. *Diss. Abst.* **26**: 1895.

Kristjansson, F. K., and Hickman, C. G. (1965). Subdivision of the allele Tf^D for transferrins in Holstein and Ayrshire cattle. *Genetics* **52**: 627.

Makarechian, M., and Howell, W. E. (1966). Improved technique for separation and identification of bovine beta globulins by starch-gel electrophoresis. *Can. J. Biochem. Physiol.* **44**: 1089.

Mann, K. G., Fish, W. W., Cox, A. C., and Tanford, C. (1970). Single-chain nature of human serum transferrin. *Biochemistry* **9**: 1348.

Parker, W. C., and Bearn, A. G. (1962*a*). Additional genetic variation of human serum transferrin. *Science* **137**: 854.

Parker, W. C., and Bearn, A. G. (1962*b*). Studies on the transferrins of adult serum, cord serum, and cerebrospinal fluid. The effect of neuraminidase. *J. exptl. Med.* **115**: 83.

Parker, W. C., Hagstrom, J. W. C., and Bearn, A. G. (1963). Additional studies on the transferrins of cord serum and cerebrospinal fluid. Variation in carbohydrate prosthetic groups. *J. Exptl. Med.* **118**: 975

Putnam, F. W. (1965). Structure and function of the plasma proteins. In Neurath, H. (ed.), *The Proteins*, Vol. III, Academic Press, New York, pp. 153–267.

Sartore, G., and Bernoco, D. (1966). Research on biochemical polymorphisms in the indigenous cattle of Piedmont, *Proc. Xth Europ. Congr. Animal Blood Groups*, Paris, pp. 283–287.

Scheidegger, J. J. (1955). Une micro-methode de l'immunoelectrophorese. *Intern. Arch. Allergy Appl. Immunol.* **7**: 103.

Schultze, H. E., and Heremans, J. F. (1966). *Molecular Biology of Human Proteins with special Reference to Plasma Proteins*, Vol. 1, *Nature and Metabolism of Extracellular Proteins*, Elsevier, Amsterdam.

Smithies, O., and Hickman, C. G. (1958). Inherited variations in the serum proteins of cattle. *Genetics* **43**: 374.

Spooner, R. L., and Baxter, G. (1969). Abnormal expression of normal transferrin alleles in cattle. *Biochem. Genet.* **2**: 371.

Spooner, R. L., Land, R. B., Oliver, R. A., and Stratil, A. (1970). Foetal and neonatal transferrins in cattle. *Animal Blood Groups Biochem. Genet.* **1**: 241.

Stratil, A. (1967). The effect of iron addition to avian egg white on the behaviour of conalbumin fractions in starch gel electrophoresis. *Comp. Biochem. Physiol.* **22**: 227.

Stratil, A. (1970). Studies on proteins of seminal fluid from the vasa deferentia of cock, *Gallus gallus* L. *Intern. J. Biochem.* **1**: 728.

Stratil, A., and Spooner, R. L. (1970). Studies on the nature of the heterogeneity of cattle transferrin. *Animal Blood Groups. Biochem. Genet.* **1**: 173.

Warner, R. C. (1954). Egg proteins. In Neurath, H. (ed.), *The Proteins*, Vol. II, Part A, Academic Press, New York, pp. 435–458.

Warner, R. C., and Weber, J. (1953). The metal combining properties of conalbumin. *J. Am. Chem. Soc.* **75**: 5094.

Wenn, R. V., and Williams, J. (1968). The isoelectric fractionation of hen's-egg ovotransferrin. *Biochem. J.* **108**, 69.

Williams, J. (1962). A comparison of conalbumin and transferrin in the domestic fowl. *Biochem. J.* **83**: 355.

Williams, J., and Wenn, R. V. (1970). Radioactive peptide "maps" of the major and minor components of hen's egg ovotransferrin. *Biochem. J.* **116**: 533.

Yphantis, D. A. (1964). Equilibrium ultracentrifugation of dilute solutions. *Biochemistry* **3**: 297.

J. WILLIAMS
C. F. PHELPS
J. M. LOWE

Ovotransferrin with One Iron Atom

TRANSFERRINS are iron-binding proteins which can carry a maximum of two atoms of iron per mole protein. If a preparation of hen ovotransferrin is incompletely saturated with iron and subjected to isoelectric focusing three main protein fractions are observed[1]. The most acidic fraction (pH$_I$ 5·78) is the protein complex with two iron atoms, and the most alkaline fraction (pH$_I$ 6·73) is the metal-free protein. In the intermediate fraction (pH$_I$ 6·25) iron and protein are present in equimolar amounts and Wenn and Williams[1] suggested that this fraction is a protein complex with one iron atom.

Woodworth, Tan and Virkaitis[2] suggest, however, that the intermediate isoelectric fraction represents a dimer composed of one molecule each of metal-free protein and iron-saturated protein. According to their interpretation of gel filtration experiments the intermediate isoelectric fraction is a labile dimer and on polyacrylamide gel electrophoresis at pH 7·5 it apparently dissociates, giving two bands which correspond to the metal-free protein and the protein complex with two iron atoms. They state they have never observed an intermediate band corresponding to a protein complex with one iron atom upon polyacrylamide gel electrophoresis.

Evidence against the proposed dimer is provided by the earlier experiments of Stratil[3]. After addition of increasing amounts of iron to whole egg white, starch gel electrophoresis gave an iron-containing band lying between the bands representing the metal-free protein and the iron-saturated protein. The intermediate band disappeared on complete saturation with iron and all the ovotransferrin was then present as the protein complex with two iron atoms. Stratil[3] suggested that the intermediate band consisted of protein molecules bearing only one atom of iron. We now report experiments on the effect of adding iron to purified metal-free ovotransferrin as determined by starch gel electrophoresis and ultracentrifugation.

Ovotransferrin bearing different amounts of iron can be resolved by starch gel electrophoresis if contaminating metals are removed from the starch powder (Connaught hydrolysed starch, lot 270–1) by washing successively with 0·02 M EDTA and deionized water. Dialysis tubing and glassware were cleaned similarly. Iron, as 100 mM iron-nitrilotriacetate[4], was added to a 2 per cent solution of the metal-free protein in 0·05 M $NaHCO_3$. Starch gel electrophoresis at pH 8·6 illustrated (Fig. 1) that in the course of converting the metal-free protein into the fully

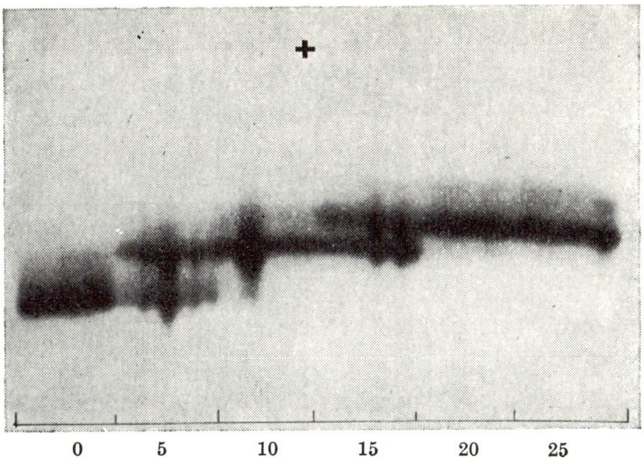

Fig. 1. Starch gel electrophoresis of ovotransferrin in the discontinuous buffer system of Poulik[7]. 11 mg of metal-free ovotransferrin was dissolved in 0·5 ml. 0·05 M $NaHCO_3$. Successive additions of 5 μl. of 100 mM iron-nitrilotriacetate were made and samples were removed for electrophoresis. The addition of 20 μl. of iron-nitrilotriacetate resulted in complete saturation.

saturated iron-transferrin complex an intermediate band exists. It seemed likely that this band would correspond to the intermediate fraction observed in isoelectric fractionation experiments[1].

Isoelectric fractionation was therefore performed on a partially iron saturated preparation of ovotransferrin as described previously[1] and the intermediate fraction (pH_I 6·25) was isolated, dialysed against deionized water (NH_4OH added to pH 9) to remove ampholytes and sucrose, and finally lyophilized. The pink coloured powder was dissolved in 0·05 M $NaHCO_3$ and examined by starch gel electrophoresis with markers of metal-free ovotransferrin and iron-saturated ovotransferrin. Fig. 2 demonstrates that the isolated fraction gives one main band whose mobility is intermediate between those of the two marker proteins; it also contains a small amount of the fully saturated protein. The electrophoretic mobility of the intermediate fraction in starch gel suggests that its molecular weight is not twice that of the marker proteins, for it would then be expected to move more slowly.

In sedimentation experiments, batches of metal-free ovotransferrin dissolved in different buffer solutions were divided into several aliquots which were then titrated with 100 mM iron-nitrilotriacetate to give different degrees of iron saturation, estimated from the $A_{470\ nm}$. In all cases the peaks were allowed to migrate at least half-way across the cell and they showed no heterogeneity. In the case of the half saturated and wholly saturated protein the absorption pattern of the sediment-

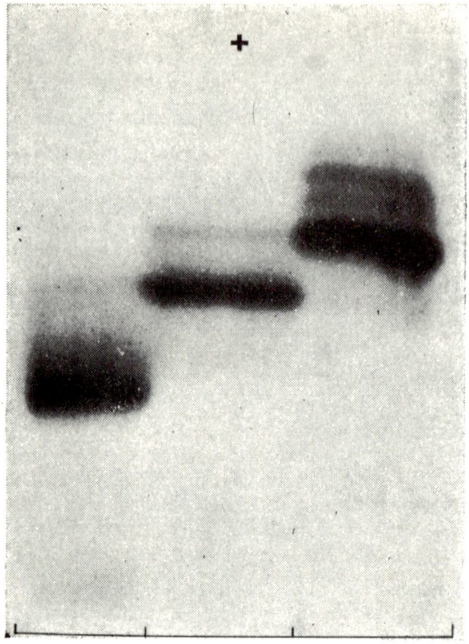

Fig. 2. Starch gel electrophoresis. Samples *a* and *c* are iron-free ovotransferrin and fully iron saturated ovotransferrin, respectively. Sample *b* is the intermediate band recovered from the isoelectric column.

ing material (as measured with an interference filter at 460 nm) coincided with the peak observed in the Schlieren experiments. In addition, in all experiments the whole of the protein could be accounted for refractively. After removal from the cell the samples showed no increase in iron content, as judged by the $A_{470\ nm}$. The sedimentation coefficients observed in three experiments are given in Table 1. In experiment 2, the buffer was the same as that used for starch gel electrophoresis. There is no increase in the sedimentation coefficient at half saturation which might have suggested the presence of a dimer. In all cases the

Table 1. SEDIMENTATION COEFFICIENTS OF OVOTRANSFERRIN SATURATED TO DIFFERENT EXTENTS WITH IRON

Buffer	Per cent iron saturation				
	0	25	50	75	100
Imidazole-HCl (0·05 M), NaCl (0·05 M), *p*H 6·8	5·1	5·0	4·9	4·8	4·9
Tris-citrate (0·076 M), *p*H 8·6	4·6	—	4·9	—	4·8
Tris (0·075 M), $NaHCO_3$ (0·05 M), HCl, *p*H 8·6	4·8	4·8	4·6	4·5	4·8

The sedimentation coefficients relate to zero protein concentration at 19° in the quoted buffer solutions.

concentration dependence of the sedimentation coefficient was greater for the fully iron-saturated protein than for the metal-free protein, which agrees with the finding by Fuller and Briggs[5] that iron-transferrin has a greater axial ratio than the metal-free protein.

The results of starch gel electrophoresis and ultracentrifugation thus support the earlier proposal[1] that the intermediate fraction observed during isoelectric fractionation is a transferrin complex with one iron atom. This implies that iron atoms are distributed among the metal-binding sites on the protein in an essentially random manner[1,6,8] and it is contrary to the view that the metal atoms bind only in pairs to the protein[4,9,10]. Many authors[1,4,6,8–10] have apparently assumed that a random distribution of metal atoms between the binding sites could only arise if the dissociation constants for the first (K_1) and second (K_2) metal atoms were approximately equal. K_2 has been variously reported to be less than K_1 (ref. 11), approximately equal to K_1 (ref. 6) or much greater than K_1 (ref. 9). It is clear, however, that the binding is effectively irreversible at alkaline *p*H (dissociation constant $\simeq 10^{36}$ M; ref. 6), and it has been shown[12] that no exchange of iron between transferrin molecules occurs at *p*H 7·3 in the absence of chelating agents. We suggest that the iron atoms are randomly distributed on the binding sites, which reflects only the availability of these sites, and we cannot draw conclusions as to the relative values of the dissociation constants.

1 Wenn, R. V., and Williams, J., *Biochem. J.*, **108**, 69 (1968).

2 Woodworth, R. C., Tan, A. T., and Virkaitis, L. R., *Nature*, **223**, 833 (1969).

3 Stratil, A., *Comp. Biochem. Physiol.*, **22**, 227 (1967).

4 Woodworth, R. C., in *Protides of the Biological Fluids* (edit. by Peeters, H.), **14**, 37 (Elsevier, Amsterdam, 1967).

5 Fuller, R. A., and Briggs, D. R., *J. Amer. Chem. Soc.*, **78**, 5253 (1956).

6 Aasa, R., Malmström, B. G., Saltman, P., and Vanngard, T., *Biochim. Biophys. Acta*, **75**, 203 (1963).

7 Poulik, M. D., *Nature*, **180**, 1477 (1957).

8 Aisen, P., Leibman, A., and Reich, H. A., *J. Biol. Chem.*, **241**, 1666 (1966).

9 Warner, R. G., and Weber, I., *J. Amer. Chem. Soc.*, **75**, 5094 (1953).

10 Schade, A. L., *Farmaco*, **19**, 185 (1963).

11 Davis, B., Saltman, P., and Benson, S., *Biochem. Biophys. Res. Commun.*, **8**, 56 (1962).

12 Aisen, P., and Leibman, A., *Biochem. Biophys. Res. Commun.*, **32**, 220 (1968).

SOME IMMUNOCHEMICAL PROPERTIES OF SUCCINYLATED HUMAN TRANSFERRIN AND RELATED PROTEINS

RAINER HANS ZSCHOCKE AND ANATOLY BEZKOROVAINY

INTRODUCTION

As early as 1934, LANDSTEINER AND VAN DER SCHEER[1] showed the ability of short-chain mono- and dibasic aliphatic acids (including succinic acid), coupled to proteins, to elicit specific antibody formation. In that work, the organic acids were attached to the protein as *p*-aminophenyl or *p*-aminoaniline derivatives *via* diazo coupling reactions, yielding mostly insoluble diazo proteins. Direct succinylation of proteins using succinic anhydride, on the other hand, yields soluble protein derivatives, and has become, in recent years, a valuable tool for the study of protein structure[2–5].

In view of the versatility of the direct succinylation technique, it seemed advisable to reinvestigate the changes in antigenicity of proteins that accompany their succinylation and, possibly, a partial unfolding. Transferrin was chosen as a model compound for these studies because of our previous experience with this protein.

We were, furthermore, interested in whether antibodies to the "active site" of transferrin could be produced in rabbits by injecting them with transferrin succinylated in the presence of iron and with the iron subsequently removed (partially

Abbreviation: AgN, antigen nitrogen.

succinylated transferrin). Previous studies indicated that the active site of transferrin was protected against losses of activity if succinylation was done in the presence of iron[3,4].

MATERIALS AND METHODS

Human apo-transferrin and human transferrin antiserum were purchased from Hoechst Laboratories. Antisera to immunoglobulin G, bovine immune globulin, and orosomucoid were obtained from Hyland Laboratories. Succinic anhydride was the product of Eastman Laboratories. Polyethylene glycol compound 20 M was kindly provided by the Union Carbide Corp.

Human transferrin was saturated with iron by the method of KORNFELD[6], and was succinylated as previously described[3]. The iron was then removed by exhaustive dialysis against 2.5% EDTA at pH 6, and the preparation was then used to immunize two albino rabbits. The immunization was done by four intramuscular injections of 5 mg protein each in complete Freund's adjuvant over a period of 1 month. After a booster injection of 5 mg protein in $Al(OH)_3$ 14 days after the last intramuscular injection, the rabbits were bled during the 10th week following the first injection. Fully succinylated transferrin, human serum and bovine colostrum 7-S globulins, and reduced-alkylated orosomucoid were prepared from the native proteins as previously described[3].

Quantitative precipitin reactions were done essentially as described by KABAT AND MAYERS[7,8]. Antigen protein solution (approx. 0.05%) in 0.1 M Tris–HCl buffer (pH 8.0) was added to 0.5-ml aliquots of antiserum. Volumes were brought to 1.0 ml with the above Tris buffer, and the precipitates were collected by centrifugation after an incubation at 37° for 60 min, and 4° for 48 h. Precipitates were washed 3 times with 0.15 M NaCl prior to Kjeldahl nitrogen analysis (Markham micro-Kjeldahl method[9]). Inhibition with sodium succinate was done by pre-incubating 0.5-ml aliquots of antiserum with 0.05 and 0.1 M sodium succinate solutions in Tris–HCl buffer (pH 8.0) at 37° for 30 min. Antigen protein was then added, precipitates were allowed to form for 30 min at 37°, and were then analyzed for nitrogen as described above.

Antigen nitrogen (AgN) was determined by precipitating the proteins with 5% phosphotungstic acid in 2 M HCl (in case of orosomucoid, 1 part of the protein solution was mixed with 1 part of the phosphotungstic acid solution). The precipitates were washed twice with the phosphotungstic acid solution and then analyzed for nitrogen by the Kjeldahl method.

Double diffusion (Ouchterlony) experiments were done on agar-coated microscope slides (1.25% Difco-Nobel agar in 0.05 M veronal buffer at pH 8.2 (ref. 10)). The intensity of the precipitin lines was increased by the repeated infusion of polyethylene glycol compound 20 M into the antibody wells after all antiserum had diffused into the agar[11].

RESULTS AND DISCUSSION

Fully succinylated transferrin, the immune globulins, and the reduced-alkylated orosomucoid failed completely to give precipitin lines in the Ouchterlony system with antisera to the native proteins. However, all the succinylated proteins

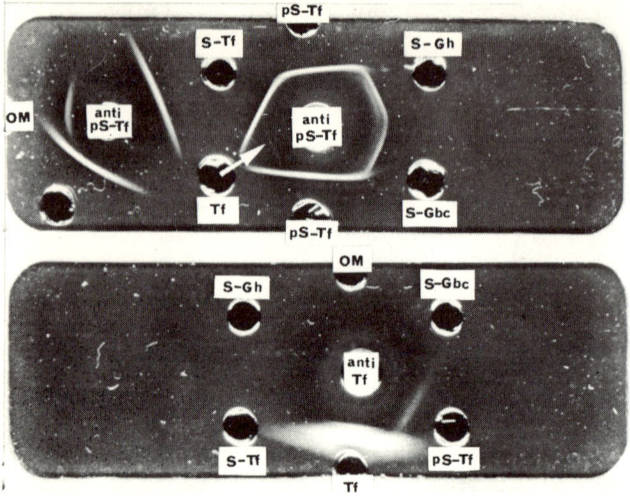

Fig. 1. Double diffusion analyses (Ouchterlony method) of succinylated proteins. Abbreviations: anti pS-Tf and anti Tf, antisera to partially succinylated and native transferrins respectively; pS-Tf, partially succinylated transferrin; S-Tf, fully succinylated transferrin; Tf, native transferrin; S-Gh, succinylated human 7-S globulin; S-Gbc, succinylated bovine colostrum immune globulin; OM, reduced-alkylated-succinylated orosomucoid.

TABLE I

CROSSREACTIVITY OF VARIOUS SUCCINYLATED PROTEINS WITH ANTISERUM TO PARTIALLY SUCCINYLATED TRANSFERRIN AND EVIDENCE FOR NON-ABSORBABLE ANTIBODIES DIRECTED AGAINST SOME NATIVE PORTION OF THE TRANSFERRIN MOLECULE

Antigen	*AgN added per 0.5 ml antiserum (µg)*	*Total nitrogen precipitated (µg)*	*Relative reactivity (%)**	*R value***	
				Found	*Expected*
Partially succinylated transferrin	3.60	71.80	100.0	10.4	10.4
Native transferrin	2.16***	25.60	16.1	5.4	—
Fully succinylated transferrin	3.20	87.86	126.4	13.7	10.8
Succinylated human serum 7-S globulin	3.44	75.68	103.5	21.0	10.5
Succinylated bovine colostrum 7-S globulin	3.28	67.10	94.5	19.5	10.7
Reduced-alkylated-succinylated orosomucoid	2.05	58.30	116.5	4.5	12.5
Experiments done with 1.5 ml antiserum absorbed with fully succinylated transferrin					
Native transferrin	0.72	10.20	17.0	6.8	—
Partially succinylated transferrin	0.72	7.60	12.6	5.0	—

* Partially succinylated transferrin is assumed to represent 100% reactivity.

** *R* values "expected" calculated from the precipitin curve given in Fig. 2. Mol. wts. used: γ-globulins: 160 000; native, partially and fully succinylated transferrins: 83 000 (ref. 3); reduced-alkylated-succinylated orosomucoid: 44 100, 41.4% carbohydrate[13]; antibody globulin: 160 000.

*** 1.5 ml of antiserum was used in this experiment.

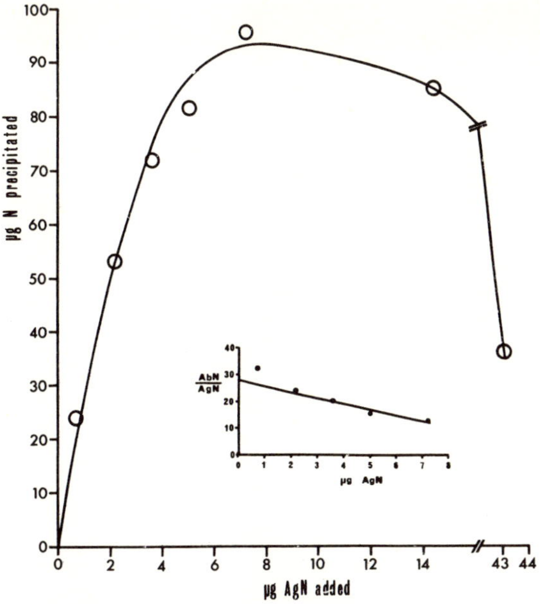

Fig. 2. Precipitin curve obtained with partially succinylated transferrin and its specific antiserum. The curve could be approximated by the relationship[12] $AbN = -mAgN^2 + bAgN$. The inserted plot of AbN/AgN *vs.* AgN served to determine m and b, where m was found to be −2.291, and b was 28.1.

showed good precipitin lines with the antiserum prepared to the partially succinylated transferrin, giving partial identity patterns. The partially succinylated transferrin, on the other hand, gave a precipitin line with both its specific antiserum and the antiserum to native transferrin, giving a partial identity pattern with native transferrin (Fig. 1).

The quantitative precipitin curve involving the partially succinylated transferrin and its specific antiserum is shown in Fig. 2. Molar antibody to antigen ratios (R values) in this system ranged from 14.5 in the extreme antibody excess region to 6.8 at equivalence to 2.6 in the moderate antigen excess region. Native apotransferrin, precipitated with its specific antiserum, gave R values of 7.2, 2.7, and 1.5 at extreme antibody excess, equivalence, and antigen excess regions respectively.

The amount of cross-reactivity of other succinylated proteins with the antiserum to partially succinylated transferrin is shown in Table I. It is seen that the R values for all succinylated proteins, except that of orosomucoid, were higher than that for the partially succinylated transferrin. Moreover, it may be noted that the R values were more dependent on the size of the proteins rather than the number of succinyl residues present in the proteins (approx. 63, 90, and 20 succinyl residues per molecule of transferrin, the immune globulins, and orosomucoid respectively). This is consistent with the view that R values depend not only on the number of antigenic determinants present in a protein molecule, but also on the maximum number of antibody molecules that can exist in physical contact with the antigen molecule. The fully succinylated transferrin had a higher R value than the partially succinylated protein, probably because of the higher Stokes radius of the former[3].

The participation of the succinyl residues in the antibody formation was confirmed by a hapten inhibition experiment using sodium succinate. These results indicated that in the presence of 0.01, 0.02, and 0.04 M succinate, percent inhibition of the precipitin reaction was 12, 24, and 35 respectively. The amount of antigen nitrogen added (partially succinylated transferrin) was 7.18 mg, corresponding to the point of equivalence (see Fig. 2).

It is clear from Fig. 1 and Table I that antibodies to partially succinylated transferrin formed precipitates with native apotransferrin, and that native transferrin antiserum reacted with the partially succinylated transferrin but not with the fully succinylated transferrin. These data were confirmed by absorbing the antiserum to partially succinylated transferrin with fully succinylated transferrin (to remove the antibodies specific for the succinyl residues), and performing the quantitative precipitin reaction with the absorbed antiserum and the partially succinylated and native transferrins. Table I (bottom portion) indicates that precipitates were still formed in this system.

Whether or not the section of native and partially succinylated transferrins reacting with the antiserum to the latter protein is indeed the active site (iron-binding site) cannot be unequivocally determined with the data obtained thus far. It is now believed, that transferrin, upon combining with iron, assumes a more compact conformation[3,14]. This change in conformation may give rise to additional antigenic (conformational) determinants (see also ref. 15). However, these determinants should, upon succinylation and the removal of iron, lose their antigenic activity, since the protein then should return to the conformation resembling that of the apotransferrin molecule. It should also be noted that the production of antisera as well as all quantitative precipitin tests and double diffusion analyses were performed with the iron-free proteins.

Alternatively, it may be argued that antigenic determinants different from those of the iron-binding site become masked following the addition of iron, and are re-exposed upon succinylation and removal of iron. Such determinants would then be expected to give precipitin lines with the native transferrin antiserum, and to elicit specific antibody formation. This and other possibilities described above are now being investigated in this laboratory.

ACKNOWLEDGEMENTS

This work was supported by U.S. Public Health Service Grant No. GM 11985-06. R.Z. is a U.S. Public Health Service trainee (Grant No. 5 TO1 GM-00471-08 BCH).

REFERENCES

1 K. Landsteiner and I. Van Der Scheer, *J. Exptl. Med.*, 59 (1934) 751.
2 I. M. Klotz and S. Keresztes-Nagy, *Biochemistry*, 2 (1963) 448.
3 A. Bezkorovainy, R. Zschocke and D. Grohlich, *Biochim. Biophys. Acta*, 181 (1969) 295.
4 R. Zschocke and A. Bezkorovainy, *Federation Proc.*, 28 (1969) 514.
5 J. Lenard and S. Singer, *Nature*, 210 (1966) 536.
6 S. Kornfeld, *Biochemistry*, 7 (1968) 945.

7 E. A. Kabat and M. M. Mayers, *Experimental Immunochemistry*, Thomas, Springfield, 2nd Ed., 1961, p. 67.
8 E. A. Kabat and M. M. Mayers, *Experimental Immunochemistry*, Thomas, Springfield, 2nd Ed., 1961, p. 72.
9 E. A. Kabat and M. M. Mayers, *Experimental Immunochemistry*, Thomas, Springfield, 2nd Ed., 1961, p. 480.
10 R. Zschocke, H. Grieble, G. Bach and T. O. Anderson, *J. Immunol.*, 102 (1969) 625.
11 M. Ceska, *Biochim. Biophys. Acta*, 177 (1969) 625.
12 E. A. Kabat and M. M. Mayers, *Experimental Immunochemistry*, Thomas, Springfield, 2nd Ed., 1961, p. 27.
13 H. E. Schultze and J. F. Heremans, *Molecular Biology of Human Proteins*, Vol. 1, Elsevier, New York, 1966, p. 188.
14 D. D. Ulmer, *Biochim. Biophys. Acta*, 181 (1969) 305.
15 F. M. Kourilsky and P. Burtin, *Nature*, 218 (1968) 375.

The Genetics of Transferrins

GEOGRAPHIC AND SPECIES VARIATION IN TRANSFERRIN AND OVOTRANSFERRIN POLYMORPHISM IN THE COLUMBIDAE

ANDREW FERGUSON

INTRODUCTION

TRANSFERRIN and ovotransferrin (= conalbumin) are iron-binding glycoproteins present in vertebrate plasma and avian egg white respectively. They have identical amino acid compositions and differ only in their carbohydrate moieties (Williams, 1962, 1968). Both transferrin and ovotransferrin appear as one or more discrete fractions on an electrophoretic gel and genetic variants show up as bands of altered electrophoretic mobility.

Genetic variants of transferrin and ovotransferrin occurring in frequencies high enough to be regarded as polymorphism have been found in a high percentage of bird species which have been examined in sufficient numbers. Alternative alleles at the locus (Tf) coding for transferrin and ovotransferrin were observed first in chicken egg white (Lush, 1961) and plasma (Ogden *et al.*, 1962). Further variants in the chicken were observed by Croizier (1966), Baker (1967) and Stratil (1968). Transferrin or ovotransferrin variation has been observed also in feral rock dove (*Columba livia*) and speckled pigeon (*Columba guinea*) (Mueller *et al.*, 1962); red-collared dove (*Streptopelia tranquebarica*) (Desborough & Irwin, 1966); muscovy duck (*Cairina moschata*), domestic goose (*Anser anser*) and laughing gull (*Larus atricilla*) (Stratil & Valenta, 1966); in several species of geese of the genus *Branta* (Baker & Hanson, 1966); ring-necked pheasant (*Phasianus colchicus*)

(Baker & Manwell, 1967); chukar partridge (*Alectoris graeca*) and red-winged blackbird (*Aegalaius phoeniceus*) (Baker, 1967); magpie (*Pica pica*), hooded crow (*Corvus cornix*), black-headed gull (*Larus ridibundus*) and common scoter (*Melanitta nigra*) (Ferguson, 1969). Of the above species, only in the chicken and the three Columbidae has the genetic control of the variation been established by breeding experiments. Here the variation is controlled by codominant alleles at an autosomal locus. The available evidence supports a similar genetic control for the other species.

The value of genetically controlled protein variants as markers in the investigation of the relationships of populations, races and species has been acknowledged for some time (for review see Sibley *et al.*, 1971). In spite of the information fundamental to evolutionary and population biology studies which can be obtained from this approach there have been to date few studies on protein polymorphisms in natural populations of birds. Differing selective pressures may result in unique alleles having evolved in geographically isolated populations. More often, however, selection results in frequency differences among populations for a particular allele. Methods of population genetical analysis such as the Hardy-Weinberg equilibrium can give information on the population structure of a species.

Milne & Robertson (1965) found evidence of partial reproductive isolation between two groups in a colony of eider ducks (*Somateria mollissima*) on the basis of allele frequencies for a variant protein—probably ovotransferrin. Brush (1968, 1970) noted that the ovotransferrin allele frequencies in the red-winged blackbird (*Aegalaius phoeniceus*) varied on a transcontinental basis.

MATERIALS AND METHODS

Plasma and egg white samples of the rock dove (*Columba livia*) were obtained from feral populations in Belfast and from wild populations in coastal areas of counties Antrim and Donegal. Plasma and egg white samples of the wood pigeon (*Columba palumbus*), barbary dove (*Streptopelia risoria*) and collared dove (*Streptopelia decaocto*) were obtained from a number of areas in north Ireland.

Samples were screened using horizontal starch gel electrophoresis with either a discontinuous tris-citrate-sodium-borate buffer system (Poulik, 1957) or a continuous borate system (Smithies, 1959). Gels were prepared with 12% hydrolyzed starch (Connaught Medical Laboratories). A sample of established phenotype was placed at each end of the gel to act as a control for the typing of unknown ones. Following electrophoresis, the gels were stained with 1% Amido Black in methanol, acetic acid and water mixture (50:10:50) or with an iron specific stain, Nitroso-R (Mueller *et al.*, 1962). Acrylamide gel electrophoresis was performed using the commercially available E–C apparatus and a discontinuous gel and buffer system as in the *E–C Technical Bulletin* Vol. 2, No. 1 (1966).

Immunoelectrophoresis, using antisera prepared by hyperimmunizing rabbits to plasma or egg white, was carried out by imbedding starch or acrylamide strips in agar (Poulik, 1964). Ouchterlony immunodiffusion plates were prepared in the standard way. Transferrin was separated from plasma by rivanol precipitation followed by chromotography on DEAE cellulose. Ovotransferrin was separated from egg white by ammonium sulphate precipitation followed by chromatography on DEAE cellulose.

The identification of certain electrophoretic fractions as transferrin or ovotransferrin was based on a number of criteria: (a) The bright green colour of these fractions after staining with the Nitroso-R salt solution. (b) Comparison with purified transferrin or ovotransferrin. (c) Immunoelectrophoresis using plasma as antigen and antiserum prepared against egg white. Immunoelectrophoresis using egg white as antigen and antiserum prepared against plasma.

RESULTS

The transferrins appeared on the electrophoretic patterns as a group of either three or four discrete fractions in the species examined. The ovotransferrins of the two *Columba* species appeared as four or five fractions in a similar position on the gell to the transferrins, but nearer to the origin. The *Streptopelia* species showed one fewer ovotransferrin fraction. The same patterns were observed with both borate and tris-citrate gel buffers and when either starch or acrylamide was used as the supporting medium.

On addition of Fe^{3+} (as ferric chloride) to the yellow plasma no change in colour was noted. By contrast, on addition of Fe^{3+}, the egg white developed a strong red-brown coloration due to the formation of the iron-ovotransferrin complex. When plasma to which iron had been added was separated alongside plasma without iron, no change in mobility of the transferrin fractions was noted. Comparison of ovotransferrin mobilities showed that this protein increased by some 6–10 per cent in its mobility upon addition of iron. In view of this change, iron was added to all samples in an amount sufficient to saturate completely the ovotransferrin molecules before individual variations were classified.

Incubation of plasma, purified transferrin, egg white and purified ovotransferrin with the enzyme neuraminidase, resulted in an overall decrease in mobility of the transferrin fractions until the mobility of these was the same as the mobility of the four major components of ovotransferrin. There was no relative change in the amount of protein in each of the transferrin fractions nor in either mobility or relative amount of the ovotransferrin fractions.

Examination of the patterns of the plasma and egg white of *Columba livia* showed that there was individual variation in the numbers and relative mobilities of the transferrin and ovotransferrin fractions. Three phenotypes were present in each. Based on their mobilities these were classed as slow, fast and slow/fast. The latter had the fractions of both the slow and fast types and could be mimicked by artificially mixing plasmas of these two types. A similar group of three phenotypes was found in the plasma and egg white of *Columba palumbus* and *Streptopelia risoria*. Only one phenotype was found in the plasma of *Streptopelia decaocto* (Fig. 1).

It was found that the transferrin type of the female was the same as the ovotransferrin type of the eggs from that female. Immunoelectrophoresis of the plasma, using antiserum to the egg white, gave precipitin lines for transferrin only. Egg white proteins developed with antiserum to the plasma revealed only ovotransferrin precipitin lines. Using purified transferrin and ovotransferrin in the Ouchterlony immunodiffusion technique, and developing with antiserum to whole plasma and egg white, the precipitin lines formed a continuous arc, indicating identity. The same immunological reactions occurred for all four species.

Genetic control of these transferrin phenotypes can be inferred from the work of Mueller *et al.* (1962) on *C. livia.* Thus the slow and fast forms are homozygotes and the slow/fast form the heterozygote under the control of two codominant alleles.

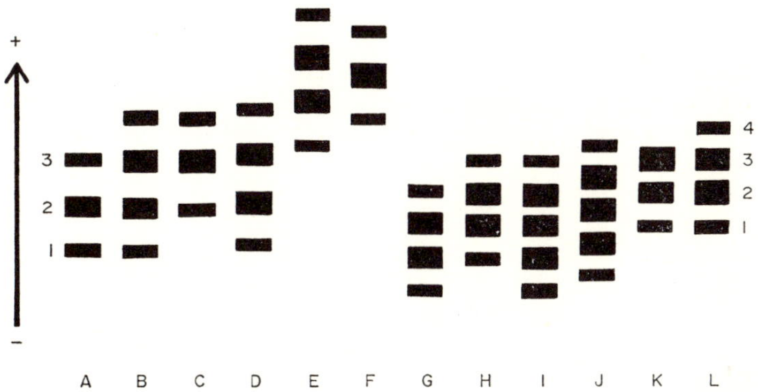

FIG. 1. Transferrin (A–F) and ovotransferrin (G–L) phenotypes as separated by horizontal starch gel electrophoresis at pH 8·6. Zymogram A—*C. livia* slow; B—*C. livia* slow/fast; C—*C. livia* fast; D—*C. palumbus* slow/fast; E—*S. risoria* slow/fast; F—*S. decaocto* fast; G—*C. livia* slow; H—*C. livia* fast; I—*C. livia* slow/fast; J—*C. palumbus* slow/fast; K—*S. risoria* slow; L—*S. risoria* slow/fast.

Baker (1967) has proposed the use of the symbol Tf for transferrin and ovotransferrin with the addition of the superscript s to denote the allele controlling the slow morph and f the allele controlling the fast one. This notation is used in Table 1 which gives the frequencies of these two alleles in different species and populations. The expected phenotype frequencies were calculated assuming Hardy-Weinberg equilibrium and tested for significance using the chi-square test (1 degree of freedom). No correlation was found between the sex of a bird and its transferrin type.

Taking the mobility of *C. livia* plasma albumin as 100 units the relative mobilities of the slowest common fractions of transferrin and ovotransferrin were calculated for each species. Table 2 gives the relative mobilities of transferrin fraction 2 in starch and acrylamide gels and of ovotransferrin fraction 2 in starch gel.

DISCUSSION

Transferrin and ovotransferrin heterogeneity

In most species, the transferrins in the plasma of an animal which is homozygous at the transferrin locus are nevertheless electrophoretically heterogeneous. For example, the transferrin of a homozygous *C. livia* consists of three electrophoretic fractions of constant relative amount. The situation is the same for ovotransferrin,

Table 1—Allele and phenotype frequencies of transferrin and ovotransferrin in various species and populations

Species	Locality	Season	Protein	N	Allele frequency		Phenotype frequency				X^2	P
					Tf^s	Tf^f		ss	sf	ff		
C. livia	Belfast	Year	Transferrin	204	0·664	0·336	O	93·0	85·0	26·0	0·88	< 0·50 > 0·30
							E	90·0	91·0	23·0		
C. livia	N. coast	Summer	Ovotransferrin	140	0·486	0·514	O	37·0	62·0	41·0	1·78	< 0·20 > 0·10
							E	33·1	69·9	37·0		
C. livia	All	Year	Transferrin and ovotransferrin	344	0·592	0·408	O	130·0	147·0	67·0	4·73	< 0·50 > 0·02
							E	120·7	166·2	57·1		
C. palumbus	All	Year	Transferrin	87	0·454	0·546	O	31·0	17·0	39·0	32·0	< 0·001
							E	17·9	43·1	25·9		
C. palumbus	All	Summer	Transferrin	24	0·687	0·313	O	13·0	7·0	4·0	6·63	< 0·01
							E	11·3	10·3	2·4		
C. palumbus	All	Winter	Transferrin	63	0·365	0·635	O	18·0	10·0	35·0	27·12	< 0·001
							E	8·4	29·2	25·4		
C. palumbus	All	Summer	Transferrin and ovotransferrin	87	0·592	0·408	O	42·0	19·0	26·0	26·52	< 0·001
							E	30·4	42·2	14·4		
C. palumbus	Antrim	Summer	Transferrin and ovotransferrin	30	0·717	0·283	O	17·0	9·0	4·0	2·08	< 0·20 > 0·10
							E	15·4	12·2	2·4		
C. palumbus	Fermanagh	Summer	Transferrin and ovotransferrin	50	0·470	0·530	O	18·0	11·0	21·0	25·55	< 0·001
							E	11·1	24·9	14·0		
S. risoria	All	Year	Transferrin	66	0·364	0·636	O	17·0	14·0	35·0	19·5	< 0·001
							E	8·7	30·6	26·7		
S. decaocto	All	Year	Transferrin	19	0·000	1·000						

Table 2—Relative mobilities of transferrin and ovotransferrin

Species	Transferrin fraction 2: Relative mobility in starch	Transferrin fraction 2: Relative mobility in 7% acrylamide	Ovotransferrin fraction 2: Relative mobility in starch
C. livia	39·06 ± 0·49	43·30 ± 0·35	32·24 ± 0·82
C. livia (age 2 days)	34·18	38·97	
C. palumbus	41·42 ± 0·68	43·53 ± 0·68	35·16 ± 0·54
S. risoria	61·73 ± 0·76	55·98 ± 0·84	43·99 ± 0·56
S. decaocto	59·65 ± 1·41	56·81 ± 0·56	

the homozygous *C. livia* having four electrophoretic fractions. Williams (1962) has shown that in the domestic fowl, treatment of the transferrin with the enzyme neuraminidase results in removal of the faster fractions with a corresponding increase in the intensity of the slowest one. Neuraminidase has been used to remove sialic acid from the transferrins of other species, but the electrophoretic result is merely a corresponding reduction in the mobility of the transferrin fractions and the heterogeneity is not removed (Lush, 1967). A similar result was obtained in this study where the transferrins decreased in mobility to that of ovotransferrin after incubation with neuraminidase.

That ovotransferrin heterogeneity can be chemically induced has been suggested by a number of authors (Bain & Deutsch, 1948; Warner & Weber, 1951; Baker & Manwell, 1962; Parker & Bearn, 1963; Baker, 1967). In the present study, electrophoresis was carried out using two different supporting media and three buffer systems with different ionic specificity, ionic strength and pH. Although the mobilities differed among the systems, the heterogeneity was constant. The addition of iron resulted in an increase in mobility of the ovotransferrin as has been noted for a number of other species by Baker (1967). Again, however, the heterogeneity was maintained.

Intraspecific polymorphism

Polymorphism of the Tf locus is present in three of the four species examined. Since both alleles at this locus are of intermediate frequencies in these three species recurrent mutation can be eliminated as a factor in the maintenance of the polymorphism. As the observed number of heterozygotes never significantly exceeded that expected, balanced polymorphism does not exist. The only viable solution is that the polymorphism is maintained by the opposing forces of selection for different alleles in different populations causing frequency divergence and gene flow between populations tending to equate the frequencies. The possibility of selectively neutral mutations and random divergence must also be borne in mind.

In Table 1 it can be seen that the Tf^s allele in the Belfast population of *C. livia* had a higher frequency than the Tf^f allele. The observed numbers of each phenotype are in close agreement with those expected assuming Hardy-Weinberg equilibrium. It is of interest that Mueller *et al.* (1962) found that the Tf^s allele was also the commoner one in their Wisconsin birds. In the thirty-nine sera which they examined, they found that the frequency of Tf^s was 0·603 (calculated from data given in their paper) as compared with 0·664 in the present study. Clearly there cannot be any gene flow between these two populations. It is of interest to question what maintains the Tf^s allele in these two isolated populations at such similar frequencies.

The frequencies of the slow and fast alleles in *C. palumbus* varied with the time of the year and the locality from whence the samples were obtained. When the transferrin phenotypes from all seasons and localities are added together there is a significant deficit of heterozygotes. It is a general principle that a lowered fitness of heterozygotes will result in selection against them and thus a decrease in the observed numbers. Manwell & Baker (1969, 1970) have discussed such negative heterosis in relation to the formation of races and species.

However, if populations of different allelic frequency are lumped together fewer heterozygotes than expected are observed—the Wahlund principle. Thus deficit of heterozygotes suggests that the individuals sampled belonged to two or more semi-isolated populations. When the *C. palumbus* transferrin phenotypes are separated into those from plasmas obtained in the summer and those from plasmas obtained in the winter (October to March), there is a significant difference between the frequencies of the Tf alleles calculated from these two groups. The summer phenotype numbers agree fairly closely with Hardy-Weinberg expectations but the winter numbers show a marked deficit of heterozygotes. In *C. palumbus* the summer breeding birds remain in the same area throughout the year. Only a small proportion of them undertake flights which could be classed as true migration and this primarily involves young birds. Ringing has shown that only about 11 per cent of the adult population and 34 per cent of the juvenile population move more than 25 miles (Murton, 1965). On the other hand, the winter birds in Ireland are probably made up of a high proportion of Continental and Scandinavian birds. That the birds in the winter sample belong to diverse populations could thus account for the lack of heterozygotes.

Egg white samples of *C. palumbus* were obtained from two areas about 100 miles apart in counties Antrim and Fermanagh. There is a significant difference between the Tf allele frequencies in these two areas. Only the phenotype numbers in the Antrim locality are in agreement with Hardy-Weinberg, however. From the large number of recent publications, it would seem that inter-population variation in allele frequency for polymorphic proteins is a common feature in all animals and represents adaptation to local environmental conditions. Geographical variation in transferrin or ovotransferrin allele frequencies has been shown in eider ducks (*Somateria mollissima*) (Milne and Robertson, 1965), red-winged blackbirds (*Aegalaius phoeniceus*) (Brush, 1968), macaque monkeys (Goodman *et al.*, 1965), lizards (Gorman & Dessauer, 1966), chimpanzees (Goodman & Tashian, 1969) and cricket frogs (*Acris*) (Dessauer & Nevo, 1969). Interpopulation variations in enzyme allele frequencies are discussed elsewhere (Sibley *et al.*, 1971).

In *Streptopelia risoria* the TF^{f} allele was found to have the higher frequency. Desborough and Irwin (1966) found only the Tf^{f} allele in their Wisconsin birds of this species (13 examined). They also found that the Tf^{f} allele had the higher frequency in the closely related *Streptopelia humilis*.

In *Streptopelia decaocto* only the Tf^{f} allele was found. Admittedly the number of specimens examined was small (19). In spite of this, if there had been a similar polymorphism as in the other *Columba* and *Streptopelia* species, the probability of having observed it would be very high. It is of interest that this species is a recent arrival in Ireland, being first noted in 1959 following a very rapid spread across Europe from Asia. In ten years it has increased dramatically in numbers and has spread to all parts of the country. Possibly the first arrivals of this species were monomorphic with regard to transferrin and since it would appear that a relatively small number of individuals colonized the country it would seem likely that this is an example of a "founder effect".

It is accepted generally that where genetic polymorphism is present to a significant degree, the condition confers some advantage on the species. However, there is little known about the effect of environmental and other factors on transferrins and ovotransferrins. Ashton (1958) has suggested that transferrin polymorphism may be correlated with climatic tolerance in cattle. Various attempts have been made to correlate transferrin and ovotransferrin types in poultry with certain economically desirable characteristics but as yet with little success (Lush, 1967). Morton *et al.* (1965) have found some evidence of an effect of the transferrin phenotype of the female on the viability of young embryos in Light Sussex hens. The elucidation of the functional significance of protein polymorphisms promises to be a most exciting area of biology during the coming decade.

Intraspecific variation

Since differences in the amino acid sequences of homologous proteins often lead to altered electrophoretic mobility, measurement of the latter should reflect the number of such substitutions and thus the phylogenetic distance. In the measurements of the electrophoretic mobility of the transferrins and ovotransferrins no significant difference (as tested by the Student *t*-test) was found between the congeneric species studied. However, between either of the *Columba* species and either of the *Streptopelia* species the mobility differences between the transferrins and ovotransferrins were found to be significant at the 1 per cent level. Since within the genera there is a greater mobility difference intraspecifically due to polymorphism than between the species, extreme caution is required in drawing taxonomic conclusions on the basis of one sample of a species. The difference in transferrin mobility due to age is a further trap for the unwary. It might be concluded that as well as being of interest in the study of populations within a species, intraspecific variability must be fully investigated in any valid interspecific study below the family level.

Acknowledgements—The author wishes to thank Drs. D. R. Bamford, E. M. Pantelouris and A. Scott for their supervision and counsel during the course of this investigation and

Professor G. Owen for providing facilities. The assistance of Helen P. Ferguson in the preparation of this manuscript is gratefully acknowledged. This work was carried out during the tenure of a Postgraduate Studentship from the Ministry of Education for Northern Ireland in the Department of Zoology, the Queen's University of Belfast, Northern Ireland.

REFERENCES

ASHTON C. G. (1958) Genetics of beta-globulin polymorphism in British cattle. *Nature Lond.* **182**, 370–372.

BAIN J. A. & DEUTSCH H. F. (1948) Separation and characterization of conalbumin. *J. biol. Chem.* **172**, 547–555.

BAKER C. M. A. (1967) Molecular genetics of avian proteins—VII. Chemical and genetic polymorphism of conalbumin and transferrin in a number of species. *Comp. Biochem. Physiol.* **20**, 949–973.

BAKER C. M. A. & HANSON H. C. (1966) Molecular genetics of avian proteins—VI. Evolutionary implications of blood proteins of eleven species of geese. *Comp. Biochem. Physiol.* **17**, 997–1006.

BAKER C. M. A. & MANWELL C. (1962) Molecular genetics of avian proteins—I. The egg white proteins of the domestic fowl. *Br. Poult. Sci.* **3**, 161–174.

BAKER C. M. A. & MANWELL C. (1967) Molecular genetics of avian proteins—VIII. Egg white proteins of the migratory quail, *Coturnix coturnix*—New concepts of "hybrid vigour". *Comp. Biochem. Physiol.* **23**, 21–42.

BRUSH A. H. (1968) Conalbumin variation in populations of the redwinged blackbird, *Agelaius phoeniceus*. *Comp. Biochem. Physiol.* **25**, 159–168.

BRUSH A. H. (1970) An electrophoretic study of egg whites from three blackbird species. *Occ. Papers Biol. U. Conn.* **1**(4), 243–264.

CROIZIER G. (1966) Polymorphismes biochimiques de la poule domestique—I. Analyse génétique des protéines du blanc d'oeuf chez des poules de races françaises et étrangères. *Annls Biol. anim. Biochem. Biophys.* **6**, 379–388.

DESBOROUGH S. & IRWIN M. R. (1966) Additional variation in serum proteins in Columbidae. *Physiol. Zool.* **39**, 66–69.

DESSAUER H. C. & NEVO E. (1969) Geographic variation of blood and liver proteins in cricket frogs. *Biochem. Genet.* **3**, 171–188.

FERGUSON A. (1969) An electrophoretic study of the blood and egg white proteins of some Columbidae. Ph.D. Thesis, the Queen's University of Belfast.

GOODMAN M., KULKARNI A., POULIK E. & REKLYS E. (1965) Species and geographic differences in the transferrin polymorphism of macaques. *Science* **147**, 884–886.

GOODMAN M. & TASHIAN R. E. (1969) A geographical variation in the serum transferrin and red cell phosphoglucomutase polymorphisms of chimpanzees. *Human Biology* **41**, 237–249.

GORMAN G. C. & DESSAUER H. C. (1966) The relationship of *Anolis* of the *Roquet* species group (Sauria: Iguanidae)—I. Electrophoretic comparisons of blood proteins. *Comp. Biochem. Physiol.* **19**, 845–853.

LUSH I. (1961) Genetic polymorphisms in the egg albumen proteins of the domestic fowl. *Nature, Lond.* **189**, 981–984.

LUSH I. (1967) *Biochemical Genetics of Vertebrates Except Man*. North-Holland, Amsterdam.

MANWELL C. & BAKER C. M. A. (1969) Hybrid proteins, heterosis and the origin of species —I. Unusual variation of polychaete *Hyalinoecia* "nothing dehydrogenases" and of quail *Coturnix* erythrocyte enzymes. *Comp. Biochem. Physiol.* **28**, 1007–1028.

MANWELL C. & BAKER C. M. A. (1970) *Molecular Biology and the Origin of Species: Heterosis, Protein Polymorphism and Animal Breeding*. Sidgwick & Jackson, London.

MILNE H. & ROBERTSON F. W. (1965) Polymorphisms in egg albumen proteins and behaviour in the eider duck. *Nature, Lond.* **205**, 367–369.

Morton J. R., Gilmour D. G., McDermid E. M. & Ogden A. L. (1965) Association of blood-group and protein polymorphisms with embryonic mortality in the chicken. *Genetics* **51**, 97–107.

Mueller J. O., Smithies O. & Irwin M. R. (1962) Transferrin variation in Columbidae. *Genetics* **47**, 1385–1392.

Murton R. K. (1965) *The Wood Pigeon.* Collins, London.

Ogden A. L., Morton J. R., Gilmour D. G. & McDermid E. M. (1962) Inherited variants in the transferrins and conalbumins of the chicken. *Nature, Lond.* **195**, 1026.

Parker W. C. & Bearn A. G. (1963) Boric acid induced heterogeneity of conalbumin by starch gel electrophoresis. *Nature, Lond.* **199**, 1184–1186.

Poulik M. D. (1957) Starch gel electrophoresis in a discontinuous system of buffers. *Nature, Lond.* **180**, 1477–1479.

Poulik M. D. (1964) Starch gel immunoelectrophoresis. *Ann. N.Y. Acad. Sci.* **121**, 470–483.

Sibley C. G., Corbin K. W., Ahlquist J. E. & Ferguson A. (1971) *Birds.* In *Biochemical and Immunological Taxonomy of Animals* (Edited by Wright C. A.). (In press.) Academic Press, London.

Sibley C. G., Wilson A. C., Brush A. H., Corbin K. W., Ferguson A. & Ahlquist J. E. (1971) Lactate dehydrogenase and esterase polymorphism in New Guinea starlings (*Aplonis*). (To be published.)

Stratil A. (1968) Transferrin and albumin loci in chickens, *Gallus gallus* L. *Comp. Biochem. Physiol.* **24**, 113–121.

Stratil A. & Valenta M. (1966) Protein polymorphism of egg white and yolk in geese and ducks. *Folia biol. Praha* **12**, 307–309.

Warner R. C. & Weber I. (1951) The preparation of crystalline conalbumin. *J. biol. Chem.* **191**, 173–180.

Williams J. (1962) A comparison of conalbumin and transferrin in the domestic fowl. *Biochem. J.* **83**, 355–364.

Williams J. (1968) A comparison of glycopeptides from the ovotransferrin and serum transferrin of the hen. *Biochem. J.* **108**, 57–67.

SELECTIVELY NEUTRAL MUTATIONS, TRANSFERRINS AND THE EVOLUTION OF NATRICINE SNAKES*

SHOU-HSIAN MAO and HERBERT C. DESSAUER

INTRODUCTION

DOES THE acquisition of selectively neutral mutations account for most of the species differences in protein structure ? Those of us versed in traditional evolutionary theory are reluctant to accept the idea that any acquired mutation is without adaptive affect. Comparative evidence at the molecular level, however, indicates otherwise. In an interpretation of the latter King & Jukes (1969) state: "There appears to be considerable latitude at the molecular level for random genetic changes that have no effect upon the fitness of the organism." We offer additional evidence on this question in the form of comparative data on the magnitude of antigenic differences between the transferrins of natricine snakes of varying degrees of morphological, physiological and ecological divergence.

The data on the transferrins were also used as the basis for speculating on the genetic affinities and evolution of modern snakes. Structural differences in such a series of homologous proteins reflect the relationships of living species and suggest times of divergence of evolutionary lines. Once two taxa are reproductively isolated their genomes evolve independently and their proteins become progressively more unlike. Transferrin, whose structures differ markedly from species to

* Supported by National Science Foundation of the United States (Grant GB-7294X) and by the National Science Council of the Republic of China.

species, appears to offer a sensitive "clock" for timing the divergence of evolutionary lines of relatively modern origin such as those of advanced snakes.

MATERIALS AND METHODS

The thirty-two species of snakes studied are classified by Underwood (1967) as members of seventeen genera and six families (Table 1). Material included two species of the *Natrix* from Asia, all named species of *Natrix* from North America and Europe and four species of genera from Asia and New Guinea that were classified as *Natrix* until recently (Malnate, 1960). These animals were either collected by professional herpetologists or purchased from commercial animal dealers. Blood was obtained from a cardiac puncture using heparin as the anticoagulant. Plasma was either processed immediately or stored in a deep freeze until needed.

Transferrins were isolated from plasma of *Natrix cyclopion, Natrix natrix, Natrix annularis* and *Xenochrophis piscator* using the "Rivanol" procedure of Sutton & Karp (1965) with minor modifications. Dilute transferrin solutions were concentrated by ultrafiltration and further purified by starch-gel electrophoresis (Smithies, 1959). Homogeneity of transferrin preparations was checked by cellulose acetate strip and starch gel electrophoresis. Transferrins were identified on gels by radioautography (Giblett *et al.*, 1959).

Antisera against transferrins of these four species were produced in adult New Zealand white rabbits of 2–4 kg body weight. Usually, 2–4 mg of purified transferrin in a 1 : 1 emulsion of saline and Freund's complete adjuvant (Difco Co.) were injected subcutaneously at multiple sites in the shoulder, flank and groin regions. One month after the initial injections the rabbit was given a second dose of antigen. A week to 10 days later blood for antiserum was collected. Thereafter, as fresh antiserum was required, the rabbit was given another priming dose of antigen and bled in a week. Rabbits were allowed to recover approximately 1 month between bleedings. Blood was drawn from an ear vein directly into a sterile syringe, allowed to clot at room temperature and refrigerated overnight to allow time for clot retraction. Antiserum was removed from clotted cells and stored frozen, without preservatives, in a number of small vials. The purity and specificity of each antiserum were analyzed using immunoelectrophoresis and radioautography (George & Dessauer, 1970).

The antisera produced against the purified transferrins were used to titrate transferrins in plasma samples from numerous species of snakes. Sarich & Wilsons' (1966) modification of Wasserman and Levines' (1961) microcomplement fixation technique (MC′F) was used. To stabilize complement (Baltimore Biological Laboratories) and other protein reactants, 1 g/l. of bovine plasma albumin (Nutritional Biochemical Co.) was added to all diluents. The dilutions of antiserum giving 50 per cent fixation of complement in homologous reactions equaled 7800 for the antiserum against the *Natrix natrix* transferrin; 5300 for that of *N. cyclopion*; 2400 for that of *Xenochrophis piscator*; and 2350 for that of *N. annularis*. Microcomplement fixation crossreactions served as the measure of index of dissimilarity (I.D.), the extent to which an antitransferrin concentration had to be raised for a particular transferrin to give a MC′F reaction equal to that of the homologous transferrin (Sarich & Wilson, 1966). The magnitude of the I.D. correlates directly with the number of sequence differences which distinguish the crossreacting antigen and the homologous antigen (Arnheim *et al.*, 1969).

RESULTS AND DISCUSSION

Transferrin has much to recommend it for use in studies of the nature of evolution at the protein level. This iron binding protein is widely distributed among vertebrates and is usually a major constituent of their plasma. When labeled with radioactive iron, transferrin is easily identified on gel electropherograms

TABLE 1—INDICES OF DISSIMILARITY BETWEEN TRANSFERRINS OF DIFFERENT SNAKES

Species*	Locality of capture	Museum No.†	Index of dissimilarity‡		
			NC	NN	NA
	Caenophidia ‖ NATRICIDAE ‖				
Natrix cyclopion	North America (Louisiana)	X	1·0	5·1	4·4
Natrix erythrogaster	North America (Louisiana)	WF3735	1·2	—	—
N. fasciata clarki	North America (Louisiana)	WF3780	1·1	—	—
N. f. confluens	North America (Louisiana)	WF5543	1·2	—	—
N. f. taeniata	North America (Florida)	WF6153	1·2	—	—
N. harteri	North America (Texas)	WF6853	1·2	—	—
N. rhombifera	North America (Louisiana)	HD1127	1·4	—	—
N. sipedon insularum	North America (Ohio)	WF6130	1·2	—	—
N. taxispilota	North America (Virginia)	WF5052	1·3	—	—
N. valida	North America (Mexico)	WF6712	1·3	—	—
N. maura	Europe§ (Spain)	HD1196	3·8	1·7	—
N. natrix	Europe§ (Italy)	HD1189	4·1	1·0	4·6
N. natrix	Europe (England)	CU9074	—	1·1	—
N. tessellata	Europe§	WF5645	4·1	1·4	—
N. tessellata	Mideast (Israel)	HD1306	—	1·4	—
N. annularis	Asia (Taiwan)	HD1203 to 1206	3·1	3·1	1·0
N. percarinata	Asia (Taiwan)	X	3·8	3·4	1·5
Adelophis foxi	North America (Mexico)	HD729	1·2	—	—
Clonophis kirtlandi	North America (Ohio)	WF5695	1·3	—	—
Regina alleni¶	North America (Florida)	WF6806	1·4	—	—
R. grahami	North America (Louisiana)	WF5705	1·3	—	—
R. rigida	North America (Louisiana)	X	1·1	—	—
R. septemvittata	North America (Ohio)	WF6695	1·5	—	—
Seminatrix pygaea	North America (Florida)	WF6715	1·2	—	—
Storeria dekayi	North America (Florida)	WF6905	1·3	—	—
Thamnophis couchi gigas	North America (California)	WF6055	1·9	—	—
T. sauritus	North America (Mississippi)	WF5880	1·6	—	—
T. sirtalis	North America (Alabama)	WF5917	1·4	—	—
Tropidoclonion lineatum	North America (Texas)	WF5077	1·4	—	—

TABLE 1 (*cont.*)

Species*	Locality of capture		Museum No.†	Index of dissimilarity‡ NC	NN	NA
		Caenophidia ‖ NATRICIDAE‖				
Xenochrophis piscator¶	Asia	(Taiwan)	HD1201	5·5	5·2	6·7
Rhabdophis swinhonis	Asia	(Taiwan)	X	8·2	6·0	6·2
Amphiesma stolata	Asia	(Taiwan)	X	5·9	5·7	5·0
A. sp.	Australia	(New Guinea)	RZ	—	5·9	5·7
		Colubridae ‖				
Coluber constrictor	North America	(California)	WF6049	—	12	—
		Viperidae ‖				
Crotalus horridus	North America	(Louisiana)	WF5073	—	18	—
		Dipsadidae ‖				
Crotaphopeltis hotamboeia	Africa	(Cape Province)	WF6679	—	10	—
Lycodonomorphus rufulus¶	Africa	(Cape Province)	WF6935	—	11	—
		Henophidia ‖ Boidae ‖				
Constrictor constrictor	South America §	(Western Brazil)	WF5562	—	71	—
		Scolecophidia ‖ Typhlopidae ‖				
Typhlops vermicularis	Middle East	(Israel)	WF6931	—	130	—

* Source of antigen.

† WF and HD specimens deposited in Louisiana State University Museum of Zoology; CU in Museum of Cornell University; RZ in American Museum of Natural History; X = specimens not available.

‡ Titrations using antibodies against: NC = transferrin of *Natrix cyclopion*; NN = transferrin of *Natrix natrix*; NA = transferrin of *Natrix annularis*.

§ Purchased from animal dealer.

‖ According to Underwood (1967).

¶ *Regina alleni* = *Liodytes alleni*; *Xenochrophis piscator* = *Fowlea piscator*; *Lycodonomorphus rufulus* = *Ablabophis rufulus*.

or in column eluates. It is readily isolated from other plasma proteins with the "Rivanol" procedure and standard physico-chemical methods (George & Dessauer, 1970). The molecule is remarkably stable, a very desirable property for the comparative biochemist who often must use tissue samples collected many years prior to their analysis. When saturated with iron, transferrins resist prolonged exposure to proteolytic enzymes and to temperatures as high as 65°C (Azari & Feeney, 1958). The electrophoretic mobility and immunological properties of transferrins did not change in plasma stored in a deep freeze for 15 yr (personal observations).

The transferrins are among the most highly variable proteins. Numerous variants, presumably inherited as multiple alleles, occur within single populations of many species (Dessauer *et al.*, 1962). The protein exhibits even more marked electrophoretic and immunological differences from species to species (Wilson & Sarich, 1969; George & Dessauer, 1970). The range of variation in transferrin structure within snakes alone is very great, as is shown in Table 1. The table lists indices of dissimilarity obtained in MC'F titrations of transferrins with antisera against the transferrins of the water snakes *Natrix cyclopion* (NC), *N. natrix* (NN) and *N. annularis* (NA). The table also gives the continent on which each species occurs, and the region of capture and museum number of the specimens examined.

Morphological, physiological and ecological divergence and transferrins

The immunological differences between transferrins do not always correlate with the degree of morphological divergence of the species compared. The gross morphology of different species of genus *Natrix* is remarkably similar. Yet when antigen and antiserum were derived from species of *Natrix* from different continents, cross reactions were relatively weak (I.D.'s ranged from 3·1 to 5·1). In contrast, the gross morphology of natricine snakes of North America varies to such a degree that the more than forty species are classified in nine genera. Yet their transferrins are of similar structure, having I.D.'s that are less than two when titrated with an antiserum against the transferrin of North American *Natrix cyclopion*.

Oviparous and viviparous species occur within genus *Natrix*, however, transferrin structure does not correlate with this character of reproductive physiology (Table 1). *Natrix cyclopion* of North America and *N. annularis* of Taiwan are both viviparous, yet their transferrins vary greatly in structure, differing by an average I.D. of 3·3. Transferrins of viviparous *N. annularis* and oviparous *N. pericarinata* from Taiwan differ by an I.D. of only 1·5; however, the transferrin of the *N. pericarinata* differs from that of *N. natrix* of Europe, which is also oviparous, by an I.D. of 3·4. Transferrins of the oviparous species of Europe differ by I.D.'s of only 1·7 or less; and those of viviparous species of North America differ by I.D.'s of 1·4 or less.

Natricine snakes of North America exhibit wide variations in ecology but have very similar transferrins (Table 1). The geographic distribution of the species examined is wide, ranging from northern Ohio to the Gulf of Mexico and from

Virginia to California (Fig. 1). Over this broad region, habitats are quite different, and the snakes must be adapted to wide ranges of temperature, rainfall and climatic cycles. Most species of *Natrix* live in fresh water, but *Natrix fasciata clarki* inhabits the salt marshes. Genera such as *Thamnophis* and *Storeria* are more terrestrial. Food may be quite varied or limited to one or two vertebrate or invertebrate species (Wright & Wright, 1957).

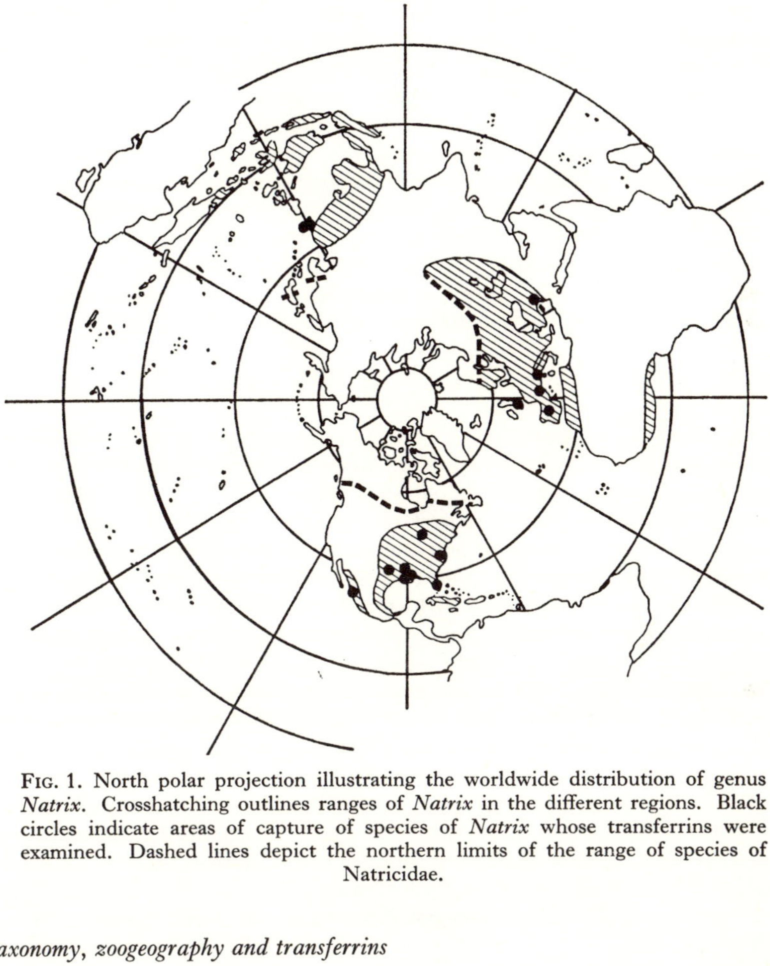

FIG. 1. North polar projection illustrating the worldwide distribution of genus *Natrix*. Crosshatching outlines ranges of *Natrix* in the different regions. Black circles indicate areas of capture of species of *Natrix* whose transferrins were examined. Dashed lines depict the northern limits of the range of species of Natricidae.

Taxonomy, zoogeography and transferrins

Transferrins of *Natrix* show a much closer resemblance to those of genera of other families of modern snakes (I.D. averaging 12·8) than to genera of families of more ancient origin such as *Typhlops* (I.D. = 130) and *Constrictor* (I.D. = 71).

The infraorders in which the latter are classified, the Scolecophidia and Henophidia, probably originated during the Mesozoic era, whereas the infraorder in which families of modern snakes are grouped, the Caenophidia, seems to date from epochs in the mid-Cenozoic (Auffenberg, 1963).

Transferrins of species of the Natricidae (as defined by Underwood, 1967) differ from each other by I.D.'s of between 1 and 8·2. An I.D. between 8 and 10 appears to mark the family level of divergence in modern snakes (see also George & Dessauer, 1970). All of the European, Asiatic and North American species had I.D.'s below 8·2 with *Rhabdophis* appearing most divergent from *Natrix*.

The transferrin I.D.'s correlate well with Malnate's (1960) systematic revision of genus *Natrix* as it was previously defined. Malnate shifted many of the species of that "unwieldly and confusing assemblage" into four other genera on the basis of the structure of the *sulcus spermaticus* and maxillary dentition. Transferrins of the three of these genera that we have examined, *Amphiesma*, *Rhabdophis and Xenochrophis* (= *Fowlea*; Malnate & Minton, 1965), have I.D.'s which vary from 5 to 8·2 when titrated with antitransferrins of *Natrix* from the three different geographic regions. The antiserum to the *Xenochrophis piscator* transferrin was a poor reagent due to its high anticomplement activity, however the antiserum gave moderate I.D.'s with plasma samples from *Natrix annularis*, *Rhabdophis swinhonis* and from species of *Amphiesma* from Taiwan and New Guinea. These titrations showed that *Xenochrophis* is as distinct from *Amphiesma* and *Rhabdophis* as it is from *Natrix*.

Natrix, even as presently defined, is one of the most widely distributed genera of modern snakes. Species occur in southeastern and central Asia, North America, Europe and in Africa north and south of the Sahara (Fig. 1). Transferrin structure reflects the geographic distribution of the many species. Immunological cross reactions were very strong when both antigens and antisera involved transferrins of species of *Natrix* from the same continent. Indices of dissimilarity for the transferrins of North American *Natrix* ranged from 1·0 to 1·4 when titrated with the *Natrix cyclopion* antitransferrin. The nine species whose transferrins were examined were collected at widely separated localities and included *N. valida*, whose range in western Mexico is disjunct from that of other North American *Natrix* (Fig. 1). The I.D.'s obtained for transferrins of three European *Natrix* ranged from 1·0 to 1·7 when titrated with *Natrix natrix* antitransferrin. The I.D. of the transferrin of Asiatic *N. pericarinata* equaled 1·5 when titrated with the antitransferrin of the sympatric species, *N. annularis*. When transferrin and antitransferrin were of species of *Natrix* from different continents, however, cross reactions between antigen and antiserum were relatively weak (I.D. ranging from 3·1 to 5·1).

Transferrins of North American natricine snakes are of very similar structure. We obtained strong cross reactions in all titrations of their transferrins with the antitransferrin of *Natrix cyclopion* (Table 1). George & Dessauer (1970, unpublished) obtained similar results using the antitransferrin of *Thamnophis couchi*, another North American natricine snake. Transferrins of twenty-one species of eight genera have been examined. I.D.'s of the titrations ranged from 1·0 to 3·6; values above 2 were obtained in cross reactions involving certain species of *Natrix* and *Thamnophis*.

The transferrin biological clock

The structural difference between the transferrins of two species of snakes probably represents selectively neutral mutations accumulated at the transferrin locus during the span of their period of reproductive isolation. Spontaneous mutations that were deleterious could not account for these differences, as selection would have eliminated them over the long periods of time involved. Likewise, spontaneous mutations that were adaptive would be expected to lead to transferrins showing some correlation with the morphology, ecology and physiology of the organism. While it is probable that some sequence changes in transferrins are adaptive, the greater number must be of the neutral variety.

The magnitude of the species differences in transferrins correlates best with the time of divergence of different evolutionary lines. The paleontological record of snakes is relatively poor, however some evidence is available on the time of divergence of animals of three evolutionary lines for which we have transferrin data (Table 1). (A) Fossils of the North American genera *Regina* and *Storeria* first appear in Pleistocene deposits (Auffenberg, 1963; Gehlbach, 1965). *Natrix cyclopion* antitransferrin gives an average I.D. of only 1·2 when tested against transferrins of these North American genera. (B) Fossils identified as *Natrix* and as *Thamnophis* appear together earlier, having been found in deposits of the North American mid-Pliocene, however the identification is not unequivocal (Auffenberg, 1963; Gehlbach, 1965). *Natrix cyclopion* antitransferrin (Table 1) and *Thamnophis couchi* antitransferrin (George & Dessauer, 1970; unpublished observations) give an average I.D. = 2·1 in cross generic titrations with transferrins of *Thamnophis* and North American *Natrix*. (C) Fossils of natricids, viperids and colubrids have been found in Miocene deposits (Auffenberg, 1963). I.D.'s of cross family titrations involving Viperidae, Colubridae and Natricidae averaged 11·2 when determined with antitransferrins of the natricids, *Natrix natrix* (Table 1) and *Thamnophis couchi*, and the colubrids, *Coluber constrictor* and *Pituophis melanoleucus* (George & Dessauer, 1970).

Measures of species differences between transferrins can serve as an evolutionary clock, if the fossil evidence on these three groups of taxa is used to calibrate the clock (Fig. 2). The logarithms of the I.D.'s distinguishing transferrins of (A) individual species of North American *Natrix*, *Storeria* and *Regina*, (B) *Thamnophis* from *Natrix* of North America, and (C) Natricidae, Colubridae and Viperidae are plotted against the estimate of the time of divergence of taxa of the three different groups as estimated from the fossil data. The absolute geological time scale (Kulp, 1961) allows us to assign dates to strata in which the fossils were discovered. The three clusters of I.D.'s fall, approximately, on a straight line, indicating a direct correlation between the log of the average I.D. of transferrins and the period of divergence of members of two evolutionary lines. Using this plot and transferrin

I.D.'s, one can estimate degrees of relationships and times of divergence of living species, thereby helping to circumvent problems caused by few fossils and uncertain anatomical conclusions (Wilson & Sarich, 1969).

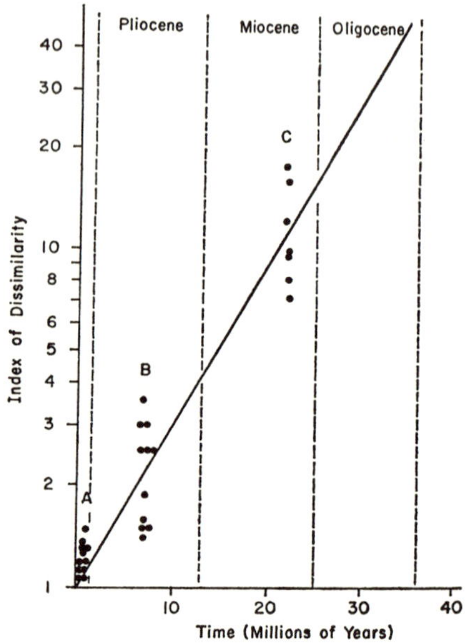

FIG. 2. Transferrin as a biological clock. Line connects averages of log I.D.'s of transferrins of species of three groups whose times of divergence are known from the fossil record: (A) I.D.'s of heterologous titrations involving antiserum against the transferrin of *Natrix cyclopion* and transferrins of North American species of *Natrix*, *Regina* and *Storeria*, divergent since the Pleistocene. (B) I.D.'s of cross generic titrations involving antisera against transferrins of *Natrix cyclopion* and *Thamnophis couchi* and transferrins of species of *Thamnophis* and of North American *Natrix*, divergent since the mid-Pliocene. (C) I.D.'s of cross family titrations involving antisera against transferrins of *Natrix natrix*, *Thamnophis couchi*, *Coluber constrictor* and *Pituophis melanoleucus* and transferrins of species of *Natricidae*, *Colubridae* and *Viperidae*, divergent since at least the early Miocene. Fossil data are from Auffenberg (1963) and Gehlbach (1965). I.D.'s involving antisera against the transferrins of *Thamnophis couchi*, *Coluber constrictor* and *Pituophis melanoleucus* are taken from George (1969) and George & Dessauer (1970).

Transferrins and the evolution of advanced snakes

Our estimate of the genetic affinities of advanced snakes (Caenophidia) based upon the transferrin evidence is summarized in Fig. 3. The Caenophidia probably diverged from primitive ancestors (Scolecophidia and Henophidia) during the Eocene. Fossils of the older infraorders are known from the late Cretaceous and early Cenozoic, but few fossils of advanced snakes are known from strata earlier than the lower Miocene. Auffenberg (1963), however, believes that modern snakes have a longer history and suggests that it probably extends to the Eocene. The transferrin I.D.'s of 71 and 130 obtained in the two cross superfamily titrations are compatible with this conclusion.

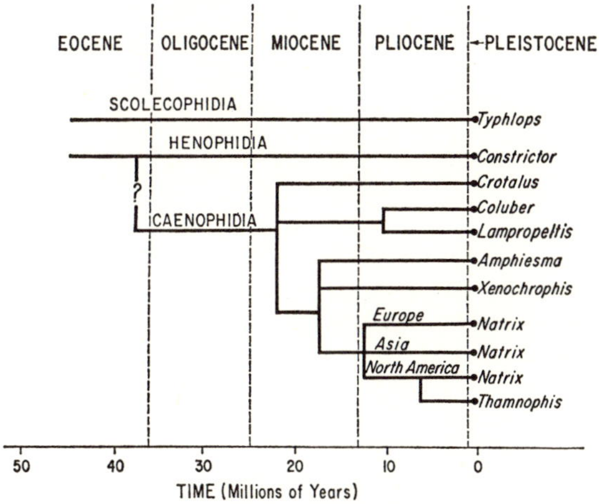

FIG. 3. Affinities of selected genera of snakes based upon transferrin structure. Scheme incorporates data from Table 1 as well as evidence from George & Dessauer (1970).

The Caenophidia apparently underwent a radiation in the early Miocene or late Oligocene. Colubrid, natricid, viperid and elapid fossils have been found in Miocene strata (Auffenberg, 1963). The I.D.'s obtained in titrations of antisera made from transferrins of species of both the Natricidae and the Colubridae (Average I.D. = 11·2; Fig. 2, Cluster C) were of the same order of magnitude when tested against transferrins of a species from another family of Caenophidia (Natricidae, Colubridae, Dipsadidae and Viperidae; Table 1, George & Dessauer, 1970).

The Natricidae apparently underwent an early radiation in Asia during which the generic lines leading to modern *Natrix*, *Xenochrophis*, *Rhabdophis* and *Amphiesma* originated. The I.D.'s obtained in heterologous titrations involving antitransferrins of species of *Natrix* and transferrins of species of these other genera averaged 6·0, suggesting that the radiation took place in the Miocene, about 17 million yr ago (Fig. 3). The immunological data show that lines leading to *Natrix* and *Xenochrophis* are clearly distinct from each other and from lines leading to *Amphiesma* and *Rhabdophis*. Without antisera to the transferrins of either *Amphiesma* or *Rhabdophis*, we are unable to comment on the affinities of these two genera to each other.

Ancestral species of *Natrix* probably dispersed northwestward across Asia into Europe and northeastward across a Bering landbridge into North America. Fossil evidence and zoogeography show that natricines are more cold-adapted than other snakes and could have spread across northern latitudes in periods having climates only slightly milder than that of the present. Natricines make up over 90 per cent of the snake fossils found in strata deposited on the high plains of western North America during glacial stages of the Pleistocene. Viperid and colubrid fossils are more common in strata of the warmer inter-glacial stages (Brattstrom, 1967). Modern species of natricine snakes range farther north than any other reptile (Fig. 1; Darlington, 1957). *Thamnophis* extends to about 60° N latitude in western North America (Wright and Wright, 1957); *Natrix* is found as far north as 65° in western Europe; and *Rhabdophis* ranges to 50° N along the eastern coast of Asia (Malnate, 1960).

Snakes of Asia, Europe and North America, ancestral to modern species of *Natrix* probably became genetically isolated near the end of the Miocene about 13 million yr ago. Heterologous transferrin titrations involving transferrins of *Natrix* from different continents averaged 3·8 (Table 1). Holman (1964) has identified fossil vertebra of natricine snakes in a Nebraska formation transitional between the Miocene and Pliocene. During the late Miocene, Bering landbridges were present and the climate of northern latitudes was milder than the present (Dunbar, 1960).

The ancestral forms of *Natrix* seem to have been aquatic or semiaquatic snakes of such generalized potential that they easily spread into terrestrial habitats (Malnate, 1960). The North American continent presented many new and unoccupied habitats to the pioneering species. Apparently, extensive speciation took place as the natricines radiated into these habitats. Transferrins of living species of North American natricine snakes differ by an average I.D. of less than 2·1, indicating that the many forms are close relatives even though they vary in morphology and ecology. The close similarities in transferrin structure also suggest that the eight genera examined are derived from a single invading species.

Ancestral *Natrix* apparently encountered areas less favorable for speciation as it penetrated into Europe. It probably was forced to move into Europe by a northern route, because homalopsine species had already saturated the semiaquatic habitats of southern Asia (Malnate, 1960). In Europe itself *Natrix* found fewer habitats available, and as a result a major radiation, similar to that which occurred in North America, did not take place. The three species of European natricine snakes are all classified as *Natrix*. Their transferrins differ by a maximum I.D. of 1·7. *Natrix natrix* occupies a more terrestrial habitat, whereas *N. tessellata* and *N. maura* occupy fresh-water habitats, as is typical for most species of the genus.

Acknowledgements—During such a project one becomes deeply indebted to many colleagues and institutions. We especially thank Caral Tate and Nicholas Nicosia for expert technical assistance. Specimens, rare or difficult to obtain, were contributed by K. K. Adler, F. Bush, R. Conant, M. B. Dunlap, H. L. Keegan, B. Kromer, E. V. Malnate, E. Nevo, F. H. Pough, D. A. Rossman, N. D. Richmond and D. E. Sutton. Other material for the study was collected during program B of the 1969 *Alpha helix* Expedition to New Guinea, financed by a grant of the National Science Foundation (United States) to the Scripps

Institute of Oceanography, University of California. The Foundation also supported the laboratory phase of this study (Grant GB 7294X). Mao was supported by a fellowship from the National Science Council of the Republic of China.

REFERENCES

ARNHEIM N., PRAGER E. M. & WILSON A. C. (1969) Immunological prediction of sequence differences among proteins. Chemical comparison of chicken, quail and pheasant lysozymes. *J. biol. Chem.* **244**, 2085–2094.

AUFFENBERG W. (1963) The fossil snakes of Florida. *Tulane Studies Zool.* **10**, 131–216.

AZARI P. R. & FEENEY R. E. (1958) Resistance of metal complexes of conalbumin and transferrin to proteolysis and thermal denaturation. *J. biol. Chem.* **232**, 293–302.

BRATTSTROM B. H. (1967) A succession of Pliocene and Pleistocene snake faunas from the high plains of the United States. *Copeia*, 188–202.

DARLINGTON P. J. JR. (1957) *Zoogeography*, p. 675. Wiley, New York.

DESSAUER H. C., FOX W. & HARTWIG Q. L. (1962) Comparative study of transferrins of Amphibia and Reptilia using starch-gel electrophoresis and autoradiography. *Comp. Biochem. Physiol.* **5**, 17–29.

DUNBAR C. O. (1960) *Historical Geology*, p. 500. 2nd Edition. Wiley, New York.

GEHLBACH F. R. (1965) Amphibians and reptiles from the Pliocene and Pleistocene of North America: a chronological summary and selected bibliography. *Texas J. Sci.* **17**, 56–70.

GEORGE D. W. & DESSAUER H. C. (1970) Immunological correspondence of transferrins and the relationships of colubrid snakes. *Comp. Biochem. Physiol.* **33**, 617–627.

GIBLETT E. R., HICKMAN C. G. & SMITHIES O. (1959) Serum transferrin. *Nature, Lond.* **183**, 1589.

HOLMAN J. A. (1964) Fossil snakes from the Valentine formation of Nebraska. *Copeia* 631–637.

KING J. L. & JUKES T. H. (1969) Non-Darwinian evolution. *Science, N.Y.* **164**, 788–798.

KULP J. L. (1961) Geologic time scale. *Science, N.Y.* **133**, 1105–1113.

MALNATE E. V. (1960) Systematic division and evolution of the colubrid snake genus *Natrix*, with comments on the subfamily Natricinae. *Proc. Acad. Nat. Sci., Philadelphia* **112**, 41–71.

MALNATE E. V. & MINTON S. A. (1965) A redescription of the natricine snakes *Xenochrophis cerasogaster*, with comments on its taxonomic status. *Proc. Acad. Nat. Sci., Philadelphia* **117**, 19–43.

SARICH V. M. & WILSON A. C. (1966) Quantitative immunochemistry and the evolution of primate albumins: micro-complement fixation. *Science, N.Y.* **154**, 1563–1566.

SMITHIES O. (1959) Zone electrophoresis in starch gels and its application to studies of serum proteins. *Adv. Protein Chem.* **14**, 65–113.

SUTTON H. E. & KARP G. W., JR. (1965) Adsorption of rivanol by potato starch in the isolation of transferrins. *Biochim. biophys. Acta* **107**, 153–154.

UNDERWOOD G. (1967) *A Contribution to the Classification of Snakes*, p. 179. Trustees British Museum Natural History, London.

WASSERMAN E. & LEVINE L. (1961) Quantitative micro-complement fixation and its use in the study of antigenic structure by specific antigen-antibody inhibition. *J. Immunol.* **87**, 290–295.

WILSON A. C. & SARICH V. M. (1969) A molecular time scale for human evolution. *Proc. natn. Acad Sci. U.S.* **63**, 1088–1093.

WRIGHT A. H. & WRIGHT A. A. (1957) *Handbook of Snakes*, 2 vols., p. 1105. Comstock, Ithaca, New York.

Abnormal Expression of Normal Transferrin Alleles in Cattle

R. L. Spooner G. Baxter

INTRODUCTION

The early reports of transferrin polymorphism in cattle detected by starch gel electrophoresis (Smithies and Hickman, 1958; Ashton, 1958) described three alleles in European breeds Tf^a, Tf^d, Tf^e.

Subsequent studies have shown that the Tf^d allele is subdivided into Tf^{d_1} and Tf^{d_2} (Kristjansson and Hickman, 1965; Jamieson, 1965). In this paper the nomenclature proposed by Jamieson is used.

The early work on transferrins utilized techniques which demonstrated three main protein bands for each allele with a faint fourth band in front. With a further refinement of technique it has been possible to subdivide these into four main bands preceded to two faint bands.This improvement in definition was developed independently in this laboratory and in Canada (Makarechian and Howell, 1966), but the exact details of technique are not identical in the two laboratories. It was clearly shown by Makarechian and Howell (1966) that all of the lines in the transferrin region in cattle detected with a protein stain were iron binding as shown by autoradiography.

An example of serum with an abnormal transferrin pattern has been described by Sartore and Bernoco (1966) and another abnormal pattern was reported by Gahne (1961).

This paper describes abnormalities in the transferrins of cattle somewhat similar to that described by Sartore and Bernoco (1966). Evidence is presented which suggests that the suppression of two protein bands is under the control of an epistatic gene, at a locus independent from the *Tf* locus.

MATERIALS AND METHODS

Starch Gel Electrophoresis

Slight modifications of the method of Kristjansson and Hickman (1965) were used. The starch batch 258/1 was used at 14.5% concentration and the tris–cacodylic acid buffer used was 0.016 M tris, *p*H 7.45. Electrophoresis of uncooled gels was carried out at 4.5 ma/cm width of gel for approximately 2 hr, and the buffer boundary allowed to travel 7.5 cm beyond the insert line. The gel dimensions were 24 × 12 × 0.6 cm and the distance between wicks 19 cm. We normally run 14 samples per gel.

Autoradiography

Fe^{59} was added at the rate of 6 μc/ml to serum and the serum incubated at 37 C for 1 hr. After electrophoresis the sliced gel was wrapped in Saran wrap and placed on Kodirex X-ray film at 4 C for 16 hr.

Neuraminidase Treatment

Three types of neuraminidase were used: (1) *Clostridium perfringens*, type V, Sigma Chemical Co. Ltd., 0.03 μmoles NANA liberated per minute from *N*-acetyl-*N*-lactose at *p*H 5.1 and 37 C by 1 mg neuraminidase. A solution of 3 mg/ml approximates to 450 Schultze units. (2) *Vibrio cholera*, Calbiochem, 500 units/ml (Schultze units). (3) *Vibrio cholera*, B.D.H., 500 units/ml (Schultze units).

Serum was dialyzed against 0.2 M acetate buffer, *p*H 5.5, with 0.04 M $CaCl_2$. Then 1 drop of neuraminidase (*V. cholera*) was added to 7 drops of serum and the mixture incubated at 37 C for 3, 6, 28, and 48 hr.

Serum was treated with *C. perfringens* type V neuraminidase after dialysis against the same acetate buffer as that used for the *V. cholera* neuraminidase. Another sample was treated after dialysis against 0.2 M phosphate buffer, *p*H 8. The concentration used for treatment was from 1 to 2 drops of a solution containing 3 mg *C. perfringens* neuraminidase per milliliter added to 0.1 ml of serum.

RESULTS

During the course of routine typing of service samples, four animals have been found where only two strong transferrin bands were seen instead of four. Figure 1 shows a starch gel containing samples from the four animals. It can be seen that for each sample there are two strong bands and two weak ones, compared with the normal four strong and two weak for each allele. This always applies to both alleles as is seen from

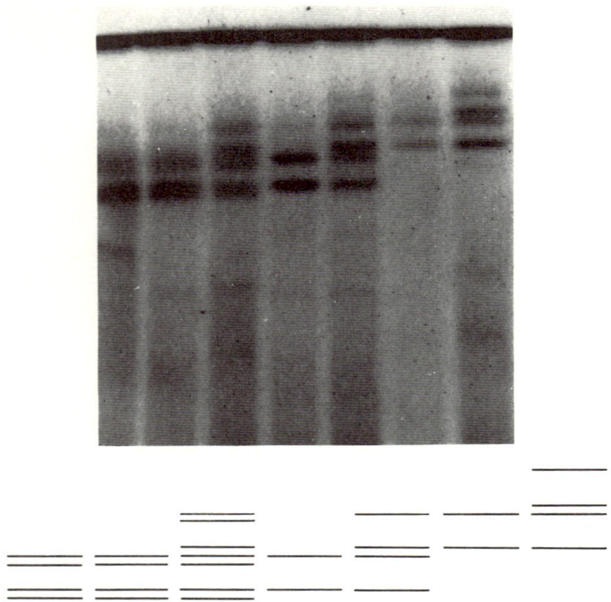

Fig. 1. Starch gel patterns of bovine transferrins, showing how the two faster strong lines for each allele are missing from the four abnormal sera, PR, BD, LHT, and RTC. PR and BD are abnormal Tfd_1d_2; LHT, abnormal Tfd_1d_1; and RTC, abnormal Tfa_2a_2. The normal transferrins are shown also.

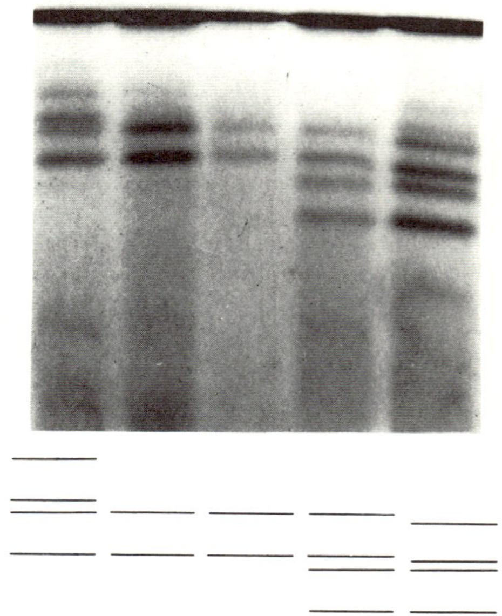

Fig. 2. Two offspring of RTC, 174 being an abnormal Tfa_2a_2 and 194 an abnormal Tfa_2d_2. RTC is weak as there was little serum left when this gel was run. A faint trace of protein can be seen in front of the two main bands of 174 and these are also seen with LHT and RTC when at equivalent concentration. They resemble the two fastest bands of the normal type which are just visible in the Tfd_2d_2 in this photograph.

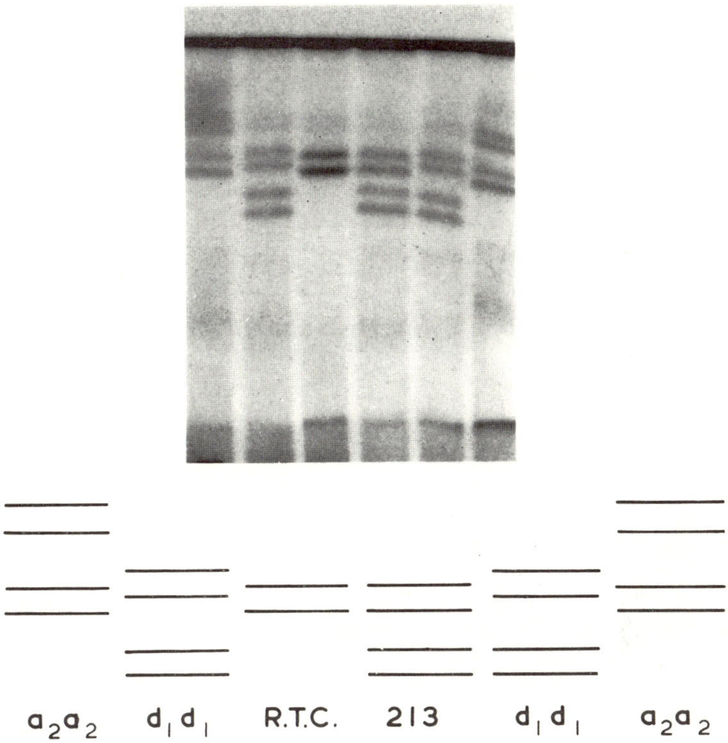

Fig. 3. Increased separation of the transferrins to show another offspring of RTC, 213, an abnormal Tfa_2d_1. The a_2a_2 to the left of the picture is rather smeared. It is, however, the same sample as the one on the right. With this degree of separation it is not easy to obtain uniformly good gels.

Table I. Transferrin Types of the Offspring of RTC

(a) Where dams known

Number of dams	Dam genotype	Number of calves — Calf genotype				
		Tf^{a_2}/Tf^{a_2}	Tf^{a_2}/Tf^{d_1}	Tf^{a_2}/Tf^{d_2}	Tf^{a_2}/Tf^{e}	Others
3	Tf^{a_2}/Tf^{a_2}	3	—	—	—	—
6	Tf^{a_2}/Tf^{d_1}	4	2	—	—	—
4	Tf^{a_2}/Tf^{d_2}	3	—	1	—	—
5	Tf^{d_1}/Tf^{d_2}	—	2+1[a]	2	—	—
2	Tf^{d_2}/Tf^{d_2}	—	—	2	—	—
1	Tf^{a_2}/Tf^{e}	—	—	—	1	—

(b) Where dams not known

Genotype of calf	Number of calves
Tf^{a_2}/Tf^{a_2}	1[a]
Tf^{a_2}/Tf^{d_1}	5
Tf^{a_2}/Tf^{d_2}	15+1[a]

[a] Represents the abnormal transferrin phenotype.

the abnormal Tfd_1d_2 samples (BD and PR) on the left of Fig. 1. (The names of the four animals are long and have been abbreviated to RTC, LHT, BD, and PR for convenience.)

The parents of two of the animals (BD and PR) were also tested and they had normal transferrins. Three of the abnormal animals were bulls and two are in use in artificial insemination. All are Herefords.

It has been possible to look at a number of offspring of the two artificially inseminated bulls. From one of these bulls (RTC), 44 offspring have now been tested (Table I) and for 22 of these their dams also. Of these samples, 31 came from pure Hereford animals in one herd where RTC had been used before he was sold for use in artificial insemination. The 13 remaining samples came from Hereford × Friesians.

All of the Friesian cross offspring of RTC had normal transferrins, i.e., they showed four dense Tf^{a_2} bands although their father had only two dense bands himself. Three of the pure Hereford offspring showed the same abnormality as their sire, while the one available dam was normal. Two of the offspring are shown in Fig. 2. It can be seen that with animal 194 only two dense lines are present but with 174 the fastest weak bands are missing and weak bands are seen in the position of the normally fast strong bands.

Sample 213 is indistinguishable from a normal Tf^{d_1}/Tf^{d_2} under the usual conditions of electrophoresis. If, however, the gel pH is dropped still further to pH 7.2, then it can be seen in Fig. 3 that the front two bands of 213 are slower than two fastest Tf^{d_1} bands and are the same as the slow A bands.Thus this is a third offspring of RTC where again faint lines are visible in the position where strong bands are normally found and the fastest weak bands are missing completely.

Repeat samples have been obtained from most of the animals showing the abnormality and on each occasion they have given results identical to those of the first samples.

In summary, therefore, it has been shown that of the 44 offspring of RTC three animals show the same abnormality as their sire and 41 are normal. In 22 of these 41 animals (i.e., where the dams were known), they must have received four strong Tf^{a_2} bands from their sire while he has only two strong bands himself, and the remainder where dams are not available possess at least one Tf^{a_2} allele.

Treatment with Neuraminidase

In an attempt to investigate further the abnormality in RTC, LHT, BD, and PR, an attempt was made to treat serum samples from these animals with neuraminidase.

Initially, samples were treated with *C. perfringens* neuraminidase (Chen and Sutton, 1967), but it was found that massive amounts of enzyme protein were needed. Approximately 1 mg of enzyme protein per milliliter of serum was required to slow the bands in electrophoresis, and the Tfa_2 phenotype was less sensitive to treatment than Tfd_2 and Tfe. On further investigation, it was found that there was no change in activity when the reaction was carried out at *p*H 5.5 or at *p*H 8.0. At *p*H 8.0, *C. perfringens* neuraminidase in phosphate buffer should have virtually no activity (Cassidy *et al.*, 1965).

Because of these difficulties, two preparations of neuraminidase obtained from *V. cholera* were used. They had identical activity. They showed much greater activity than the *C. perfringens* preparation, although large concentrations of enzyme were

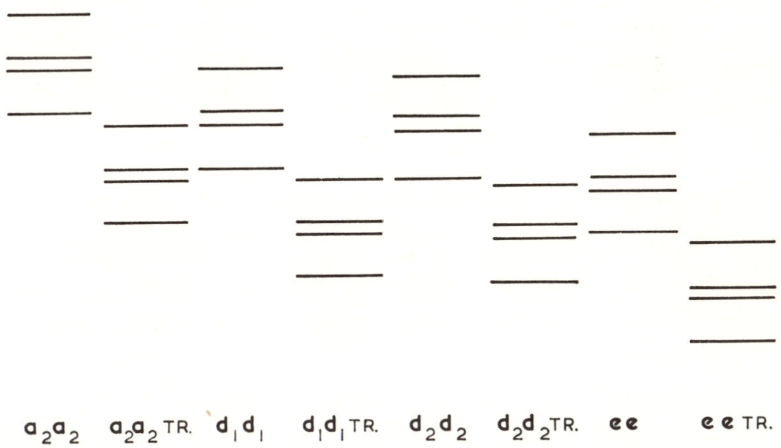

Fig. 4. Diagram to show the effect of the treatment of bovine transferrins with neuraminidase for 48 hr.

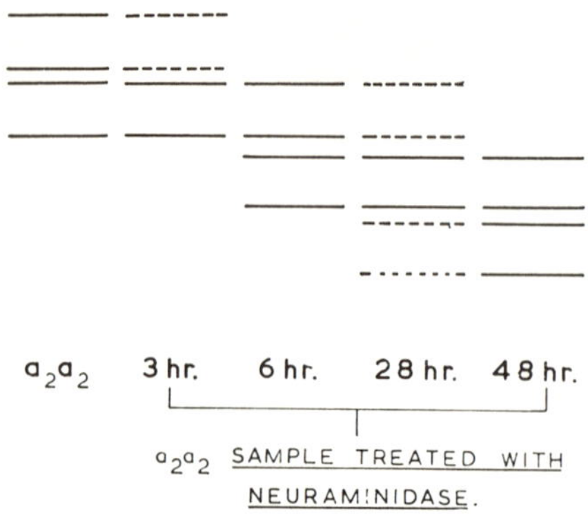

Fig. 5. Diagram to show the progressive slowing of transferrin bands on treatment with neuraminidase.

still necessary, i.e., 60 units per ml. The enzyme activity was greater at *p*H 5.5 than at *p*H 7.5 and also was completely destroyed in the presence of 0.01 M EDTA, which is consistent with the characteristics of *V. cholera* neuraminidase (Cassidy *et al.*, 1965). Within 6 hr there was marked slowing of the transferrin bands when using serum dialyzed against 0.2 M acetate buffer, *p*H 5.5, but the reaction was less marked at *p*H 7.4. The results of a 48-hr treatment of the four homozygous transferrin phenotypes found in our cattle are shown in Fig. 4. It can be seen that all four bands of the transferrin are apparently slowed and that their resulting position does not correspond to that of one of the normal slower phenotypes. The positions of each band in a homozygous transferrin type were, however, not significantly altered relative to each other. If, however, the serum samples are treated for only 3 hr, then a different picture is seen (Fig. 5). The two faster protein bands are slowed down, but the two slower bands are not altered. This produces an appearance in the stained gel virtually identical with that seen with untreated RTC. Further treatment produces more slowing of the bands. The progress is shown in Fig. 5. This has a similar time scale to the results described by Chen and Sutton (1967) but clearly the process is operating on at least four bands for each *Tf* allele and no band in any allele corresponds to a band in any other *Tf* allele. Treatment of RTC and LHT with neuraminidase during the first 4 hr produces no effect, but after longer incubation there is slowing of the bands, the results for RTC being indistinguishable from those for a normal Tfa_2a_2 treated with neuraminidase and for LHT indistinguishable from a normal Tfd_1d_1 treated with neuraminidase. They are seen in Fig. 6 where only the 48-hr picture has been shown.

Test for Neuraminidase-Like Activity in the Serum of Affected Animals

To test for the presence of enzyme activity or some inhibitor in the serum of RTC, serum from RTC was mixed with an equal volume of serum from an animal with a normal transferrin pattern. The mixture was incubated at 37 C for 24 hr, and then run in a starch gel. Apart from the dilution, there was no detectable effect on the normal pattern.

Autoradiography

Using Fe^{59} citrate it was shown that iron binding corresponded exactly with the protein bands seen after Nigrosin staining. With RTC and LHT and the other abnormal samples, the only iron binding was in the region of the two slower protein bands. The missing bands were not therefore running with greatly altered mobility such as with albumin.

DISCUSSION

In this paper examples of an abnormal transferrin pattern are described. All are from Herefords and four are from a bull and three of its offspring.

The technique of electrophoresis is critical to the investigation of the abnormality. It was found that by slight alterations to the concentration and *p*H of the gel buffer the degree of separation of the different bands of transferrin could be increased. Shortly after the increased resolution was developed here, Makarechian and Howell (1966) described a similar separation in Canada. They, however, defined the *p*H as 7.3–7.35. It has been found here that slight reduction in the buffer concentration has an effect similar to dropping the *p*H, and in this laboratory the gels are normally run at *p*H 7.4–7.5. Makarechian and Howell (1966) describe, in fact, six bands per allele, but the two fastest moving bands are very faint, and it has not always been possible to detect them. They have been ignored in this investigation.

The abnormality appears as the absence of the two fastest moving protein bands of the six controlled by each *Tf* allele and two weak bands in place of the two fastest strong bands. No case has been found where the faster bands of only one allele were involved. The abnormality has been found only in the Hereford breed. There is the definite impression, though at the moment no quantitative evidence, that there is double the normal amount of transferrin in the two slow bands of the affected animals. The finding that mild treatment of normal transferrin with neuraminidase produces slowing of the fast bands only, resulting in a picture very like the actual cases found, suggests that the first sialic acid residues to be removed by neuraminidase are more weakly attached to the faster two strong protein bands than to the slower bands. Mild treatment of RTC with enzyme has no effect and it is only after more prolonged treatment with enzyme that bands are slowed and four instead of two are produced. The neuraminidase-treated RTC is indistinguishable from a treated Tfa_2a_2 and similarly the treated LHT is indistinguishable from a treated Tfd_1d_1. This would suggest that in these abnormal transferrins the two faster bands have mobilities in starch gel identical to the two slower bands, because they lack the sialic acid which these particular proteins normally carry.

Difficulty was experienced with the *C. perfringens* neuraminidase. This was of the same type and source as that used by Chen and Sutton (1967). They reported that they were using the technique of Blumberg and Warren (1961), but the latter workers used a different *p*H and used neuraminidase from *V. cholera* not from *C. perfringens.* The lower resolution of the acrylamide gel electrophoresis of Chen and Sutton (1967)

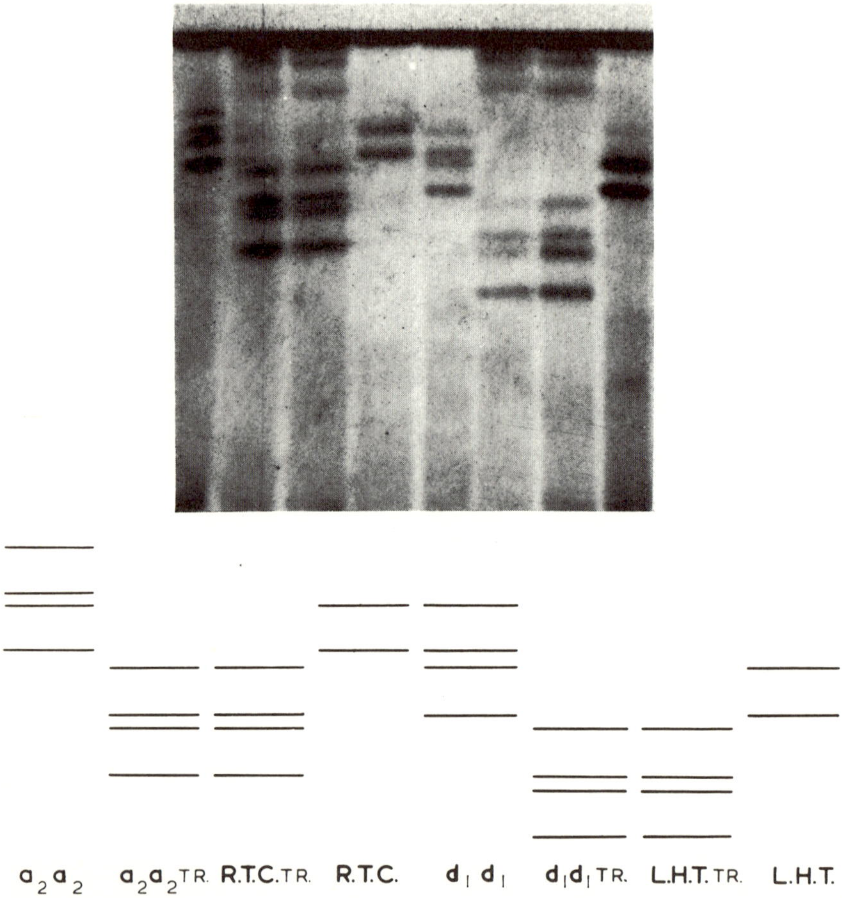

Fig. 6. Effect of 48-hr treatment of RTC and LHT with neuraminidase compared with its effect on the corresponding normal transferrin.

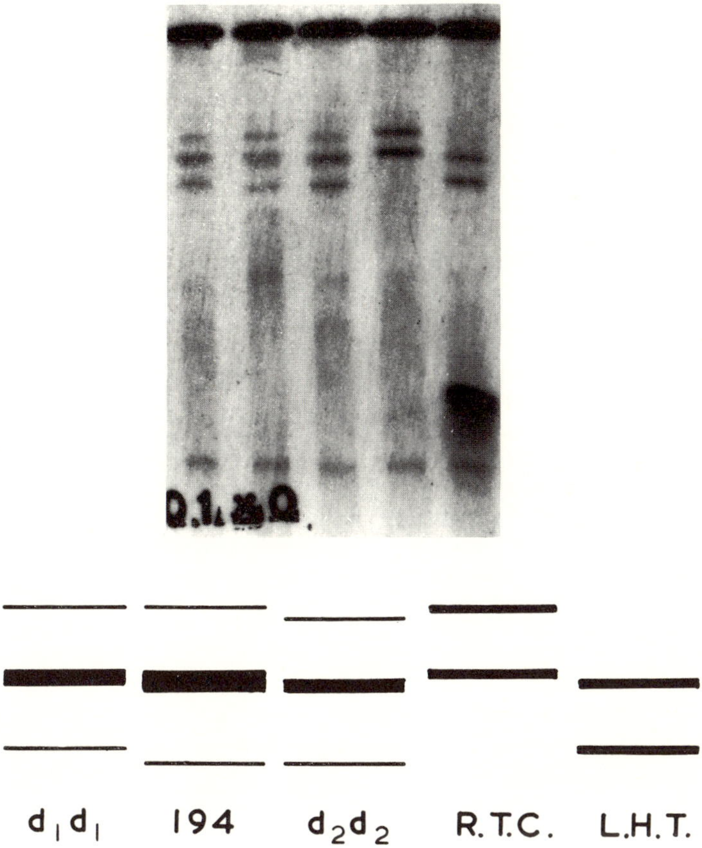

Fig. 7. To show how with a less discriminating technique the abnormality is more difficult to detect in the heterozygous transferrin, e.g., 194.

makes it difficult to interpret their results in the light of the findings presented here. In our studies, treatment of Tfa_2 with neuraminidase produced slowing of the bands (as found by Chen and Sutton, 1967) but none of these bands corresponded in mobility to any bands of slower normal alleles or any bands of other alleles after treatment with enzyme, indicating variation in the protein as well as in the sialic acid binding. Earlier work had suggested that there was no simple relationship between the decrease in sialic acid content as the mobility of the protein decreased (Parker and Bearn, 1962). This was also the case in pigs (Kristjansson and Cipera, 1963). Moreover the presence of at least 16 major protein bands in the four alleles common in this country, with the distance between each varying greatly, makes a simple explanation of decreasing sialic acid levels seem unlikely.

Whatever the exact explanation for the action of neuraminidase on bovine transferrins, the findings fit with the hypothesis that in these abnormal types the two fastest strong transferrin bands are slowed to an intermediate position and on treatment with neuraminidase they and the normally two slower bands are slowed still further. We would like to suggest that the affected animals are homozygous for a recessive epistatic gene at a locus distinct from and not linked to the *Tf* locus, and that this gene affects the sialic acid binding to the two faster transferrin bands. Other explanations do not appear to fit the findings and, if the above hypothesis is correct, this is the first example of an epistatic gene affecting a protein variation of this type. It is hoped to cross a large number of the offspring of one of these abnormal bulls with one of the other abnormals and to determine the segregation ratios in the resulting offspring. A direct back cross is not feasible for commercial reasons. Experiments are also envisaged aimed at discovering how the linkage of sialic acid to the two faster strong protein bands differs from its linkage to the two slower bands.

It may be that the abnormality described here is not the only one in which the relative proportion of the different protein bands varies. Other abnormalities which appear to occur in several individuals in the same form are currently being studied to establish whether they are related to the abnormality described in this paper.

Finally, it should be noted that, although this abnormality can be seen in a homozygous transferrin whatever the starch gel technique, when some Tf heterozygotes are studied they could be overlooked if the electrophoretic discrimination is poor. Figure 7 shows an example where there are only three bands of protein per allele. The middle sample is 194, the abnormal Tfa_2d_2. It would easily be read as a Tfd_2d_2. An abnormality of this nature may be more widespread than this communication would indicate, though it is unlikely that any cases have been overlooked in the samples tested in this laboratory in the past year during which time the major British breeds have been surveyed.

ACKNOWLEDGMENTS

We wish to thank in particular Dr. Gareth Williams of the English Milk Marketing Board for his assistance in obtaining samples from the offspring of RTC and also the former owner of RTC, Mr. J. R. H. Jones, and RTC's present owners, Horlicks Farms and Dairies Limited.

REFERENCES

Ashton, G. C. (1958). Genetics of β-globulin polymorphism in British cattle. *Nature* **182**: 370.

Blumberg, B. S., and Warren, L. (1961). The effect of sialidase on transferrins and other serum proteins. *Biochim. Biophys. Acta* **50**: 90.

Cassidy, J. T., Jourdain, G. W., and Roseman, S. (1965). The sialic acids. VI. Purification and properties of sialidase from *Clostridium perfringens*. *J. Biol. Chem.* **240**: 3501.

Chen, S., and Sutton, H. E. (1967). Bovine transferrins: Sialic acid and the complex phenotype. *Genetics* **56**: 425.

Gahne, B. (1961). Studies of transferrins in serum and milk of Swedish cattle. *Animal Prod.* **3**: 135.

Jamieson, A. (1965). The genetics of transferrins in cattle. *Heredity* **20**: 419.

Kristjansson, F. K., and Cipera, J. D. (1963). The effect of sialidase on pig transferrins. *Can. J. Biochem. Physiol.* **41**: 2523.

Kristjansson, F. K., and Hickman, C. G. (1965). Subdivision of the allele TfD for transferrins in Holstein and Ayrshire cattle. *Genetics* **52**: 627.

Makarechian, M., and Howell, W. E. (1966). Improved technique for separation and identification of bovine beta globulins by starch-gel electrophoresis. *Can. J. Biochem. Physiol.* **44**: 1089.

Parker, W. C., and Bearn, A. G. (1962). Alterations in sialic acid content of human transferrin. *Science* **133**: 1014.

Sartore, G., and Bernoco, D. (1966). Research on biochemical polymorphisms in the indigenous cattle of Piedmont. *Proc. Xth Eur. Congr. Anim. Blood Grps* (Paris), 283–287.

Smithies, O., and Hickman, C. G. (1958). Inherited variations in the serum proteins of cattle. *Genetics* **43**: 374.

Foetal and neonatal transferrrins in cattle

R. L. Spooner, R. B. Land, R. A. Oliver and A. Stratil

Introduction

In a study of sera from newborn calves it was found that the transferrin genotype was sometimes difficult to ascertain until the animals were several weeks old. It was therefore decided to investigate the ontogeny of bovine transferrins from fairly early foetal life to attempt to trace the reason for this neonatal change. Earlier studies on transferrins from bovine foetuses were carried out by Buschmann and Schmid (1961), but their work was performed before the developments in starch gel technique which are now available (Makarechian and Howell, 1966; Spooner and Baxter, 1969).

Materials and methods

Samples

Blood was collected directly from the heart of 38 abattoir foetuses. In many cases the foetuses had been dead for several hours when the blood was sampled. In some of the later cases cows carrying foetuses of known genotype were slaughtered intentionally to aid the identification of the foetal transferrin, and in these cases blood was collected within 10 minutes after death. The crown-rump length of the foetus was measured and its age assessed from tables prepared by Lyne (1960). Samples were also collected shortly after birth and over the first weeks of life. All samples were stored at —30°C.

Starch gel electrophoresis

As described previously (Spooner and Baxter, 1969) 0.016 *M* Tris-cacodylic acid buffer, pH 7.4 or 7.25, and Connaught Starch Lot No 262/1 was used. For some purposes, 0.0143 *M* Tris-citric acid buffer, pH 7.6, was used in the gel, and 0.3 *M* boric acid - NaOH buffer, pH 8.0, for electrode vessels (Dr J. G. Hall, personal communication).

Autoradiography

10 μl ^{59}Fe citrate (activity 0.7 to 1.0 μCi) were added to 120 μl serum. The mixture was incubated for 1 hour at room temperature before electrophoresis. The sliced gel was wrapped in Saran Wrap and placed directly on Kodirex X-ray film for 48 to 72 hours at —23°C.

Results and discussion

The normal adult homozygous transferrin has four major bands of protein with two minor faster bands as shown in Fig. 1. As has been shown previously (Spooner and Baxter, 1969) this normal picture is made up of two major pairs and one minor pair of bands. The foetal transferrin corresponding to this adult type has only the slower band of each pair present and the slower band of the fastest pair is very much stronger in the foetus than in the adult. It can be seen in Fig. 1, however, that although the

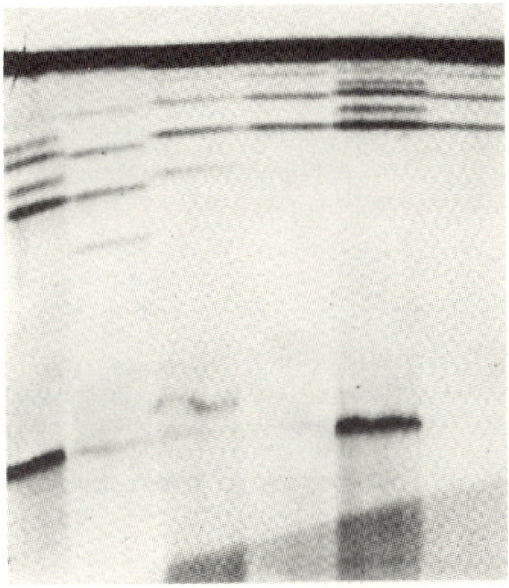

Fig. 1. Starch gel electrophoretic separation of several foetal sera to compare the foetal transferrin with its adult equivalent.

D_2	—	—	—	A	—	Adult Tf
—	D_2E	AD_1	A	—	A	Foetal Tf

slowest band of each variant has identical mobility in the foetal and adult sera, the two faster foetal bands are slightly slower than the bands in the adult transferrin to which they appear to correspond. This situation applies in all of the foetal variants that have been compared with their adult equivalents. In the 38 samples tested the numbers of the various transferrin phenotypes encountered was A 6, AD_1 8, AD_2 9, AE 3, D_1D_2 4, D_1E 5, D_2 2 and D_2E 1.

Towards the end of gestation the faster band of each pair begins to appear and before term there are usually three pairs of bands of about equal intensity. At the same time the intensity of the existing fastest foetal band begins to decrease and the transferrin phenotype approaches the adult type usually before or less commonly within a few weeks of birth. The time of change-over from the foetal to adult picture is somewhat variable and exceptionally one can even obtain neonatal animals with only three main transferrin bands. These are, however, rare and probably represent premature calves.

It can be difficult to read the transferrin phenotype in neonatal calf sera if the fastest pair of bands remain at high concentration. It is possible to obtain a picture in the heterozygote that could be taken as a mosaic. For example in a D_1D_2 heterozygote if the fastest pairs of bands are still present, the phenotype appears as if three alleles — A, D_1 and D_2 — are all present. Similarly a D_1E appears as if alleles A, D_1 and E are present. If present, this confusing picture disappears within at most six weeks.

Autoradiography (Fig. 2) confirms that the β protein bands corresponding in position on starch gel to some of the bands of adult transferrin are in fact iron-binding and that the degree of iron binding is proportional to the intensity of staining as detected with a protein stain. In this figure some of the samples show evidence of ^{59}Fe ahead of transferrin but this appears to be free iron at the buffer boundary. It is not

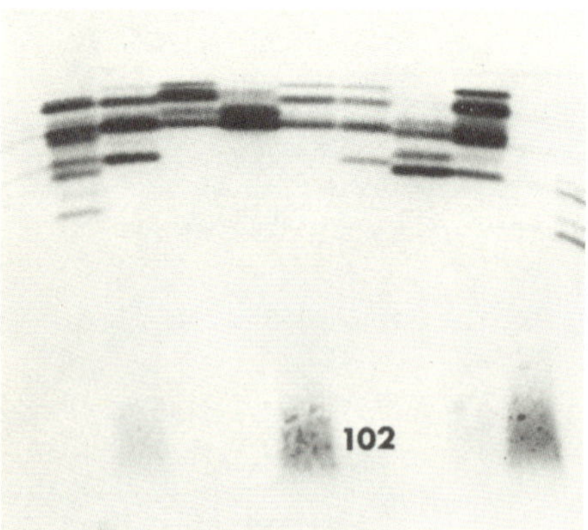

Fig. 2. Autoradiograph of a starch gel separation of foetal and adult sera to which ^{59}Fe citrate has been added. The trailing from the origin and the very fast band in some samples represent unbound iron. In Sample 2, which is from a 35-week-old foetus, it can be seen that the second band of each pair is already appearing. Abnormal Tf A sample run for comparison; it shows that most of the ^{59}Fe is bound by the two slowest bands.

E_1 — — A Abn.A — — D_2 — — E Adult Tf

— D_1E AD_1 — — A AD_2 — AD_2 D_2E — Foetal Tf

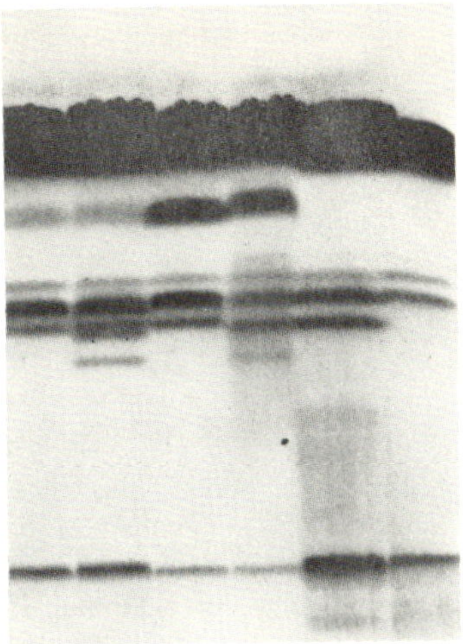

Fig. 3. Starch gel electrophoretic separation of foetal and adult sera using a Tris-citrate buffer pH 7.6. Note that the differentiation of D_1, D_2 and D_1D_2 is not possible under these conditions.

—	—	—	—	D_2	A	Adult Tf
D_1D_2	D_1E	AD_1	AE	—	—	Foetal Tf

^{59}Fe bound by albumin or other protein as autoradiography of gels run in Tris-citrate buffer where the buffer boundary is well ahead of albumin, still show some iron at and in front of the buffer boundary and none in the position of albumin or α_1 protein.

The method of starch gel electrophoresis is critical for the study of foetal transferrins. Only those buffer systems which separate transferrin homozygous types into 6 bands can provide satisfactory and convincing results. In other buffer systems, e.g. in Tris-

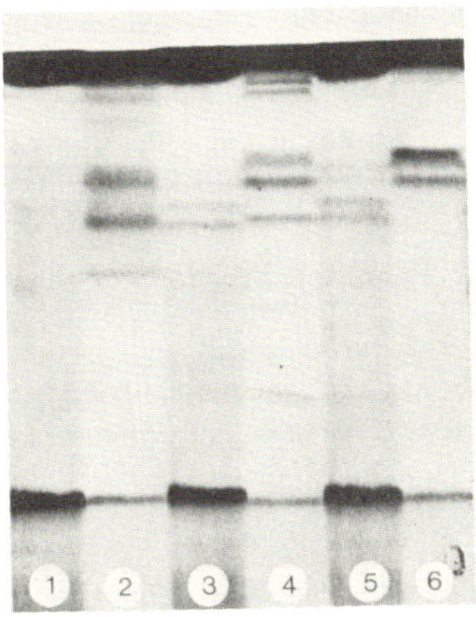

Fig. 4. Starch gel separation of three foetal (2, 4 and 6) and three adult sera (1, 3 and 5) with a Tris-cacodylic acid buffer to show individual variation in the α_1 protein (between albumin and transferrin).

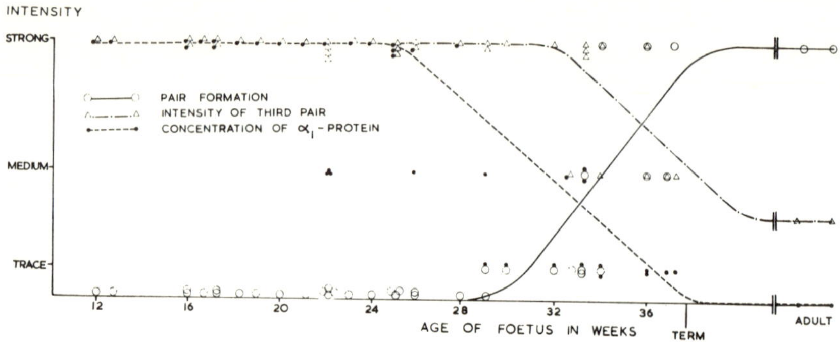

Fig. 5. Schematic diagram to show the approximate time relations of the various changes taking place in the embryonic development of bovine transferrin and α_1 protein.

citrate, pH 7.6, the foetal transferrins are undistinguishable from adult transferrins (Fig. 3).

It can be seen from Fig. 4 that another protein migrating between transferrin and albumin is present until some 200 days of foetal life. The mobility of this α_1 protein in starch gel corresponds to the migration rate of fetuin (see Schultze and Heremans, 1966, for review). The gradual disappearance of this protein between 180–250 days fits with the results of Barboriak et al. (1958), who showed that fetuin levels fall off after mid-term in goats, when electrophoretic methods of estimation are used. Progressive decrease in the concentration of foetal protein was also observed during human embryonic development (Bergstrand and Czar, 1957). However these results do not fit with the evidence of Bergmann et al. (1962), who showed that fetuin levels measured by a complement fixation test rose slowly to term. Further studies are needed to clarify these differing conclusions. It may be that fetuin is only a part of the α_1 protein detected by electrophoretic methods.

The α_1 protein appears as a diffuse broad band when Tris-citrate buffer system is used (Fig. 3) but forms 2–3 clear-cut fractions in a Tris-cacodylic acid buffer (Fig. 4). Evidence from the small number of samples that have been collected here shows definite evidence of individual variation (Fig. 4).

In Fig. 5 the time of appearance and relative intensities of the various protein fractions described here are shown diagrammatically. It can be seen that the decrease in the concentration of the fastest foetal band of each variant corresponds in time to the appearance of the second band of each pair and when this second band has formed, then the mobility of the slower band of the two fastest pairs is the same as that in the adult transferrins. It can also be seen that although there is considerable variation in the exact time of disappearance of the α_1 protein it is only present in trace quantities by seven months of foetal life.

The results presented here particularly the evidence for the formation of a second transferrin band in each of the three pairs of any variant, are relevant to the understanding of the heterogeneity of bovine transferrins, and the genetic control of that variation. Studies aimed at explaining this heterogeneity are described elsewhere (Stratil and Spooner, 1970).

Acknowledgments

We are most grateful to our farm managers, Mr J. C. Harris and Mr J. S. Tavernor, for their help in collecting samples, and also to Mr J. Norval of the Gorgie Abbattoir Edinburgh, for permission to bleed foetuses.

References

Barboriak, J. J., G. Meschia, D. H. Barron & G. R. Cowgill, 1958. Blood plasma proteins in fetal goats and sheep. *Proc. Soc. exp. Biol. Med.* 98: 635–637.

Bergmann, F. N., L. Levine & R. G. Spiro, 1962. Fetuin: Immunochemistry and quantitative estimation in serum. *Biochim. biophys. Acta* 58: 41–51.

Bergstrand, C. G. & B. Czar, 1957. Paper electrophoretic study of human fetal serum proteins with demonstration of a new protein fraction. *Scand. J. clin. Lab. Invest.* 9: 277–286.

Buschmann, H. & D. O. Schmid, 1961. Transferrin - groups of foetal calf serum. *Nature* 190: 1209–1210.

Lyne, A. G., 1960. Pre-natal growth of cattle. *Proc. Aust. Soc. Anim. Prod.* 3: 153–161.

Makarechian, M. & W. E. Howell, 1966. Improved technique for separation and identification of bovine beta globulins by starch - gel electrophoresis. *Can. J. Biochem. Physiol.* 44 :1089.

Schultze, H. E. & J. F. Heremans, 1966. Molecular biology of human proteins with special reference to plasma proteins. Vol. 1: Nature and metabolism of extracellular proteins. Elsevier, Amsterdam, pp. 904.

Spooner, R. L. & G. Baxter, 1969. Abnormal expression of normal transferrin alleles in cattle. *Biochem. Genetics* 2: 371–382.

Stratil, A. & R. L. Spooner, 1970. Studies on the nature of the heterogeneity of cattle transferrin. *Anim. Blood Grps biochem. Genet.* 1: 173–174.

MICROTUS POPULATION BIOLOGY.
II. GENETIC CHANGES AT THE TRANSFERRIN LOCUS IN FLUCTUATING POPULATIONS OF TWO VOLE SPECIES[1]

Robert H. Tamarin[2] and Charles J. Krebs

In recent years, a great emphasis has been placed on the necessity of considering the genetics and the ecology of natural populations as a unified approach to the study of the problems of population biology (Birch, 1960; Ford, 1964; Lerner, 1965). We report here an attempt to study the population genetics of natural populations of voles (*Microtus*) whose ecology is reasonably well known (Krebs, Keller and Tamarin, MS).

The phenomenon of interest in this study is the 3–4 year cycle in numbers exhibited by microtine rodents. Chitty (1967) has proposed that these populations are self-regulated, the mechanism being a genetic-behavioral polymorphism. Detailed demographic studies (Chitty, 1952; Chitty and Chitty, 1962; Chitty and Phipps, 1961; Kalela, 1957; Krebs, 1964*a* and 1966) have demonstrated qualitative changes during a cycle in numbers (changes in body weight distributions, length of breeding season, mortality rates). In addition, Krebs (1964*b*) has demonstrated a change in the regressions of skull size on body size during a cycle. There is at present no evidence that these qualitative changes are expressions of a basic genetic change during these population cycles, and while it has seemed highly unlikely a priori that genetic changes play a large role in such short-term events (Christian and Davis, 1964; Wilbert, 1963; Pitelka, 1964), the possibility must be investigated (Thoday, 1963). Semeonoff and Robertson (1968) have demonstrated that gene frequencies at a serum esterase locus change significantly during the population decline in *Microtus agrestis*.

In this study, five populations of two vole species (*Microtus ochrogaster*, the prairie vole, and *M. pennsylvanicus*, the meadow vole) were studied in southern Indiana from June 1965 to September 1967. For these same populations, detailed demographic data have been gathered (Krebs et al., MS).

Materials and Methods

Demographic Data

Live trapping was carried out from June 1965 to August 1967 on old fields in south-

[1] This work has been supported by National Science Foundation Grants GB-3509 and GB-6273 and U.S. Public Health Service Genetic Training Grants 20-82(C2) and GM 82.

[2] Parts of the paper were submitted as a thesis in partial fulfillment of the degree, Doctor of Philosophy, Department of Zoology, Indiana University. Present address: Department of Genetics, University of Hawaii, Honolulu, Hawaii 96822.

ern Indiana, on the Grasslands Research Area of Indiana University, about 7 miles east of Bloomington. Three contiguous grids (A, B, and D) of approximately 2 acres each were live-trapped for a 2-day period every 2 weeks. Each grid was a 10 by 10 checkerboard of 100 points, 25 feet apart, each point having one Longworth live trap (or two when numbers became high). The trapping regime was designed to enumerate all animals present and thus avoid the sampling difficulties inherent in capture-recapture methods.

When a mouse was caught for the first time, a numbered fingerling fish tag was placed in the right ear. In addition, the location on the grid, sex, species, and external reproductive condition were noted.

The following is a description of each grid:

Grid A. This grid was unfenced and surrounded on three sides by gravel roads and the fourth side by the fence on Grid B. It had populations of both species present and was treated as a control grid.

Grid B. This grid, and the remaining one, were surrounded by fencing to prevent the mice moving on and off the area. The fencing consisted of hardware cloth extending 2 feet into the ground and 2 feet above. This was covered by V-shaped aluminum sheeting to prevent animals from climbing over the fence. This grid contained populations of both species and acted as a control for the effects of fencing.

Grid D. This grid was also surrounded by fencing and contained an introduced population of *Microtus ochrogaster.* This population was started in February 1966 with 18 voles removed from a peak population 3 miles northeast of the main study area.

Populations in the two fenced grids were followed until August 1967, when the experiments were terminated and the populations trapped out. Data were punched on IBM cards, and analyzed on the CDC 3400–3600 computer at the Indiana University Research Computing Center. For a more detailed account of the area and methodology, see Keller and Krebs (MS) and Krebs et al. (MS).

The Transferrin System and Sampling Mortality

Transferrin is an iron-binding β-globulin, found in the serum of vertebrates and easily detected by means of electrophoresis. Variant forms show up as bands with different relative mobilities on an electrophoretic gel. Maurer (1967) has demonstrated the heritability of the transferrin system in both *Microtus pennsylvanicus* and *M. ochrogaster*, and each variant form is controlled by an allele at a single locus. This interpretation is further supported by breeding data from our laboratory (Gaines, unpublished) and from a large amount of published data in other species (see Lush, 1967 for a summary). In this study we have used the allelic nomenclature of Maurer (1967). Each of the three alleles found in this study produced two zones on the electrophoretic gel, one major and one minor (resolved to one major and two minor under certain conditions). The allele producing the slowest group of zones is Tf^F, the intermediate group is produced by Tf^E, and the fastest group is produced by Tf^C. Each population had two alleles. The *M. pennsylvanicus* populations had the Tf^E and Tf^C alleles, while the *M. ochrogaster* populations had the Tf^E and Tf^F alleles.

Serum samples were taken by toe-clipping mice in the field. Mice were released immediately. Survival rate was measured as the number known alive at week t + 2 divided by the number released at week t. Table 1 shows survival rates of bled and non-bled mice of the two species on Grid A. Survival rates of the bled mice were lower in all the *M. ochrogaster* samples (averaging 15–20% lower) and 8 of 10 *M. pennsylvanicus* samples (averaging 5–10% lower). These survival rates were compared within periods with a sign test (Siegel, 1956) and only two periods showed significantly lowered survival in the bled group (*M. ochrogaster* males, period III,

TABLE 1. *Average unweighted mean survival rates per 14 days for voles bled by toe-clip technique and those not bled, grouped over the five periods of the cycle for the two species on Grid A.*

	Period = I Summer 1965		II Winter 65–6		III Summer 1966		IV Winter 66–7		V Summer 1967		Pooled	
	Male	Female	Male	Female	Male	Female	Male	Female	Male	Female	Male	Female
M. ochrogaster												
Bled	.61	.60	.65	.89	.57	.77	.43	.56	.50	—	.56	.71
Not Bled	.66	.95	.84	.94	.80	.86	.66	.66	.55	—	.74	.85
M. pennsylvanicus												
Bled	.46	.83	.93	.75	.65	.80	.77	.83	.58	.76	.68	.80
Not Bled	.80	.95	.80	.86	.75	.86	.82	.89	.72	.74	.77	.85

$p = .019$; *M. pennsylvanicus* males, period I, $p = .016$).

This unfortunate mortality will not invalidate our conclusions if it is distributed randomly over the various genotypes. The frequency of genotypes which disappeared within 2 weeks of bleeding was compared with the frequency of genotypes which were bled. If mortality falls randomly, we expect these frequencies to be the same. There was no significant difference in either species when survival rates were compared by a chi-square contingency test. The data also were broken down into the periods of the cycle, and the same comparison was made, with no significant differences. Thus we conclude that although bleeding seems to lower the survival of the bled mice, this effect is distributed randomly over the various genotypes. In the three fenced populations, toe-clipping did not cause additional mortality.

The serum sample was taken in a small quantity of sodium citrate to prevent clotting. The sample was centrifuged and the supernatant serum pipetted off and frozen. For most samples, electrophoresis was carried out within 2 weeks of bleeding.

During the first year of this study, electrophoresis was carried out with the polyacrylamide disc procedure of Ornstein (1964) and Davis (1964). The iron-binding capacity of the transferrins was verified by staining with the Canalco 800 series iron stain kit (Canal Industrial Corp., Bethesda, Maryland). After the first year of this study we used a vertical method of acrylamide electrophoresis. Gels were run on the E-C 470 vertical electrophoresis apparatus (E-C Apparatus Corp., Philadelphia, Penn.). A tris-glycine pH 9.3 buffer was used (E-C bulletin, 1965), and the prescribed method was followed with the exception that an albumin marker (bromphenol blue) was added prior to electrophoresis, and the gels were stained with a 1% amidoblack solution in 7½% acetic acid. The gels were destained electrophoretically in a 15% acetic acid solution using the E-C 479 Electrophoretic Destainer.

To demonstrate the iron-binding capacity of the transferrins in this system, the iron-binding stain system of Mueller, Smithies and Irwin (1962, modified by Koehn, 1967) was used.

In the course of this study, 3526 individuals were trapped, of which 2311 (65.5%) were bled.

RESULTS

Gene frequencies were determined on a bi-weekly basis by direct enumeration of voles known to be alive. Figures 1–5 show Tf^E frequency and population density for the voles on Grids A, B and D. Two points should be noted from the gene frequency graphs. First, the polymorphism is maintained at a high Tf^E frequency in the *M. ochrogaster* populations (c. 75–90%) and at an intermediate level in the *M. pennsylvanicus* populations (c. 45–55%). Second, males and females do not follow the same trend in terms of gene frequency. Evidence

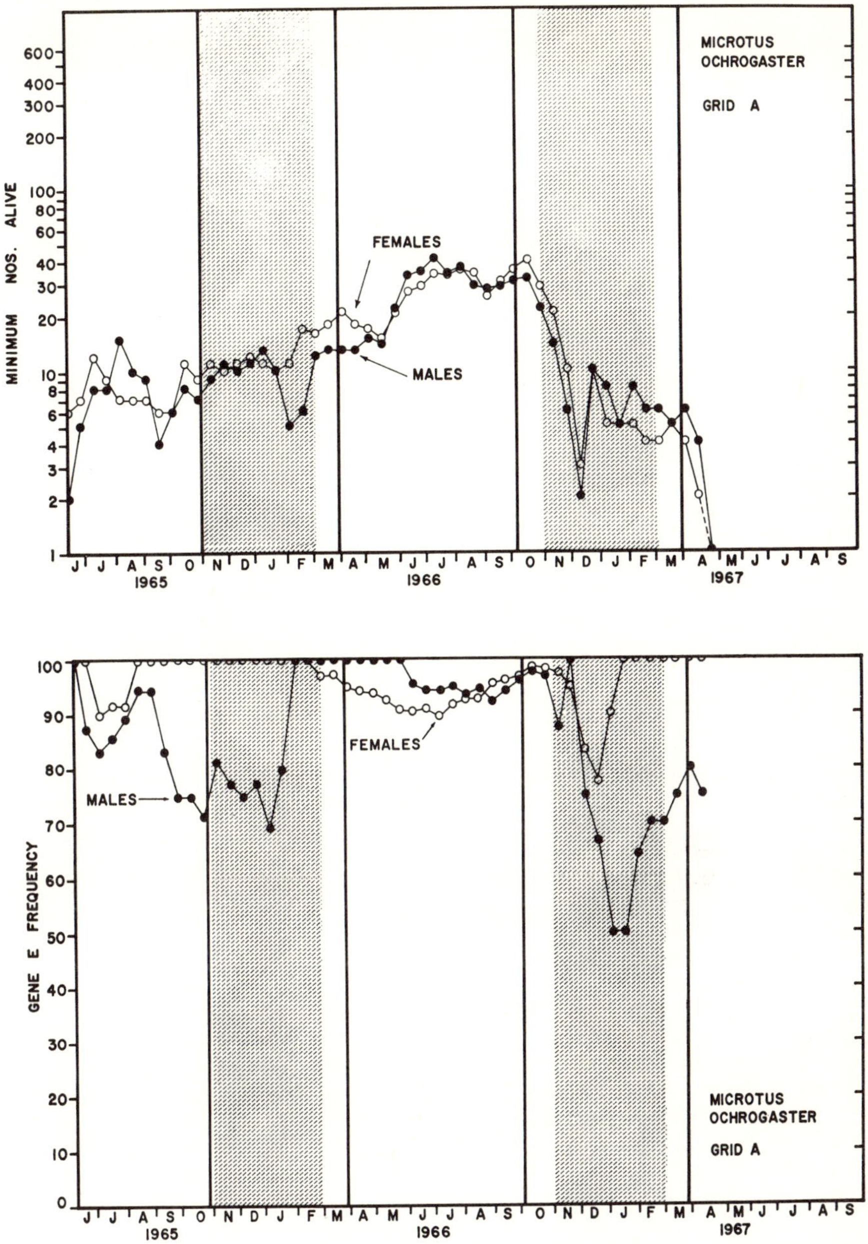

FIG. 1. *M. ochrogaster*, Grid A, population density (upper graph) and Tf^E frequency (lower graph). The four vertical lines divide the study into five periods on the basis of seasonal reproductive changes. The shaded areas are the four winter months (November to February).

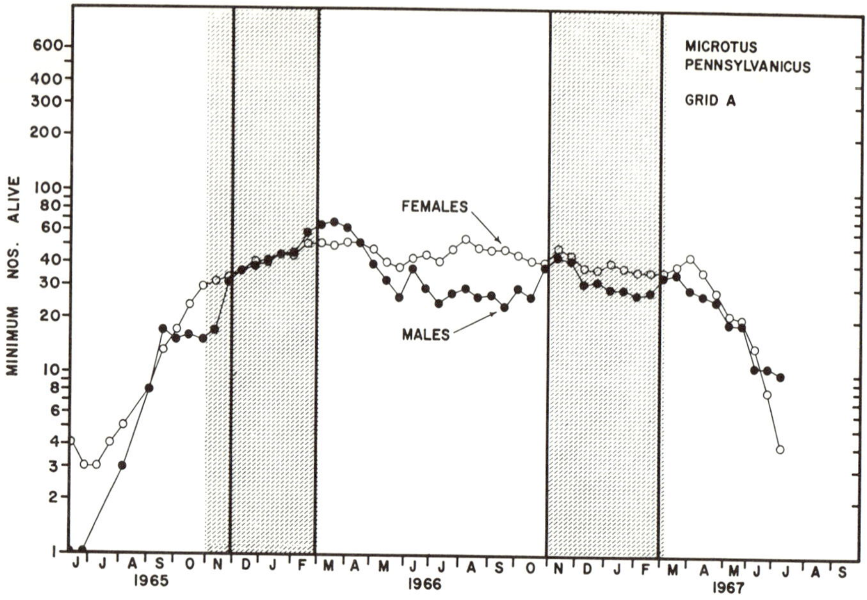

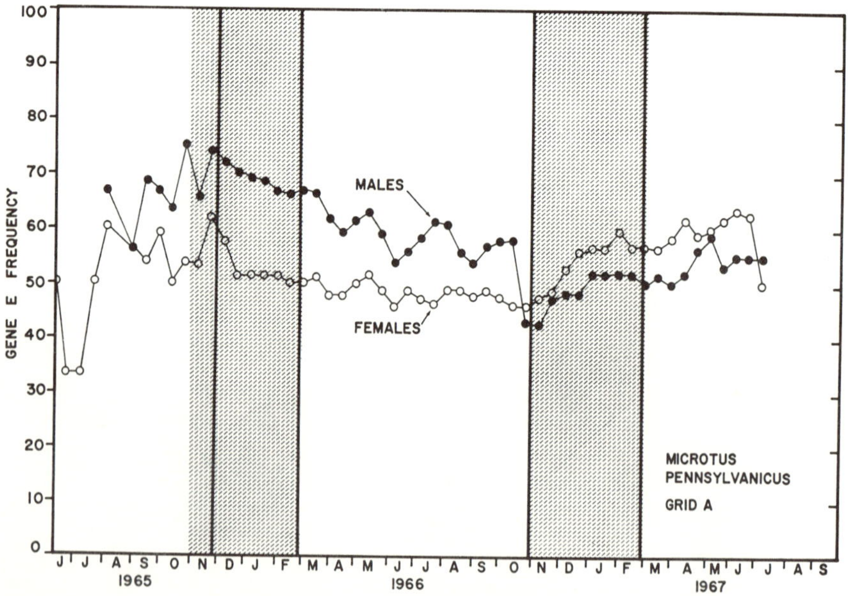

FIG. 2. *M. pennsylvanicus*, Grid A. See legend for Fig. 1.

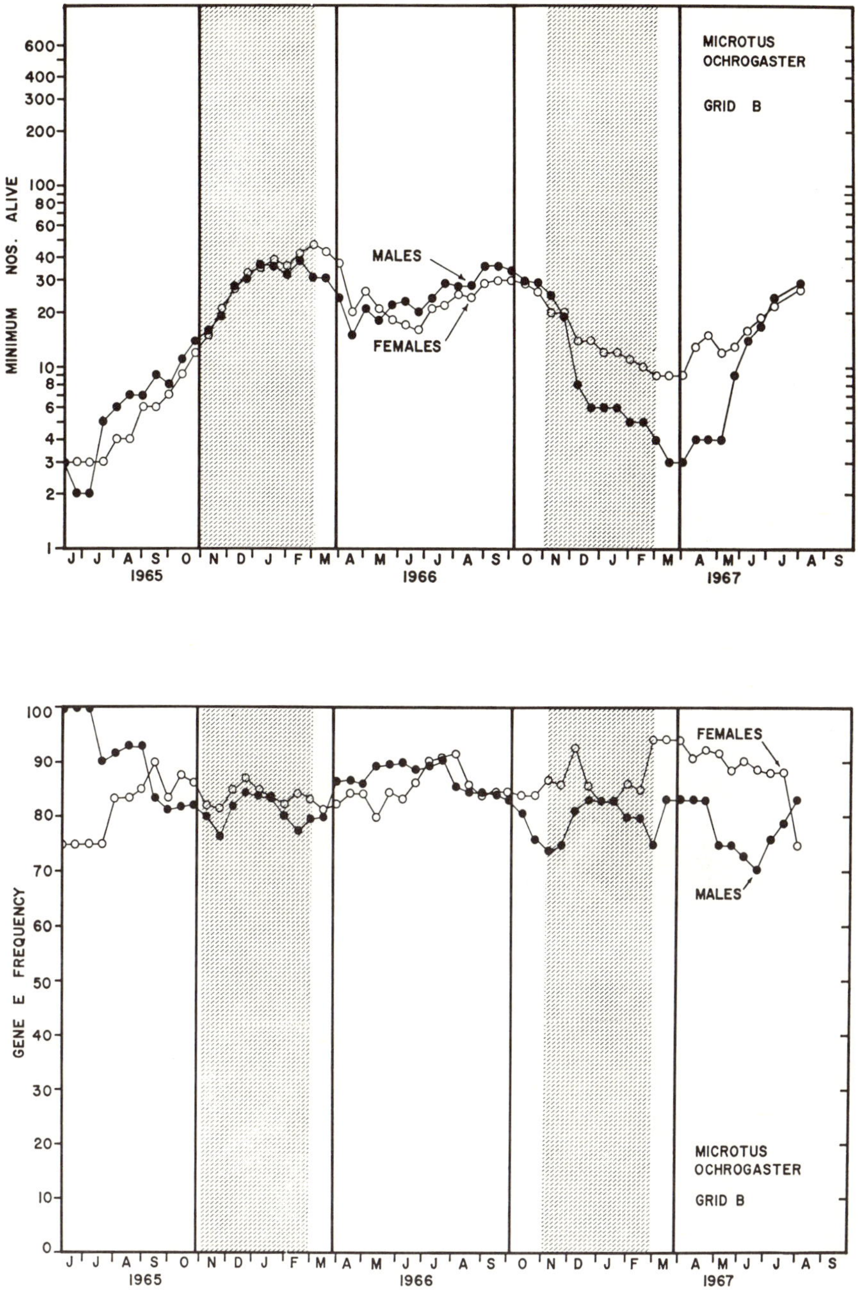

FIG. 3. *M. ochrogaster,* Grid B. See legend for Fig. 1.

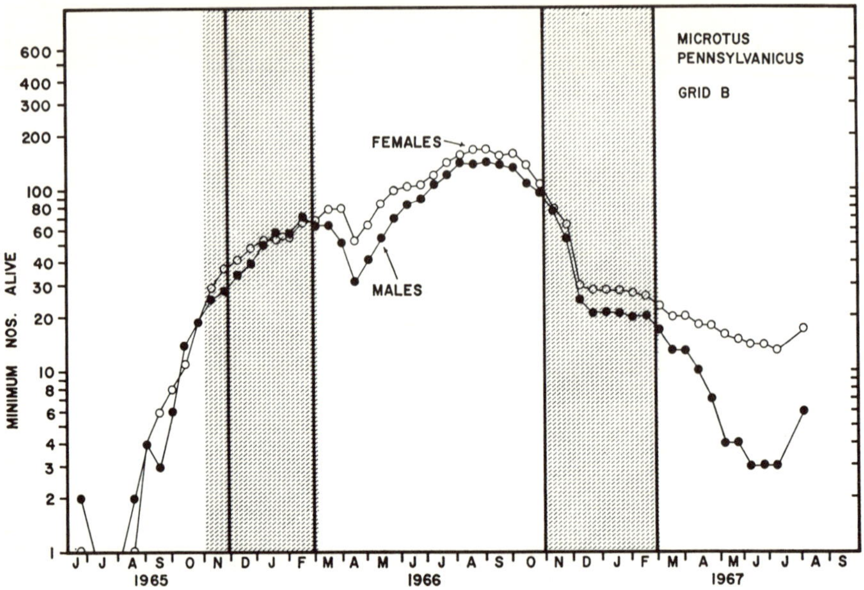

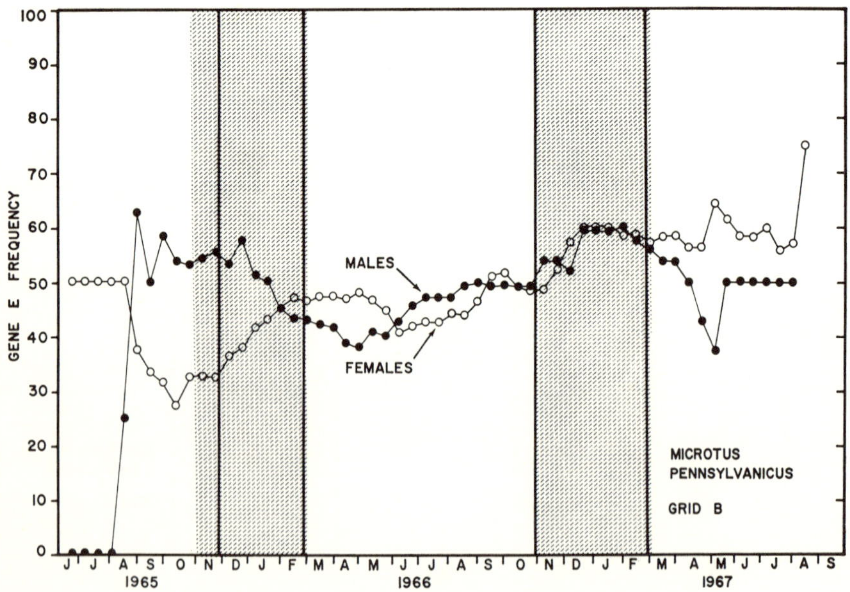

FIG. 4. *M. pennsylvanicus*, Grid B. See legend for Fig. 1.

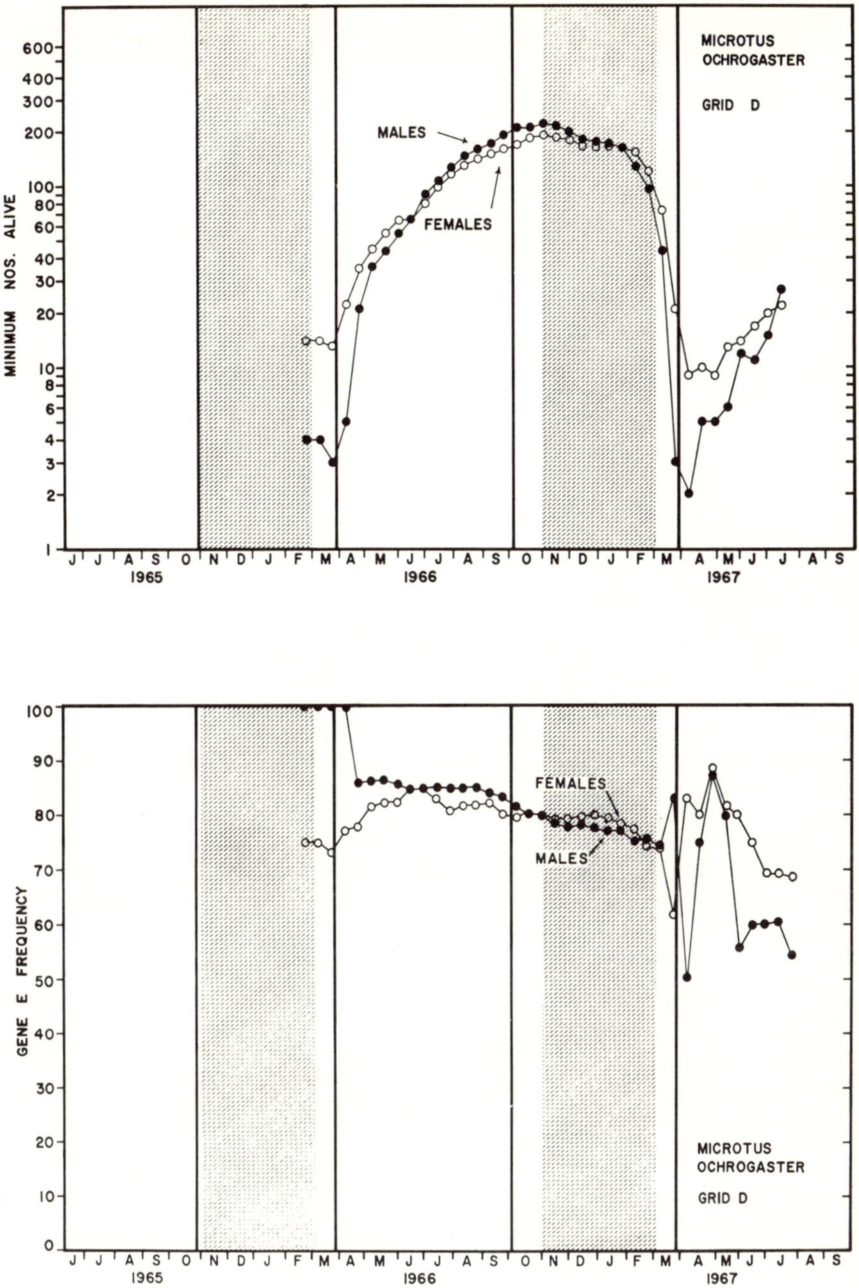

FIG. 5. *M. ochrogaster,* Grid D. See legend for Fig. 1.

TABLE 2. *Equilibrium* Tf^E *frequencies, selection coefficients (*s *and* t*), and related data obtained from the regression of* Δp *on* p *for the five populations. See text for further details.*

	Microtus ochrogaster						*Microtus pennsylvanicus*			
	Grid A		Grid B		Grid D		Grid A		Grid B	
	Male	Female	Male	Female	Male	Female	Male	Female	Male	Female
N[1]	52	50	53	53	36	36	49	49	46	46
F-Value	12.36	48.73	7.53	10.45	6.53	10.06	4.54	6.79	5.13	1.46
Probability	<0.005	<0.001	<0.01	<0.005	<0.025	<0.005	<0.05	<0.025	<0.05	<0.25
Equilibrium Tf^E Frequency	0.83	0.94	0.81	0.86	0.77	0.79	0.58	0.52	0.50	0.61
95% Confidence Interval	0.78–0.88	0.91–0.97	0.79–0.83	0.85–0.87	0.73–0.81	0.78–0.80	0.56–0.60	0.51–0.53	0.48–0.52	0.58–0.64
$b_{\Delta p \cdot p}$ (Slope)	−0.198	−0.504	−0.096	−0.144	−0.161	−0.250	−0.084	−0.114	−0.096	−0.023
s	0.20	0.36	0.11	0.15	0.18	0.25	0.13	0.20	0.18	0.04
t	0.98	>1.00	0.47	0.92	0.60	0.94	0.18	0.22	0.18	0.06

[1] N = Sample size (trapping periods).

will be presented in the following sections to demonstrate the nature of the polymorphism and to show that the observed changes in transferrin gene frequency are not merely random effects, but are correlated with demographic changes, and that different effects are occurring in the two sexes.

The Nature of the Polymorphism

In a balanced polymorphism where fitnesses are constant, the relationship of gene frequency (p) and change in gene frequency (Δp) is a defined curve with one non-trivial stable equilibrium point (Li, 1955*a*, p. 283). If fitnesses are not constant, then the relationship of Δp and p does not have a unique explanation (Wright and Dobzhansky, 1946). Constant fitnesses would imply heterosis; however, changing fitnesses, such as frequency-dependent selection, without heterosis, could also account for this relationship (Li, 1955*a*; Tobari and Kojima, 1967).

If data are confined to the portion of the curve near the equilibrium point, then a straight line relationship is approximated. With this assumption, the regression of Δp (change in Tf^E frequency) on p (Tf^E frequency) was calculated separately for the five populations treating the sexes separately. The only case where this regression was not found to be significant was that of the female *M. pennsylvanicus* on Grid B. In the males of this population, and in all the other populations, the significance of this regression demonstrates stability of the polymorphism.

Confidence limits for this stable point were calculated by inverting the regression to make p the dependent variable. Table 2 presents these data for the five populations. The only case where the confidence limits for the equilibrium gene frequency of the two sexes overlapped is the *M. ochrogaster* population on Grid D. In the four other populations, the two sexes maintained separate equilibrium Tf^E gene frequencies over the cycle.

If we assume that the polymorphism in these species is maintained by heterosis, selection coefficients can be calculated. A serious difficulty arises in that the breeding structure of these species does not conform to any of the standard population genetics models. Thus selection coefficients can

TABLE 3. *Equilibrium* Tf^E *frequencies for the five populations calculated from the regression of* Δp *on* p. *Where the 95% confidence limits for the two sexes do not overlap, the numbers are in boldface.*

	Period = I Summer 1965		II Winter 65–6		III Summer 1966		IV Winter 66–7		V Summer 1967	
	Male	Female	Male	Female	Male	Female	Male	Female	Male	Female
M. ochrogaster										
Grid A	**.77**	**.97**	.97	$>$ 1.00	.95	.94	**.72**	**.96**	.56	.67
Grid B	.82	.86	.81	.83*	**.77**	**.86**	**.80**	**.89**	**.75**	**.90**
Grid D					.83	.82	.78	.80*	.66*	.79*
M. pennsylvanicus										
Grid A	**.67***	**.56**	**.64**	**.50***	**.54**	**.48***	.53	.59	**.54**	**.59**
Grid B	**.55***	**.31**	**.37**	**.56**	.50	.46	.58	.61	**.49**	**.59***

* Regression of Δp on p significant at the 0.05 level.

only be very rough estimates, but useful for comparative purposes. A model in which the whole cycle is considered as one generation is assumed in order to calculate selection coefficients. Note that the two species have different alternatives to the Tf^E allele.

If the assumption of a straight line relationship between p and Δp holds, then the slope of the line, $b_{\Delta p.p}$, approximates the slope of the tangent of the theoretical curve ($d\Delta p/dp$) at the equilibrium value of p.

Δp can be represented as follows (Falconer, 1964, p. 30):

$$\Delta p = -pq \quad (sp - qt)/(1 - p^2 s - q^2 t).$$

By differentiating this equation and setting it equal to the slope ($b_{\Delta p.p}$), we get (letting the subscript 'e' represent the equilibrium condition):

$$s \simeq b_{\Delta p.p}/(b_{\Delta p.p} \cdot p_e - p_e)$$
$$t \simeq s \cdot p_e/q_e.$$

Further violations of the underlying assumptions do not justify the use of more sophisticated iterative methods. These selection coefficients are given at the bottom of Table 2; they quantify the assumption that the heterozygote is at an advantage and show that in the *M. ochrogaster* populations the Tf^E/Tf^E homozygote is at a greater advantage than the rare Tf^F/Tf^F homozygote. In all *M. ochrogaster* populations the fitnesses of the homozygotes were lower in the females than in the males. In the *M. pennsylvanicus* populations the two homozygotes were at a relatively equal disadvantage, and the fitnesses of the two sexes seemed about equal.

The same type of analysis was performed on the data broken down into the five periods of the cycle (shown by the vertical lines in Figs. 1–5). This resulted in a reduction of sample size to the point where most individual regression lines were not significant. However, confidence limits were put on these equilibrium values, and in many cases there was non-overlap (Table 3). This is an indication that perhaps the equilibrium points change during the cycle, owing to changing fitnesses. These equilibrium gene frequencies from Table 3 for the *M. ochrogaster* population on Grid A were plotted against phase of the cycle to try to discern any cyclical trends if present (Fig. 6). Although these data suggest a cyclic variation in gene frequency in step with population density changes, we can draw no firm conclusions about the cyclic aspects of this graph. There is unfortunately no replication in this study. The fenced populations (Grids B and D) show anomalous demographic changes (Krebs et al., MS) and are not replicates of unfenced Grid A. The fenced populations decimated their habitats and declined. After the habitat was naturally renewed in the spring of 1967, these fenced mice went directly into an increase phase. On the unfenced grid, the habitat was not

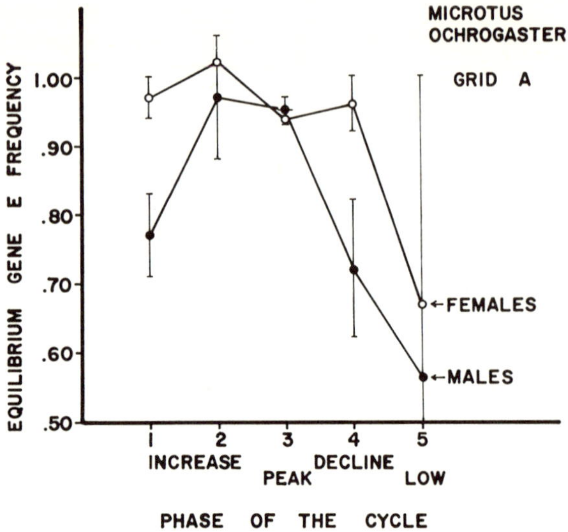

FIG. 6. Equilibrium Tf^E frequency with 95% confidence interval vs. phase of the cycle for the *M. ochrogaster* population on Grid A.

decimated and yet the mice declined to low numbers and stayed there in the spring of 1967.

Analysis of Genotypic Frequencies

If the polymorphism is maintained by heterosis, one would expect to find an excess of heterozygotes. However, this may be an oversimplification of a very complex situation. Ashton (1965) presented a model for a heterotically maintained transferrin polymorphism in cattle, involving the interplay of four parameters, of which two, fertility in males and females, showed a heterozygous disadvantage. Similarly, Fujino and Kang (1968) presented evidence for a balance of fertility and viability in the transferrin system in skipjack tuna. This balance resulted in a heterozygous excess at birth, but none at maximum size. Thus, although heterosis may be a significant phenomenon, it may be obscured by opposite effects in different population parameters and further obscured by inbreeding, subdivision, and possible cyclic trends.

There is a further difficulty in determining heterozygous excess in species which have continuous overlapping generations. Since sampling involved enumeration and was carried out bi-weekly, a large number of the animals contribute to the gene pool for several weeks, and therefore the heterozygote estimates for each sample are not independent.

First, deviations from the Hardy-Weinberg equilibrium were looked at in the data broken down into the five periods of the cycle. In computing the expected values, we used Levene's exact probabilities (Levene, 1949), and found no obvious trends. There existed cases of heterozygote deficiency, heterozygote excess, and cases of no deviations from the expected. Thus we conclude that no consistent heterozygote excess existed.

An O/E ratio (observed heterozygotes/expected heterozygotes) was calculated for the bi-weekly data. As expected from the non-independence of the samples, a graph of the O/E ratio with time tends to produce a smooth curve. This is shown in

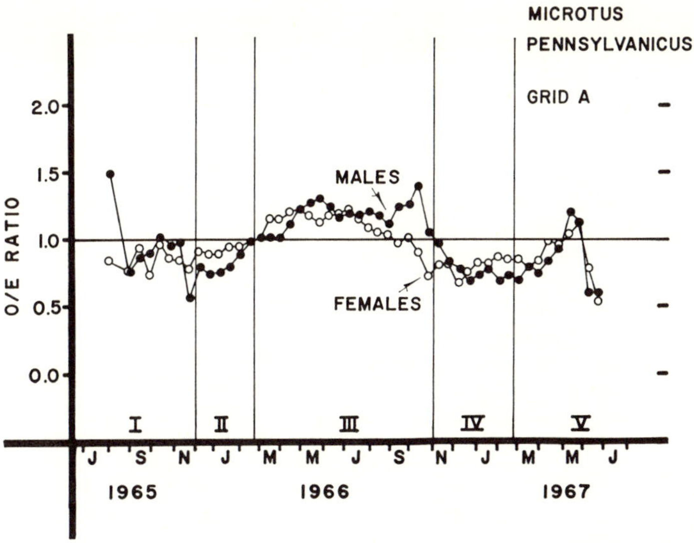

FIG. 7. *M. pennsylvanicus*, Grid A, changes in the ratio of (Observed no. heterozygotes/Expected no.) during the population cycle. An O/E ratio of 1.0 occurs when the observed number of heterozygotes equals the expected number. When the ratio is greater than one, there is a heterozygote excess, when less than one, a deficiency.

Figure 7 for the *M. pennsylvanicus* population on Grid A.

In order to study the relationship of change in gene frequency with change in genotype frequency, the O/E ratio was correlated with gene frequency for the biweekly sampling periods (for details, see Tamarin, 1968, Table 5).

For the populations of *M. ochrogaster* from Grids A and B, the Tf^F/Tf^F homozygote was very rare, and thus any increase in Tf^E would have to be a result of decreased heterozygotes. The other three populations, however, had both types of homozygotes in relatively high numbers.

The Grid A populations of *M. pennsylvanicus* showed a negative relationship of the O/E ratio and Tf^E frequency similar to the Grid A and B populations of *M. ochrogaster*. The remaining two populations showed a positive relationship of the O/E ratio with Tf^E frequency. Thus an increase in Tf^E frequency came at the expense of heterozygotes in the Grid A population of *M. pennsylvanicus*, but was due to an increase in heterozygotes and a decrease in the rarer homozygote in the Grid D population of *M. ochrogaster* and Grid B population of *M. pennsylvanicus*. This is not necessarily a result of selection, because the same factors that influence heterozygote frequency also influence the O/E ratio.

To summarize, we have demonstrated that the polymorphism is a balanced one; however, owing to the lack of a clear heterozygote excess we cannot be sure what the mechanism of maintenance is. It may be heterosis with constant fitnesses or some mechanism of changing fitnesses such as frequency-dependent selection. By comparing the O/E ratio with Tf^E frequency we found out what types of genotypic changes caused the observed Tf^E frequency changes. We will now proceed to investigate the relationship of gene frequency and genotype frequency with the population parameters of density and survival rate.

Population Parameters

Are changes in gene frequencies at the transferrin locus associated with population processes involving changes in density and survival? If not, we must assume that random events are the driving forces behind the changes shown in Figures 1–5. Note here that the populations of greatest interest are those of unfenced Grid A, which we assume are representative of natural conditions.

Density.—Two problems arise here. First, we assume that the populations we are talking about have been completely enumerated from a standpoint of density and almost completely so from a standpoint of gene frequency. Thus, gene frequency data represent the exact situation rather than a statistical statement of the data. In other words, we are using the "local" approach of Lloyd and Ghelardi (1964) where we do not consider our measurements of density and gene frequency as samples but as exact measurements of what is occurring on this particular piece of grassland. Although we do realize that each new generation is a "sample" of the genes of the parents, statistical treatment of gene frequency change is almost impossible due to the second point. This second point is the non-independence of sampling due to overlapping generations. Many of the same individuals are represented in many bi-weekly samples. This violates the assumption of independence required for analysis of gene frequency change by standard statistical methods. With this in mind, we are forced to present many of the changes in gene frequency in a descriptive manner.

Table 4 presents the correlation coefficients for the relationship of Tf^E frequency and population density. For the Grid A population of *M. ochrogaster* there was a negative relationship between these two variables during the increase and peak (first three periods). The relationship was positive during the decline and low phases.

Two periods of remarkably rapid gene frequency change are evident in Figure 1. During January 1966, the males showed a very rapid rise in Tf^E frequency associated with a temporary decline in population density of males. During November and December 1966, a very rapid drop in numbers was correlated with an equally substantial drop in Tf^E frequency, an effect opposite to that just described from the previous winter. From the middle of December 1966 and thereafter, Tf^E frequency and density rose in both sexes. This was due to migration onto the grid, and explains the sudden reversal of demographic and genetic events. It demonstrates that Tf^E was more frequent in the gene pool of the migrants than of the residents, which may in itself be of interest.

The *M. pennsylvanicus* population on Grid A, on the other hand, shows mainly negative correlations with density. Thus in this species, density changes seem to select against the Tf^E allele when numbers are increasing and to favor the Tf^E allele when numbers decline. As is evident from Figure 2, Tf^E frequency fell steadily during the first three periods, more so in the males, and rose thereafter. It is remarkable that the Tf^E frequency remained separate and distinct in the two sexes through these first three periods, even though breeding was occurring throughout. In the last two periods, the Tf^E frequency again remained separate in the two sexes, in this case males having the lower Tf^E frequency. This clearly indicates differential selective effects in the two sexes.

For the three fenced populations, the results are more difficult to interpret, and this difficulty is primarily due to what we believe are demographic disturbances that fencing has introduced (see Krebs et al., MS).

For the *M. ochrogaster* population on Grid B, the predominant correlation is in a negative direction similar to that in the *M. pennsylvanicus* population on Grid A. Note the increase in Tf^E frequency accompanying the decline in numbers in the males in February–April 1966 and November–December 1966. The only significant positive correlation is in period I for the

TABLE 4. *Correlation coefficients for the relationship of Tf^E frequency with density.*

	Period = I Summer 1965		II Winter 65–6		III Summer 1966		IV Winter 66–7		V Summer 1967		Totals	
	Male	Female	Male	Female	Male	Female	Male	Female	Male	Female	Male	Female
M. ochrogaster												
Grid A	N[1] = 10	10	11	11	13	13	13	13	5	3	52	50
	r = –0.01	–0.54	–0.23	–0.77**	–0.87**	–0.23	0.64*	0.18	0.78	—	0.43**	0.10
Grid B	N = 10	10	11	11	13	13	12	12	7	7	53	53
	r = –0.91**	0.78**	0.24	–0.14	–0.69**	–0.14	–0.53	–0.45	–0.84*	–0.66	–0.20	–0.04
Grid D	N = —	—	—	—	16	16	12	12	8	8	36	36
	r =				–0.72**	0.61*	0.87**	0.92**	–0.42	–0.93**	–0.02	0.22
M. pennsylvanicus												
Grid A	N = 7	7	6	6	18	18	8	8	10	10	49	49
	r = 0.35	–0.67	–0.97**	–0.93**	0.73**	0.28	–0.88**	–0.73*	–0.67*	–0.78**	0.06	–0.67**
Grid B	N = 5	5	6	6	17	17	8	8	10	10	46	46
	r = 0.06	0.20	–0.82*	0.95**	0.94**	0.06	–0.80*	–0.96**	0.71*	–0.30	–0.30*	–0.16

[1] N = Sample size (trapping periods). r = Correlation coefficient.
* Significant at the 0.05 level. ** Significant at the 0.01 level.

TABLE 5. *Correlation coefficients for the relationship of Tf^E frequency with survival. Data for the periods of population decline are in boldface.*

	Period = I Summer 1965		II Winter 65–6		III Summer 1966		IV Winter 66–7		V Summer 1967		Totals	
	Male	Female	Male	Female	Male	Female	Male	Female	Male	Female	Male	Female
M. ochrogaster												
Grid A	N[1] = 10	10	11	11	13	13	13	13	3	2	50	49
	r = –0.16	0.74*	0.27	–0.17	0.11	0.29	**–0.57***	**0.65***	**0.82**	—	–0.11	0.41**
Grid B	N = 10	10	11	11	13	13	12	12	7	7	53	53
	r = –0.28	–0.32	–0.03	0.07	0.33	0.49	**0.64***	**0.42**	0.27	0.46	0.32*	0.02
Grid D	N = —	—	—	—	16	16	12	12	8	8	36	36
	r =				–0.09	–0.39	**0.72****	**0.93****	–0.33	0.44	0.14	0.42*
M. pennsylvanicus												
Grid A	N = 7	7	6	6	18	18	8	8	6	6	42	42
	r = –0.74	0.14	–0.50	–0.73	0.34	–0.29	0.65	0.59	**–0.72**	**–0.70**	–0.05	0.02
Grid B	N = 5	5	6	6	17	17	8	8	6	6	45	45
	r = 0.10	0.91*	–0.44	0.55	–0.12	–0.63**	**0.74***	**0.77***	0.54	–0.18	0.14	–0.20

[1] N = Sample size (trapping periods). r = Correlation coefficient.
* Significant at the 0.05 level. ** Significant at the 0.01 level.

females. Period I for the three fenced populations (period III for the *M. ochrogaster* on Grid D) is similar in that in all three cases, the males and females started from small numbers with widely differing gene frequencies that appeared to equilibrate after a number of weeks (5–16 weeks, see Figs. 3–5). This is probably a "founder" phenomenon, a result of the genotypes of those animals that happened to be present at low numbers at the start of this study.

On Grid D, the *M. ochrogaster* females showed a positive relation between density and gene frequency through a rapid increase, peak and decline of numbers, and then as numbers rose again, Tf^E frequency fell. For the males, Tf^E frequency fell as numbers rose, and continued to fall as numbers peaked and then declined. Then, in line with the females, gene frequency dropped as numbers began to rise again.

For the female *M. pennsylvanicus* on Grid B, Tf^E frequency rose significantly with numbers during the late increase phase (period II), and then rose as numbers fell. For the males, Tf^E frequency fell as numbers rose in the late increase, fell significantly during the spring 1966 drop-off in numbers and increased as the population approached peak numbers in late summer 1966. Tf^E frequency continued to rise as numbers declined, but then fell during the spring 1967 decline in numbers.

To summarize, increasing *M. pennsylvanicus* populations showed selection against the Tf^E gene, while when these populations declined selection reversed and favored the Tf^E gene. During the increase and peak phases in *M. ochrogaster* selection acts against the Tf^E gene, at least in males. There is not, however, complete agreement among these different populations, and this may be explained by the effects of fencing Grids B and D on population processes.

The unfenced Grid A populations (Figs. 1–2), after the peak in numbers, declined and maintained declining numbers until the end of the study. This is presumably a typical pattern for these 3–4 year cycles. The fenced populations, on the other hand, typically increased at a more rapid rate than the unfenced ones. These rapid population increases carried Grids B and D to densities three to four times what is normal for this area. The *M. ochrogaster* population on Grid D is especially atypical in that the peak went to very high numbers and the whole cycle lasted only 1 year. This rapid increase in fenced populations was achieved through very high survival rates in the trappable populations. Having reached very dense levels, these populations typically proceeded to devastate their habitat and suffer a catastrophic decline (Grid B, fall 1966; Grid D, spring 1967). These catastrophic declines may not be a complete analog to "normal" cyclic declines in these species. This is suggested by the too rapid return of these populations to the increase phase (e.g. *M. ochrogaster*, Grids B and D, summer 1967). For a more detailed description of these events, see Krebs et al., (MS).

Thus, from an ecological standpoint we can see that the fenced populations were atypical in their demography, and that this is probably because of high survival and therefore lower selection. These populations nevertheless do show some of the facets of a true cycle such as winter breeding during the increase and high adult body weights at the peak, and for these reasons their further analysis will be continued.

Survival.—Survival rates of marked animals between trapping periods were obtained by direct enumeration. This parameter was correlated to Tf^E frequency, and the correlation coefficients are presented in Table 5.

We are interested in the correlation of Tf^E frequency and survival throughout the whole cycle, but especially during the periods of decline in numbers, where survival is the poorest. This occurs in period IV (winter 1966–7) for all but the unfenced populations. The Grid A population of *M. ochrogaster* continued to decline into period V, and the Grid A population of *M.*

pennsylvanicus did not decline until period V (summer 1967). During these periods of decline most of the significant correlations are observed.

For the *M. ochrogaster* population on Grid A, period IV shows significant correlations of survival and Tf^E frequency with both sexes, but in opposite directions. This difference in direction is due primarily to the effect of migration onto the grid when both sexes reached very low numbers (2 males, 3 females). As can be seen from Figure 1, low survival rate in both sexes (declining numbers) is accompanied by a decrease in Tf^E frequency, with a slight lag in the males, implying that decreased survival of the resident voles puts the Tf^E allele at a relative disadvantage, thus favoring the heterozygotes.

The *M. ochrogaster* populations on Grids B and D show this positive relation in period IV and in these populations all high correlations are in the positive direction, implying that here, too, decreased survival puts the Tf^E allele at a disadvantage in both sexes.

In the *M. pennsylvanicus* population on Grid A, no correlations are significant. It is interesting to note however that in the decline (period V), both sexes show high negative correlations of Tf^E frequency and survival, implying that lower survival favors the Tf^E allele. For the fenced-in *M. pennsylvanicus* population (Grid B), the correlations for the decline (period IV) are both positive and significant, similar to those for the other fenced-in populations.

In summary, Tf^E frequency has been correlated to the population parameters of density and survival rate in order to determine what relationship exists between demographic parameters and gene frequency. In the unfenced *M. pennsylvanicus* population and the Grid B population of *M. ochrogaster*, density had a negative correlation with Tf^E frequency. Thus in the increase phases the Tf^E allele was selected against, and during the decline, favored. In the unfenced *M. ochrogaster* population, the relationship was consistently in the negative direction. In the Grid B population of *M. pennsylvanicus* and the Grid D population of *M. ochrogaster* the relationship of density and Tf^E frequency was very complex.

Tf^E frequency and survival rate were usually correlated during the decline periods. In the fenced populations the relationship was positive. Thus lowered survival rates selected against the Tf^E allele. This same effect was found in the unfenced population of *M. ochrogaster.* The unfenced *M. pennsylvanicus* population showed the opposite relationship where lowered survival rates favored the Tf^E allele. We now turn our attention to a study of some of the components of fitness.

Individual Parameters

Individual parameters are those components of fitness measured in this study that could be compared on a genotypic basis. They are: weight at first capture, reproductive condition, survival rate, body weight distribution, and growth rate.

Since the Tf^F/Tf^F homozygote was almost non-existent in the *M. ochrogaster* populations, most of the analyses for these populations will compare the common homozygote (Tf^E/Tf^E) and the heterozygote (Tf^E/Tf^F). Two genotypes were compared by the Mann-Whitney U test (Siegel, 1956), and for the case of three genotypes, the Kruskal-Wallis one-way analysis of variance was used (Siegel, 1956). Nominal data were compared with contingency chi-square tests.

Weight at first capture.—This parameter was examined as an index of whether animals of differing genotype entered the trappable population at the same size. Two to four weeks usually elapse between weaning and the time when juveniles enter the trappable population, females usually entering at slightly lighter weights than males.

The data for the five populations were broken down by sexes into the periods of the cycle and analyzed. For weight at first

TABLE 6. *Genotypic differences in intensity of adult breeding measured by external sexual characters on live-trapped voles for the five populations. Data summed over the entire cycle. Total sample size in parentheses.*

M. ochrogaster	Tf^E/Tf^E		Tf^E/Tf^F		Tf^F/Tf^F
Grid A					
Testes Scrotal*	92% (319)	$>$	79% (48)		
Nipples Medium + Large	52% (372)		63% (27)		
Vagina Perforate[1]	50%		52%		
Pubic Symphysis Open[1]	15%		11%		
Grid B					
Testes Scrotal**	86% (403)	$>$	76% (174)		
Nipples Medium + Large	46% (396)		48% (170)		
Vagina Perforate*	46%	$>$	34%		
Pubic Symphysis Open	15%		14%		
Grid D					
Testes Scrotal	75% (1284)		73% (624)		64% (50)
Nipples Medium + Large*	31% (1109)	$<$	36% (516)	$>$	20% (91)
Vagina Perforate*	50%	$<$	57%	$>$	51%
Pubic Symphysis Open	8%		10%		5%
M. pennsylvanicus	Tf^C/Tf^C		Tf^C/Tf^E		Tf^E/Tf^E
Grid A					
Testes Scrotal	89% (108)		90% (298)		89% (228)
Nipples Medium + Large	43% (180)		40% (395)		36% (221)
Vagina Perforate	65%		62%		55%
Pubic Symphysis Open**	14%	$<$	26%	$<$	27%
Grid B					
Testes Scrotal	90% (173)		89% (287)		87% (135)
Nipples Medium + Large	44% (236)		39% (316)		49% (144)
Vagina Perforate	51%		53%		52%
Pubic Symphysis Open	17%		20%		17%

[1] Sample size same as nipple category above.
* Significant at the 0.05 level.
** Significant at the 0.01 level.

capture, few groups showed significant differences, and among those that did there was no pattern present. Thus we concluded that the different transferrin genotypes enter the trappable populations at the same body weights.

Reproduction.—Reproduction was studied by a genotypic comparison of the field observations on reproductive condition of voles. For males, one measure of reproduction was used, testes position (abdominal, non-breeding; scrotal, breeding). These data were broken down into the five periods of the cycle for each population and within periods the genotypes were compared by contingency chi-square tests.

For males, over the whole cycle, the populations of *M. ochrogaster* on Grids A and B showed a significant excess of the Tf^E/Tf^E homozygote in breeding condition as compared to the heterozygote Tf^E/Tf^F (Table 6). For the population of *M. ochrogaster* on Grid D there were no significant differences; however, over the whole cycle the trend was in the same direction as the other populations—an excess of Tf^E/Tf^E homozygotes in breeding condition. The heterozygote here was intermediate. The *M. pennsylvanicus* males showed no significant differences nor any trends.

For the females four field measures were taken as an index to breeding condition: obvious pregnancy; vagina perforate or not (perforate indicating breeding); nipple size small, medium or large (medium and large indicating lactation); and pubic symphysis

TABLE 7. *Minimum survival rates per 14 days of transferrin genotypes,* M. ochrogaster. *Data summed over periods, sample size in parentheses. Periods with survival rates differing among genotypes by 0.10 or greater are in boldface.*

	Grid A		Grid B		Grid D*	
	Males	Females	Males	Females	Males	Females
Period I (Summer 1965)						
Tf^E/Tf^E	0.72 (43)	**0.89** (57)	0.98 (51)	1.00 (26)		
Tf^E/Tf^F	0.79 (19)	**0.50** (2)	0.94 (17)	0.92 (13)		
Period II (Winter 65–6)						
Tf^E/Tf^E	**0.92** (65)	0.94 (109)	0.91 (148)	0.93 (152)		
Tf^E/Tf^F	**0.79** (14)	—	0.89 (92)	0.97 (79)		
Period III (Summer 1966)						
Tf^E/Tf^E	**0.84** (262)	**0.92** (244)	0.91 (180)	0.85 (156)	0.96 (606)	0.95 (540)
Tf^E/Tf^F	**0.69** (16)	**0.78** (32)	0.87 (60)	0.84 (58)	0.96 (233)	0.97 (225)
Period IV (Winter 66–7)						
Tf^E/Tf^E	**0.62** (58)	**0.70** (110)	0.80 (74)	0.92 (119)	0.86 (883)	0.89 (813)
Tf^E/Tf^F	**0.75** (32)	**0.33** (6)	0.86 (43)	0.88 (32)	0.87 (511)	0.88 (394)
Period V (Summer 1967)						
Tf^E/Tf^E	0.38 (8)	0.29 (7)	**0.97** (34)	0.93 (75)	1.00 (20)	0.86 (43)
Tf^E/Tf^F	0.33 (3)	—	**0.85** (27)	0.95 (20)	0.94 (18)	0.85 (26)

* Grid D Tf^F/Tf^F survival rates: Period III, males 1.00 (9), females 0.95 (41); Period IV, males 0.85 (54), females 0.90 (80); Period V, males 1.00 (4), females 1.00 (3).

closed, slightly open or open (open indicating near term in pregnancy). No autopsy data on genetically known mice were available for more detailed aspects of breeding.

What is sought here is an index that is both accurate and non-biased from a genetic sense. Of these four indices, obvious pregnancy is perhaps the poorest, because it is very subjective in the early stages of pregnancy. The size of the nipples (medium and large indicating lactation) is probably the best for our purposes. However, obvious trends should be supported by all the indices. The females in the unfenced *M. ochrogaster* population basically show no pattern of differences when compared genotypically within periods (Table 6). Neither does the population of *M. ochrogaster* on Grid B. The Grid D population of *M. ochrogaster*, however, shows significant trends of a breeding advantage to the Tf^E/Tf^F heterozygote. If lactation is used as the index, the increase and peak phases and the total data for the whole cycle show significant advantage to the heterozygote over both homozygotes. This is supported by the other measures of reproduction.

For the female reproductive data both *M. pennsylvanicus* populations showed no obvious patterns.

We can, therefore, conclude that in the *M. ochrogaster* populations, the male Tf^E/Tf^E homozygotes have a breeding advantage, while the only obvious trends in the females occur in the *M. ochrogaster* population on Grid D where the Tf^E/Tf^F heterozygote holds the breeding advantage. It must be remembered that these reproductive indices, both in males and females, are basically on a gross level, and more refined data certainly are needed here.

Survival rate.—Survival rate is defined as the number of mice alive at week (t + 2) divided by the number released

TABLE 8. *Minimum survival rates per 14 days of transferrin genotypes,* M. pennsylvanicus. *Data summed over periods, sample size in parentheses. Periods with survival rates differing among genotypes by 0.10 or greater are in boldface.*

	Grid A		Grid B	
	Males	Females	Males	Females
Period I (Summer 1965)				
Tf^C/Tf^C	**0.85** (13)	**0.82** (33)	**0.67** (12)	0.95 (38)
Tf^C/Tf^E	**0.64** (33)	**0.95** (58)	**1.00** (28)	0.96 (45)
Tf^E/Tf^E	**0.81** (47)	**0.90** (42)	**0.88** (24)	1.00 (8)
Period II (Winter 65–6)				
Tf^C/Tf^C	0.94 (16)	0.91 (44)	0.95 (41)	0.88 (58)
Tf^C/Tf^E	0.90 (50)	0.88 (66)	0.94 (77)	0.96 (73)
Tf^E/Tf^E	0.85 (46)	0.94 (48)	0.90 (40)	0.92 (26)
Period III (Summer 1966)				
Tf^C/Tf^C	0.72 (54)	0.93 (120)	0.84 (211)	0.89 (278)
Tf^C/Tf^E	0.81 (194)	0.88 (261)	0.86 (361)	0.87 (374)
Tf^E/Tf^E	0.75 (117)	0.86 (103)	0.87 (157)	0.85 (206)
Period IV (Winter 66–7)				
Tf^C/Tf^C	**0.89** (53)	0.89 (57)	0.71 (24)	**0.60** (25)
Tf^C/Tf^E	**0.79** (57)	0.90 (86)	0.75 (76)	**0.83** (69)
Tf^E/Tf^E	**0.94** (51)	0.95 (58)	0.77 (43)	**0.85** (46)
Period V (Summer 1967)				
Tf^C/Tf^C	0.69 (42)	0.76 (42)	**0.80** (10)	**0.71** (7)
Tf^C/Tf^E	0.69 (68)	0.77 (90)	**0.86** (29)	**0.83** (47)
Tf^E/Tf^E	0.77 (48)	0.78 (77)	**0.58** (12)	**0.88** (26)

at week (t). This is calculated separately for each genotype and summed, within sexes, over the periods of the cycle. Since these data represent almost the whole population of survival rates and are subject to a systematic bias because they are minimum survival rates, they have not been treated statistically. We will, however, consider those values differing by 0.10 or greater as biologically significant. These data refer to animals in the trappable population (2 to 4 weeks or more old), and migration from the unfenced grid is also included as mortality.

Table 7 presents these data for the *M. ochrogaster* populations. The biologically significant differences for the Grid A males occur in the middle three periods. The second and third periods favor the homozygote in survival and the fourth period favors the heterozygote. The females also show three periods of biological significance, all showing increased survival for the homozygote. However, two of these periods have very small sample sizes for the heterozygotes. The fenced grids show virtually no differential genotypic survival and this indicates that there is no selection on this component of fitness in the fenced *M. ochrogaster* populations.

Table 8 presents these same data for the *M. pennsylvanicus* populations. In the Grid A males, periods I and IV showed superior survival for the homozygotes, while period I in the females showed superior survival for the heterozygote. The Grid B males showed better survival for Tf^E carriers in period I, and Tf^C carriers in period V. The females had better survival for the Tf^E carriers in periods IV and

TABLE 9. *Number of male voles observed above 45.5 grams for the different transferrin genotypes, compared with number expected if body weight is independent of genotype.*

		Tf^E/Tf^E	Tf^E/Tf^F	Tf^F/Tf^F	Chi-square
M. ochrogaster					
Grid A	Observed	41	0		
	Expected	34.3	6.7		7.40**
Grid B	Observed	136	39		
	Expected	117.3	57.7		11.15**
Grid D	Observed	407	170	17	
	Expected	380.6	195.6	17.8	6.94*
		Tf^C/Tf^C	Tf^C/Tf^E	Tf^E/Tf^E	Chi-square
M. pennsylvanicus					
Grid A	Observed	52	120	75	
	Expected	49.3	112.4	85.3	2.61
Grid B	Observed	72	110	64	
	Expected	63.9	123.5	58.6	3.83

* Significant at the 0.05 level.
** Significant at the 0.01 level.

V. Thus, effects not found in the fenced populations of *M. ochrogaster* are found in the fenced populations of *M. pennsylvanicus*. In the fenced *M. ochrogaster* populations, selective effects must be occurring prior to the animals reaching the trappable population, or in other components of fitness such as differential reproduction. Biologically significant effects are found in both unfenced populations.

Body weight distribution.—Growth rates and body weight distributions will be considered only in the males, due to the confounding effects of pregnancy in females. High body weights are of interest because they are characteristic of peak and expanding populations in other microtine rodents studied (Krebs, 1964*a*, 1966; Chitty and Chitty, 1962).

High body weight males were considered to be 46 grams and above. Therefore the body weight distributions for the different periods for the different male populations were grouped into two classes: below and above 45.5 grams.

The results of this analysis in the population of *M. ochrogaster* are quite striking (Table 9). The unfenced Grid A population had no heterozygote males over 45.5 grams. All the heavy males were homozygous Tf^E/Tf^E and occurred in the first three periods (increase and peak). This was highly significant when the data were totalled. The same trend was evident in the two fenced populations of *M. ochrogaster* where there were always excesses of the homozygote in the over-45.5-gram category. This proved significant in their totals. For Grid D, the number of the rare Tf^F/Tf^F homozygotes in the above 45.5-gram class did not deviate appreciably from the expected number.

In the *M. pennsylvanicus* populations, the results were not clear-cut. On the unfenced grid, Grid A, the Tf^C/Tf^C homozygote dominates the excess, and this is significant only in the last period of the cycle (chi-square (2 df) = 13.256, $P < .005$). On the fenced grid, Grid B, there seems to be no clear-cut trend in the heavy-weight males; however, the Tf^C/Tf^C homozygotes over 45.5 grams are in excess of expected in the totals.

High body weight is actually a composite index of growth rate and survival. Therefore, we will look at the last individual parameter, that of growth rate.

Growth rate.—Growth rates, like body weight distributions, were considered only for the males. Growth rates were calculated as instantaneous relative growth rates and were adjusted to body weights by re-

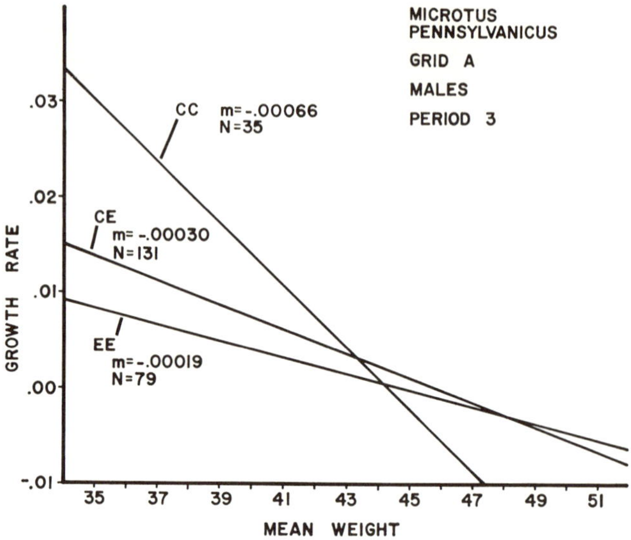

FIG. 8. Regression of growth rate on body weight for the two homozygotes (Tf^E/Tf^E, Tf^C/Tf^C) and the heterozygote (Tf^C/Tf^E) Grid A *M. pennsylvanicus* males during the peak phase (period III). The slope is designated as "m" and the sample size as "N." Mean weight is in grams and the growth rates are instantaneous relative growth rates.

gression. The regression lines for the individual genotypes were compared by covariance analysis (Dixon and Massey, 1957).

This analysis pointed to four periods of significantly different growth rates among the genotypes. Period V (return to increase phase) for the *M. ochrogaster* males on both fenced grids showed significant differences, and both the unfenced populations during the peak phase (period III) showed highly significant differences in growth rate among the genotypes.

Figure 8 shows the growth regressions for Grid A *M. pennsylvanicus* males during the peak phase (period III). The genotypic relationship of high body weight follows this same pattern ($Tf^C/Tf^C > Tf^C/Tf^E > Tf^E/Tf^E$). Thus differential growth may account for the excess of Tf^C/Tf^C homozygotes in the high body weight category in this population.

The *M. ochrogaster* males of both genotypes (Tf^E/Tf^E, Tf^E/Tf^F) reached growth plateaus at both high and low body weights (cf. Krebs et al., MS, Fig. 22). Thus the difference in growth regressions appears to be only a statistical difference probably due to the small sample size of the Tf^E/Tf^F heterozygote. Although these genotypes do not seem to have different growth asymptotes, the Tf^E/Tf^E homozygote has greater survival during the increase and peak phases (Table 7), and thus this homozygote dominates the heavy weight class.

DISCUSSION

A tremendous amount of variation exists in natural populations (Lewontin and Hubby, 1966). Shaw (1965, p. 942), for example, states, "Almost all enzymes thus far studied have shown electrophoretic variation." What is striking is that the selective basis or the ecological function of these polymorphisms is virtually unknown. An even moderately complete explanation is seldom available. The abnormal hemoglobins associated with sickle-cell anemia in humans form a balanced polymorphism maintained by heterozygote advantage in malaria resistance (Harris, 1959). The industrial melanism found in British moths (Kettlewell, 1961), the color and banding polymorphism in snails (*Cepaea*) (Cain and Sheppard, 1952), and the t-allele polymorphism in house mice (Lewontin and Dunn, 1960; Petras, 1967) are also understood reasonably well. Beyond these few examples little is known.

The transferrin polymorphism in *Microtus* may be viewed in two ways. First, we may consider it as a marker system not in itself of primary importance but perhaps linked in a supergene complex with some ecologically relevant loci. Second, we may consider the polymorphism itself to have ecological significance directly through the mechanism of iron transport in the blood, even though we cannot at present trace this complex chain from the level of the gene products to the level of the population. There is no operational way of distinguishing these two viewpoints with our present findings, and the results of this study must be viewed with this in mind.

The existence of a polymorphism immediately raises two questions (Ford, 1964): (1) is the polymorphism stable or transient? (2) if stable, how is the polymorphism maintained without going to fixation? The transferrin polymorphism in *M. ochrogaster* and *M. pennsylvanicus* exists in a balanced state. This was demonstrated earlier by the regression of Δp on p (Table 2). Further, this polymorphism has been found in all the populations we have sampled in southern Indiana and also in vole populations from Wisconsin to New England (Maurer, pers. comm.).

Li (1955*b*) mentions three basic ways of maintaining a balanced polymorphism: (1) heterosis with constant fitnesses, (2) different local environments with different constant fitnesses in each niche, and (3) frequency-dependent selection. For our purposes, (2) does not apply and (3) may be subdivided into any mechanism involving variable fitnesses. We then recognize the following four categories as applicable in our study: (1) heterozygote advantage with constant fitnesses; (2) heterozygote advantage with fluctuating fitnesses; (3) frequency-dependent selection (Kojima and Yarbrough, 1967) in which the fitness of a genotype is a function of its relative frequency; and (4) cyclic selection alternatively favoring one homozygote, then the other. It is not easy to distinguish these mechanisms operationally. The first explanation, heterosis with constant fitnesses, is the classic explanation (Fisher, 1958). If this explanation held here, we would expect to find a clear heterozygote excess and relatively constant equilibrium gene frequencies in the various phases of the cycle. We found neither. If genetic changes at this locus are important in causing these population cycles, this explanation *cannot* hold. The second explanation allows fluctuating fitnesses, as we have observed here, but it also predicts heterozygote excess, which we did not find. Nevertheless, we cannot reject this proposed mechanism conclusively because other factors such as inbreeding could obscure heterozygote excess. Frequency-dependent selection, the third possible mechanism, could be involved. The fourth mechanism, cyclic selection, might involve seasonal effects of the type described by Semeonoff and Robertson (1968) or longer-term effects associated with these 3–4 year population fluctuations. Further difficulties are that other mechanisms involving heterosis could be superimposed on this mechanism. Thus three possible mechanisms as well as complex interactions, could be involved in maintenance of this transferrin polymorphism, and present information is inadequate to distinguish among them.

Note that we may be working with two entirely different mechanisms in the two species. In the *M. ochrogaster* populations the Tf^E allele exists at a very high frequency but is intermediate in the *M. pennsylvanicus* populations. Both species have different alternative alleles to the Tf^E allele

(Tf^C in *M. pennsylvanicus* and Tf^F in *M. ochrogaster*).

Selection may operate at a number of points in the life history of these voles. A great deal of mortality always occurs before young voles reach trappable size. An approximate estimate of these losses can be obtained from the number of embryos produced by pregnant females. Averaged over the three summer breeding periods (April–September 1965, 1966, and 1967) these values are 3.4 for *M. ochrogaster* and 5.0 for *M. pennsylvanicus* (Keller and Krebs, MS, data from snap-trapped animals). These can be compared to a mean index of early juvenile survival (Krebs et al., MS). This index is computed by comparing the number of newly tagged animals in week t + 4 with the number of lactating females in week t and estimates how many young per litter entered the trappable population. This index averaged 1.16 in *M. pennsylvanicus* and 0.64 in *M. ochrogaster* over the whole cycle. By multiplying the mean number of embryos by the number of lactating females we can estimate roughly how many young should have been recruited and then compare this to the number of juveniles which actually entered the trappable population.

Summing all the data for all the populations to get a crude estimate, we find that 1569 of a possible 7586 juveniles were recruited into the populations. This is a loss of almost 80% or over 6000 young that never reached the trappable population. For the different populations, the following losses were found: *M. ochrogaster*, Grid A, 78% (687 young) lost; Grid B, 80% (773 young) lost; Grid D, 84% (1879 young) lost; and *M. pennsylvanicus*, Grid A, 85% (1436 young) lost; Grid B, 69% (1243 young) lost. Thus there is ample opportunity for selection, in terms of reproductive and survival differences, to act before young reach the trappable population.

We may now briefly summarize our findings to this point:

The *M. ochrogaster* on Grid A maintained a balanced polymorphism, the mechanism of which may be some form of frequency-dependent or cyclic selection. During the increase phase, the Tf^E/Tf^E homozygote was at an advantage in both sexes. This homozygote was selected against in both sexes during the decline.

The *M. pennsylvanicus* population on Grid A maintained a balanced polymorphism which, again, may be maintained by heterosis, but the mechanism is not clear. The increase and peak phases favored the heterozygote, while in the decline phases the heterozygotes were selected against.

The major changes introduced by fencing seem to be the introduction of a different type of mortality. Low survival rates in the fenced populations usually resulted from habitat damage, and this type of mortality may not be ecologically comparable to normal episodes of low mortality in unfenced populations which do not overgraze the habitat. Also, the relationship of change in gene frequency with change in genotype frequency differs in the fenced populations as shown by the relationship of the O/E ratio and Tf^E frequency. Lastly, the effect of density on gene frequency is much more complex and less understandable in the fenced populations. Individual parameters for the most part agree in both types of populations.

Non-selective Factors

We must now determine what effect the non-selective factors of founder effects, random drift and inbreeding have had on the changes we have described. Apparent effects of founders seem obvious in the early periods of Figures 3–5. These effects are the result of unequal gene frequencies in the two sexes requiring several months to equilibrate. The unfenced populations, however, do not show this to any great extent, and several observations preclude a determining importance to this phenomenon in unfenced vole populations, especially after the start of the increase phase. First, these species are highly mobile (Hamilton, 1937; Fitch, 1958). This mo-

TABLE 10. *Mean density, effective population size* (N_e), *and* $1/(4N_e)$ *for the five populations.*

	Period = I Summer 1965	II Winter 65–6	III Summer 1966	IV Winter 66–7	V Summer 1967	N_e	$1/(4N_e)$
M. ochrogaster							
Grid A	15.4	22.6	53.7	22.1	5.5	14.1	0.018
Grid B	10.8	59.7	49.9	27.8	18.2	24.8	0.010
Grid D	—	—	152.5	305.1	24.7	60.0	0.004
M. pennsylvanicus							
Grid A	34.6	85.0	79.7	72.1	47.0	56.2	0.005
Grid B	34.6	105.7	202.2	71.1	24.8	51.0	0.005

bility almost insures that a newly founded population will get the various alleles if a polymorphism is maintained in the species. Second, although there is a phase of very low numbers after a decline, we do not know to what extent populations do go to extinction, or at least to fixation of alleles at very low numbers. Third, the five populations showed roughly uniform levels of the polymorphism within species, indicating an ability to overcome founder phenomena to whatever extent they occur.

Inbreeding may occur, but the degree is not known. We need to know more about family structure and breeding structure in these voles. Some weak indirect evidence suggests that inbreeding is probably a negligible factor to consider in these populations. An inbreeding coefficient was calculated after Li and Horvitz (1953, p. 108). This inbreeding coefficient was not correlated with density in any of the populations of either species, as we would expect if inbreeding were a major factor at low numbers. Thus either the effects of inbreeding are not significant in these voles, or they are confounded by selective effects.

Random genetic drift occurs in small populations, and the question here is whether these vole populations are on the order of size where random drift might be the decisive factor. According to Wright (1931), selection is the over-riding factor when the selection coefficient is of the order of magnitude of $1/(4N_e)$, where N_e is the effective population size. In a population undergoing large fluctuations over several generations where sexes are present in about equal numbers, the effective population size is defined as the harmonic mean of the population numbers over the various generations (Wright, 1939).

If we assume each period is a generation and use the mean number of individuals alive as the population number, then we can calculate effective numbers for the five populations. The mean number alive, the effective number (N_e) and the value $1/(4N_e)$ are given in Table 10 for the five populations. By comparing the value of $1/(4N_e)$ with the selection coefficients (s and t) given in Table 2, we can see that the mean of the male and female selection coefficients are, on the average, at least an order of magnitude above the value $1/(4N_e)$. We may thus conclude that the effect of selection is the dominant force acting to change gene frequency.

There is ample opportunity in all these populations for selection to act. Note that previously we calculated that about 6000 young, or about 80%, die before recruitment into the populations. Along with random deaths, there seems to be sufficient room for selection to act at this point alone. Mortality in the trappable population was typically 30–40% per month in the unfenced area, and even under the excellent survival rates of the fenced grids the loss was still 5–20% per month. Selection also probably acts through reproductive mechanisms which we could not study in live-trapped voles.

Table 11. *Genotypes at a selective advantage during the phases of the cycle in the five populations. Unfenced populations and fenced populations which showed the same type of selection are in boldface.*

		Increase	Peak	Decline
M. ochrogaster				
Grid A				
	Males	$\mathbf{Tf^E/Tf^E}$	$\mathbf{Tf^E/Tf^E}$	$\mathbf{Tf^E/Tf^F}$
	Females	$\mathbf{Tf^E/Tf^E}$	$\mathbf{Tf^E/Tf^E}$	$\mathbf{Tf^E/Tf^F}$
Grid B				
	Males	Tf^E/Tf^F	$\mathbf{Tf^E/Tf^E}$	$\mathbf{Tf^E/Tf^F}$
	Females	$\mathbf{Tf^E/Tf^E}$	$\mathbf{Tf^E/Tf^E}$	$\mathbf{Tf^E/Tf^F}$
Grid D				
	Males	Tf^E/Tf^F	$\mathbf{Tf^E/Tf^E}$	Tf^E/Tf^E
	Females	$\mathbf{Tf^E/Tf^E}$	$\mathbf{Tf^E/Tf^E}$	$\mathbf{Tf^E/Tf^F}$
M. pennsylvanicus				
Grid A				
	Males	$\mathbf{Tf^C/Tf^E}$	$\mathbf{Tf^C/Tf^E}$	$\mathbf{Tf^E/Tf^E}$
	Females	$\mathbf{Tf^C/Tf^E}$	$\mathbf{Tf^C/Tf^E}$	$\mathbf{Tf^E/Tf^E}$
Grid B				
	Males	Tf^E/Tf^E	$\mathbf{Tf^C/Tf^E}$	Tf^C/Tf^E → $\mathbf{Tf^E/Tf^E}$
	Females	$\mathbf{Tf^C/Tf^E}$	$\mathbf{Tf^C/Tf^E}$	Tf^C/Tf^E

Effect of Selection on Population Fluctuations

Given that selective effects are correlated with demographic parameters, we now ask the critical question: what relation does selection at the transferrin locus have to demographic events, or more generally, what role does natural selection play in determining demographic changes in fluctuating vole populations?

To begin with, there is general disagreement on what is the controlling factor in microtine cycles. Several theories have been put forth linking the microtine cycle to food shortage (Pitelka, 1958) and endocrine stress (Christian and Davis, 1964). Most hypotheses do agree, however, that genetic changes play no part in these demographic events. We discuss here one alternative view, the genetic-behavioral hypothesis postulated by Chitty (1960, 1967). Briefly, this theory proposes that during the increase and peak phases, selection occurs for more aggressive animals. These selected types, although they have increased fitness as far as aggressiveness is concerned, have lowered fitness in other components, perhaps through greater susceptibility to common mortality factors. This paves the way for the population decline. We now ask whether changes at the transferrin locus support this idea. In other words, is there a genotype that is selected for during the increase and peak and is then subsequently selected against through the decline?

A transferrin genotype exists that fits this pattern in each species. In the unfenced *M. pennsylvanicus* population, the heterozygote Tf^C/Tf^E is favored during the increase and peak. In the decline, the Tf^E/Tf^E homozygote is most fit. In the unfenced *M. ochrogaster* population, the Tf^E/Tf^E homozygote is most fit in the increase and peak, and the Tf^E/Tf^F heterozygote is most fit in the decline.

The fenced populations show to some extent the same pattern (Table 11). At the present time, the only way we can explain the discrepancies between the fenced and unfenced populations is the change in selection regime brought on by fencing.

Thus we have a pattern of selection at

the transferrin locus where different genotypes in the two species act as "increase" genotypes, being most fit during increase and peak phases and less fit in the decline. A similar pattern was found by Semeonoff and Robertson (1968) in *Microtus agrestis* populations in Scotland, where an esterase genotype, E_1 negative, corresponds to the "increase" genotype.

If Chitty's hypothesis is true, and if selection occurs at the organismal level, we would expect that many loci are involved in the "increase" genotype, and our results and those of Semeonoff and Robertson (1968) support this. If many loci were not involved, the probability of picking a genetic marker which showed correlations with population processes would be very low.

The next step is to study the behavior of these organisms to see if aggressive behavior varies in the predicted manner among these transferrin genotypes. This is being done (Krebs, MS), and the results will be reported elsewhere.

Prediction of Demographic Events

A genetic system intimately involved with demographic processes should provide us with some predictive insight. Two levels of prediction might be considered. First, absolute prediction would allow us to take a genetic profile of a population at any moment in time and from this to determine from what phase of the cycle the sample was drawn and what the course of future events would be. We do not think that this level of prediction can be achieved primarily because of the great variety of environmental factors impinging on these populations. Absolute peak densities vary considerably from place to place and also from time to time on the same area. There is also reason to expect that the gene pool of a species will vary geographically, being integrated with climatic and other environmental variables. Thus a genetic profile may not contain sufficient information to provide absolute predictive powers.

A second level of prediction, relative prediction, should be attainable. This would involve comparative studies on paired populations having many environmental variables in common. For example, we can predict that for two adjacent populations of *M. pennsylvanicus* at low density, the population with the higher Tf^E frequency will have the higher rate of increase. Or conversely for *M. ochrogaster* for two adjacent peak populations, the population with the lower Tf^E frequency should decline less rapidly. Note that we can make these predictions only for these two vole species in southern Indiana at present. We do not necessarily expect that the "increase" genotypes will be the same specific transferrin type throughout the species' range, nor do we expect that the transferrin locus will always be involved in demographic processes in other species of voles and lemmings.

Summary

1) A 26-month study of the population dynamics of two species of microtine rodents, *Microtus ochrogaster* and *M. pennsylvanicus*, in southern Indiana was accompanied by serum sampling to observe genetic changes at the transferrin locus. The results from the analysis of one unfenced and two fenced populations of *M. ochrogaster* and one unfenced and one fenced population of *M. pennsylvanicus* are reported here.

2) Changes in gene frequency and genotype frequency were measured throughout a complete cycle in the unfenced populations and at least one cycle in the fenced populations—which exhibited atypical fluctuations with declines caused by habitat destruction.

3) The transferrin polymorphism was balanced in both species: at a high Tf^E frequency in the *M. ochrogaster* populations and an intermediate Tf^E frequency in the *M. pennsylvanicus* populations. The two species had different alternative alleles to Tf^E. The mechanism of the maintenance of the polymorphism could not be determined. There was no clear heterozygote

excess, and the fitnesses of the different genotypes did not remain constant.

4) Deviations from the Hardy-Weinberg equilibrium were studied with an O/E ratio (observed heterozygotes/expected heterozygotes). By a correlation of this ratio with Tf^E frequency, changes in Tf^E frequency could be related to changes in relative numbers of heterozygotes and homozygotes.

5) Tf^E frequency was correlated with the population parameters of density and survival rate. Density was associated with decreased Tf^E frequency in the unfenced *M. ochrogaster* population. In the unfenced *M. pennsylvanicus* population and one of the fenced populations (Grid B, *M. ochrogaster*), increasing density was associated with decreased Tf^E frequency and decreasing density was associated with increased Tf^E frequency. In the remaining two fenced populations, the relationship of density and Tf^E frequency was complex.

6) Tf^E frequency and survival rate were usually correlated during decline phases. In the unfenced *M. pennsylvanicus* population, the Tf^E allele was favored at times of low survival. In the unfenced *M. ochrogaster* population, and the fenced populations, low survival selected against the Tf^E allele.

7) The individual parameters of weight at first capture, reproduction, survival rate, body weight distribution, and growth rate were compared for the different genotypes. Weight at first capture showed no obvious pattern. The Tf^E/Tf^E homozygote *M. ochrogaster* males were in breeding condition to a greater extent than were the other genotypes. The females showed little in the way of significant differences in reproduction. Usually the Tf^E/Tf^E homozygote had a better survival; however, exceptions occurred. The Tf^E/Tf^E homozygotes dominated the heavy weight class in the *M. ochrogaster* males. In the unfenced *M. pennsylvanicus* males, the Tf^C/Tf^C homozygote dominated the heavy weight group. Differences were found in growth regression on body weight for the males in four of the five populations.

8) With the available knowledge, inbreeding, founder effects and random genetic drift were ruled out as sufficient explanations for the observed changes in gene frequency. Inbreeding was ruled out because no correlation was found between an inbreeding coefficient and density, and also because there was no consistent deficiency of heterozygotes at low numbers. Founding effects were ruled out because of the homogeneity between populations of the same species. Random drift was ruled out because the selection coefficients were an order of magnitude larger than $1/(4N_e)$, where N_e is the effective population size. Selection is apparently the driving force, and an 80% loss of young provides ample room for selection to act before animals reach the trappable population. Once the young are in the trappable population, selection acts on the components of fitness we have measured: survival, reproductive condition, body weight, and growth rate.

9) The genetic changes found in this study (especially in the unfenced populations) were discussed with reference to Chitty's genetic-behavioral hypothesis of population regulation, and our results tend to support this hypothesis. An "increase" genotype exists which is selected for during increase and peak phases and in turn is selected against during the decline. This genotype is Tf^E/Tf^E in *M. ochrogaster* and Tf^C/Tf^E in *M. pennsylvanicus*.

Acknowledgments

We would like to gratefully acknowledge the field assistance of Barry L. Keller and Michael S. Gaines. Robert Tompkins donated technical assistance and equipment in the laboratory, and Dr. Robert Semeonoff aided in the preparation of a selection model. Professor Dennis Chitty critically reviewed the manuscript, and Professors James F. Crow and Yuichiro Hiraizumi gave many helpful comments. Ginger Tamarin gave technical aid in the preparation of this manuscript.

Literature Cited

Ashton, G. C. 1965. Cattle serum transferrin: a balanced polymorphism? Genetics 52:983–997.

Birch, L. C. 1960. The genetic factor in population ecology. Amer. Natur. 94:5–24.

Cain, A. J., and P. M. Sheppard. 1952. The effects of natural selection on body color in the land snail *Cepaea nemoralis*. Heredity 6: 217–231.

Chitty, D. 1952. Mortality among voles (*Microtus agrestis*) at Lake Vyrnwy, Montgomeryshire in 1936–39. Phil. Trans. Roy. Soc. London, Ser. B, 236:505–552.

——. 1960. Population processes in the vole and their relevance to general theory. Canadian J. Zool. 38:99–113.

——. 1967. The natural selection of self-regulatory behaviour in animal populations. Proc. Ecol. Soc. Australia 2:51–78.

Chitty, D., and E. Phipps. 1961. A declining vole population. J. Anim. Ecol. 30:490–491.

Chitty, H., and D. Chitty. 1962. Body weight in relation to population phase in *Microtus agrestis*. Symposium Theriologicum, Brno, p. 77–86.

Christian, J. J., and D. E. Davis. 1964. Endocrines, behavior, and population. Science 146:1550–1560.

Davis, B. J. 1964. Disc electrophoresis—II. Method and application to human serum proteins. N. Y. Acad. Sci., Ann. 121:404–427.

Dixon, W. J., and F. J. Massey, Jr. 1957. Introduction to statistical analysis. Second ed. McGraw-Hill Book Co., N. Y. 488 p.

E-C Bulletin. 1965. Electrophoresis in synthetic gels. E-C Apparatus Corp., 222 S. 40th St., University City, Phila., Pa. 19104.

Falconer, D. S. 1964. Introduction to quantitative genetics. Second reprinting. The Ronald Press Co., N. Y. 365 p.

Fisher, R. A. 1958. The genetical theory of natural selection. Second revised ed. Dover Publications, Inc., N. Y. 291 p.

Fitch, H. S. 1958. Home ranges, territories, and seasonal movements of vertebrates of the natural history reservation. Univ. Kansas Publ. Mus. Nat. Hist. 11:63–326.

Ford, E. B. 1964. Ecological genetics. Methuen, London. 335 p.

Fujino, K., and T. Kang. 1968. Transferrin groups of tuna. Genetics 59:79–91.

Hamilton, W. J., Jr. 1937. Activity and home range of the field mouse, *Microtus pennsylvanicus pennsylvanicus* (Ord). Ecology 18: 255–263.

Harris, H. 1959. Human biochemical genetics. Cambridge Univ. Press, London. 310 p.

Kalela, O. 1957. Regulation of reproduction rate in subarctic populations of the vole *Clethrionomys rufocanus* (Sund.). Ann. Acad. Sci. Fenn., Ser. A, 4:1–60.

Keller, B. L., and C. J. Krebs. MS. *Microtus* population biology. III. Reproductive changes in *M. ochrogaster* and *M. pennsylvanicus* populations in southern Indiana, 1965–68. To be submitted to Ecological Monographs.

Kettlewell, H. B. D. 1961. The phenomenon of industrial melanism in Lepidoptera. Ann. Rev. Ent. 6:245–262.

Koehn, R. K. 1967. Blood proteins in natural populations of catostomid fishes of western North America. Ph.D. Thesis, Arizona State Univ. 153 p.

Kojima, K., and K. M. Yarbrough. 1967. Frequency-dependent selection at the esterase 6 locus in *Drosophila melanogaster*. Proc. Nat. Acad. Sci. U.S. 57:645–649.

Krebs, C. J. 1964*a*. The lemming cycle at Baker Lake, Northwest Territories, during 1959–62. Arctic Inst. North Amer., Tech. Paper No. 15. 104 p.

——. 1964*b*. Cyclic variations in skull-body regressions of lemmings. Canadian J. Zool., 42:631–643.

——. 1966. Demographic changes in fluctuating populations of *Microtus californicus*. Ecol. Monographs 36:239–273.

——. MS. *Microtus* population biology. IV. Behavioral changes associated with the population cycle in *M. ochrogaster* and *M. pennsylvanicus*. In prep.

Krebs, C. J., B. L. Keller, and R. H. Tamarin. MS. *Microtus* population biology. I. Demographic changes in fluctuating populations of *M. pennsylvanicus* and *M. ochrogaster* in southern Indiana, 1965–67. To be submitted to Ecology.

Lerner, I. M. 1965. Synthesis. Genetics Today 2:489–494.

Levene, H. 1949. On a matching problem arising in genetics. Ann. Math. Stat. 20:91–94.

Lewontin, R. C., and L. C. Dunn. 1960. The evolutionary dynamics of a polymorphism in the house mouse. Genetics 45:705–722.

Lewontin, R. C., and J. L. Hubby. 1966. A molecular approach to the study of genic heterozygosity in natural populations. II. Amount of variation and degree of heterozygosity in natural populations of *Drosophila pseudoobscura*. Genetics 54:595–609.

Li, C. C. 1955*a*. The stability of an equilibrium and the average fitness of a population. Amer. Natur. 89:281–295.

——. 1955*b*. Population genetics. Univ. Chicago Press, Chicago. 366 p.

Li, C. C., and D. G. Horvitz. 1953. Some methods of estimating the inbreeding coefficient. Amer. J. Human Genet. 5:107–117.

Lloyd, M., and R. J. Ghelardi. 1964. A table for calculating the 'equitability' component of species diversity. J. Anim. Ecol. 33:217–225.

Lush, I. E. 1967. The biochemical genetics of vertebrates except man. A. Neuberger and

E. L. Tatum [ed.] Frontiers of Biology, Vol. 3. North-Holland Publ. Co., Amsterdam. 118 p.
MAURER, F. W. 1967. Heritability of the plasma transferrin protein in three species of *Microtus*. Nature 215:95–96.
MUELLER, J. O., O. SMITHIES, AND M. R. IRWIN. 1962. Transferrin variation in Columbidae. Genetics 47:1385–1392.
ORNSTEIN, L. 1964. Disc electrophoresis—I. Background and theory. N. Y. Acad. Sci., Ann. 121:321–349.
PETRAS, M. L. 1967. Studies of natural populations of *Mus*. II. Polymorphism at the T locus. Evolution 21:466–478.
PITELKA, F. A. 1958. Some aspects of population structure in the short-term cycle of the brown lemming in northern Alaska. Cold Spring Harbor Symp. Quant. Biol. 22:237–251.
——. 1964. The nutrient-recovery hypothesis for arctic microtine cycles. I. Introduction, p. 55 to 56. *In* D. J. Crisp [ed.] Grazing in terrestrial and marine environments. Brit. Ecol. Soc. Symp. No. 4. Blackwell Sci. Publ., Oxford.
SEMEONOFF, R., AND F. W. ROBERTSON. 1968. A biochemical and ecological study of plasma esterase polymorphism in natural populations of the field vole, *Microtus agrestis* L. Biochem. Genet. 1:205–227.
SHAW, C. R. 1965. Electrophoretic variation in enzymes. Science 149:936–943.
SIEGEL, S. 1956. Non-parametric statistics for the behavioral sciences. McGraw-Hill Book Co., N. Y., 312 p.
TAMARIN, R. H. 1968. Genetic changes at the transferrin locus in fluctuating populations of two vole species (*Microtus ochrogaster* and *M. pennsylvanicus*) in southern Indiana. Ph.D. Thesis, Indiana University. 108 p.
THODAY, J. M. 1963. Correlation between gene frequency and population size. Amer. Natur. 97:409–412.
TOBARI, Y. N., AND K. KOJIMA. 1967. Selective modes associated with inversion karyotypes in *Drosophila ananassae*. I. Frequency-dependent selection. Genetics 57:179–188.
WILBERT, H. 1963. Können Insektenpopulationen durch Selektionsprozesse reguliert werden? Z. ang. Entomologie 52:185–204.
WRIGHT, S. 1931. Evolution in Mendelian populations. Genetics 16:97–159.
——. 1939. Statistical genetics in relation to evolution. Actualités Scientifiques et Industrielles, No. 802. Paris: Hermann et Cie. 63 p.
WRIGHT, S., AND TH. DOBZHANSKY. 1946. Genetics of natural populations. XII. Experimental reproduction of some of the changes caused by natural selection in certain populations of *Drosophila pseudoobscura*. Genetics 31:125–156.

The Physiology of Transferrins

Elevated Serum Iron, Low Unbound Transferrin and Candidiasis in Acute Leukemia

By LEONA CAROLINE, FRED ROSNER AND PHILIP J. KOZINN

TRANSFERRIN OR SIDEROPHILIN is the iron binding protein of human plasma and has the electrophoretic mobility of a beta-l-globulin. Normally only about one third of the transferrin is saturated with iron.[1] In 1946, Schade and Caroline[2] demonstrated the bacteriostatic effect of transferrin. This in vitro antimicrobial power is depressed by free iron and enhanced by an increase in iron-binding capacity.[3] Fresh human serum has also been shown to be fungistatic.[4-6] This inhibition of fungal growth can be overcome by the addition of iron.[7,8] Thus, the fungistatic principle in normal human serum may be transferrin.

Serum from patients with acute leukemia has been shown to have a markedly reduced capacity to inhibit the growth of yeasts such as Candida.[9,10] The present report demonstrates that many patients with acute myeloblastic leukemia have elevated serum iron levels and nearly totally saturated serum iron-binding capacities. Some of these patients had systemic candidiasis, elevated Candida agglutination titers and positive anticandidal precipitin tests. It is postulated that these aberrations in iron metabolism in patients with acute leukemia may be causally related to the development of candida and other fungal infections.[11] In vivo and in vitro studies support this hypothesis.

MATERIALS AND METHODS

A. *Clinical Studies*

Patients with the following diseases were studied: acute myeloblastic leukemia (34 patients): acute lymphoblastic leukemia (6 patients): chronic lymphocytic leukemia (13 patients): chronic myelogenous leukemia (10 patients): polycythemia vera (12 patients): lymphoma (14 patients): multiple myeloma (11 patients). Unequivocal diagnoses were established in each patient on the basis of clinical, peripheral blood, and bone marrow findings and/or tissue sections and other laboratory determinations such as serum and urine protein analyses in patients with multiple myeloma and blood volume determinations in

Supported by grants from the National Institute of Child Health and Human Development HD 02029, the National Cancer Institute CA 05923 and the Jewish Philanthropic League and the Squibb Institute for Medical Research.

patients with polycythemia vera.

Serum iron and iron binding capacity were measured by the method of Schade, Oyama, Reinhart and Miller.[12] Candida agglutination titers were determined by a slight modification of the method of Thjotta, Jansen and Rasch.[13] Precipitin bands against candidal antigen were measured by the immunodiffusion technic.[14]

B. *In Vitro Studies*

Materials: Glassware—All glassware was rendered iron-free by soaking in nitric acid for 18 hours. Sterile demineralized water was used throughout.

Leukemic Sera—Serum from three patients with acute myeloblastic leukemia in whom the transferrin was 96 per cent saturated (one patient) or 100 per cent saturated (2 patients) were employed.

Normal Serum—A single healthy man was used as a source of normal serum. His serum iron was 100 μg. per cent and his iron binding capacity 30 per cent saturated.

High Unbound Iron Binding Capacity Serum—Pooled serum obtained from patients with iron deficiency anemia was used. This serum had an iron level of 80 μg. per cent and an unbound iron binding capacity of 266 μg. per cent (23 per cent saturated).

Glucose—A 1 per cent solution was prepared, sterilized by filtration and the pH verified at neutrality with a glass electrode.

Ascorbic Acid—An aliquot of 12.5 mgm ascorbic acid was dissolved in 5 ml. of iron free water immediately before use. This solution was then diluted with 9 parts of 1 per cent glucose. The addition of .06 ml. of this ascorbate-glucose mixture to 0.5 ml. of serum brought the final concentration of ascorbic acid to 0.0025 mgm per cent and that of glucose to 100 mgm per cent.

Human Transferrin—Iron-free, undenatured, purified human transferrin (Behringwerke, Germany) was obtained through the courtesy of Dr. A. L. Schade of the National Institute of Allergy and Infectious Diseases, Bethesda, Maryland. Ten milligrams of this substance was dissolved in 1 ml. of iron-free water. Thus 0.1 ml. of solution contained 1 mgm transferrin.

Iron Standard—A stock solution containing 702 mg. of $(NH_4)_2 Fe (SO_4)_2 .6 H_2O$ dissolved in 100 ml. of 0.06 N HCl was made and 15 mgm of ascorbic acid added. This solution containing 1 mg. iron per ml. was stored at 4 C. A fresh 1:20 dilution was made immediately before use and this final working solution thus contained 50 μg. iron per ml.

Candida Albicans Inoculum—An 18 hour culture of *C. albicans* Tyson grown at 37 C. on 4 per cent glucose, 1 per cent neopeptone agar (Difco) was used. This organism is a laboratory strain originally isolated from a patient with a positive blood culture and conforms to the cultural identification criteria of *Candida albicans.* A 10^6 suspension of the organism was made in sterile, demineralized water and a chamber count was performed on an aliquot. The organism suspension was diluted to contain 5000 viable *C. albicans* per ml. or 150 units in 0.03 ml.

Method of Procedure

All sera were collected aseptically using iron-free glassware. The sera were stored at 20 C. until used. The various components of the test system were added to 13 × 100 mm. sterile pyrex test tubes according to the schema outlined in Table 1. All tests were performed in duplicate. Test tubes 1 and 2 were aimed at examining the growth of *Candida albicans* in serum from normal and leukemic patients respectively in the presence of glucose and ascorbic acid. Tube 3 tested the effect of exogenously added iron sufficient to saturate fully the endogenous transferrin in normal serum to determine whether the known fungistatic effect of normal serum could be overcome. Tube 4 combined leukemic serum (100 per cent saturation of transferrin) with a serum containing high unbound iron binding capacity to determine whether the expected growth of yeast in the leukemic serum could be overcome by the addition of unsaturated transferrin. Tube 5 was identical to tube 4 except exogenous iron was added to saturate fully the previously added high unbound iron binding capacity serum. Tube 6 determined the ability of exogenous purified human trans-

Table 1.—Experimental Schema for in vitro Studies. Each + represents the presence of the material indicated in the left hand column. Blank spaces indicate absence of these substances.

CONTENTS of TUBES	TEST TUBE NUMBERS						
	1	2	3	4	5	6	7
Normal Serum (30% Saturation of transferrin)	+		+				
Leukemic Serum (100% Saturation of Transferrin)		+		+	+	+	+
High U.I.B.C.* Serum (23% Saturation of Transferrin)				+	+		
Human Transferrin (1 mg)						+	+
Iron Standard (2.5 μgm)			+		+		+
Ascorbic Acid (.0025 mg% final concentration)	+	+	+	+	+	+	+
Glucose (100 mgm % final concentration)	+	+	+	+	+	+	+
Candida Albicans Inoculum (150 organisms)	+	+	+	+	+	+	+

* U.I.B.C. Unbound Iron Binding Capacity

All tubes are subjected to a stream of CO_2 in air for 1 minute and then incubated at 20°c. for 48 hours.

ferrin to reverse candidal growth in leukemic serum. Tube 7 was identical to tube 6 except iron was added to neutralize the effect of the added purified human transferrin. All tubes contained equal volumes of total contents at pH 7.3.

After the additions were made according to the schema outlined in Table 1, all the tubes were shaken by hand and equilibrated with a stream of 5 per cent CO_2 in air for one minute. Tubes were closed with sterile rubber stoppers and incubated at 20 C. for 48 hours. Wet mount examinations and viable plate counts were made at 24 and 48 hours as described below.

Viable Plate Counts—There was little filamentation or germ tube formation by the *Candida albicans* under all the conditions described. In some cases, small clumps of yeast cells were noted. In other tubes, large aggregates appeared, as if the yeast cells were not released following budding. A semi-quantitative estimation of the total yeast growth was made, using a uniform method of dilution and plating.

Serial dilutions were made in sterile demineralized water to yield approximately 100 colonies per plate. Aliquots of final dilution were measured into sterile petri dishes. Melted

Table 2.—Increased Serum Iron Levels and Complete Saturation of the Iron Binding Capacity in Patients with Leukemia, Polycythemia Vera, Lymphoma and Multiple Myeloma.

Disease	No. of Patients	No. with High Serum Iron (>120 μg%)	No. with Fully Saturated Transferrin
Acute Myeloblastic Leukemia	34	21**	17**
Acute Lymphoblastic Leukemia	6	2*	2*
Chronic Myelocytic Leukemia	10	2	2
Chronic Lymphocytic Leukemia	13	0	0
Polycythemia Vera	12	0	0
Lymphoma	14	2	2
Multiple Myeloma	11	0	0

* 1 Patient had Systemic Candidiasis

** 2 Patients had Systemic Candidiasis

4 per cent glucose, 1 per cent neopeptone agar at 46 C. was added and the plate contents mixed well. Plates were allowed to harden, inverted and then incubated at 37 C. for 48 hours. The colonies were counted and appropriate calculations were made.

Results of Clinical Studies (Table 2)

A. Acute Leukemia

Twenty-one (64 per cent) of the thirty-four patients with acute myeloblastic leukemia in relapse had elevated serum iron levels (greater than 120 μg. per cent; normal range in this laboratory is 70–120). In seventeen of these twenty-one patients, the iron binding globulin was fully saturated (UIBC equals 0) on at least one occasion and usually repeatedly on several determinations. In an additional ten patients, the per cent saturation of transferrin was greater than 50 per cent. Normally, transferrin is only one third saturated (normal range of TIBC in this laboratory is 270–330 μg. per cent). Seven patients in the total group of acute myeloblastic leukemia patients had significant *Candida* agglutination titers (1:320 or greater) and two of these patients had proved systemic candidiasis including positive blood cultures. Both latter patients also had positive precipitin bands against candidal antigen and both were successfully treated with amphotericin B.

Two of six patients with acute lymphoblastic leukemia had elevated serum iron levels (226 μg. per cent and 149 μg. per cent) and very low or absent unbound transferrin (4 μg. per cent and 0 μg. per cent). One of these patients had systemic candidiasis proved at autopsy. In the other patient, both serum iron and unbound transferrin reverted to normal when clinical and hematologic remission was achieved. A third patient had normal serum iron and unsaturated transferrin values but developed systemic candidiasis with positive agglutination titers, precipitin tests and *Candida* cultures from throat, stool and urine.

B. Chronic Leukemia

In two of ten patients with chronic myelogenous leukemia, there were elevated serum iron levels (184 μg. per cent and 144 μg. per cent) and near or complete saturation of transferrin (96 per cent and 100 per cent respectively). Neither patient had clinical or laboratory evidence of candidiasis.

In none of the thirteen patients with chronic lymphocytic leukemia was the serum iron increased or the unbound transferrin level decreased. None of these patients had signs of candidal infection.

C. Other Disorders

None of the patients with multiple myeloma or polycythemia vera had abnormalities in serum iron or iron binding capacity. Among the fourteen patients with lymphoma, one patient with reticulum cell sarcoma and another with lymphosarcoma had increased serum iron levels (214 μg. per cent and 125 μg. per cent) and low or absent unbound transferrin values (30 μg. per cent and 0 μg. per cent respectively). Neither patient had clinical or laboratory evidence of candidal infection.

Results of In Vitro Studies

Three separate but identical sets of experiments were conducted as decribed above, using sera from three patients with acute myeloblastic leukemia during relapse. In two of the patients, transferrin was completely saturated and in the third it was 96 per cent saturated. Similar results were obtained in all three instances (Table 3). Mean values for the three sets of experiments are graphically represented and summarized in Figure 1.

Growth of *Candida albicans* in the leukemic sera was approximately 1000 times greater than in normal serum. This marked enhancement of growth occurred when only 150 units of *Candida albicans* were inoculated into each serum and incubated at 20 C. for 48 hours. Addition of iron sufficient to saturate fully the transferrin in normal serum permitted growth of *Candida albicans* comparable to that in serum of the leukemic patients. (Table 3 and

Table 3.—Growth of Candida Albicans in Serum from Normal and Leukemic Subjects.

	Test Mixtures	Patient's % Saturation of Transferrin: A 100%	B 100%	C 96%
		Viable Units of Candida Albicans per ml after 48 hours incubation at 20 C.		
1)	Normal Serum (30% saturation of transferrin)	36,500	16,900	17,675
2)	Leukemic Serum (96% or 100% saturation of transferrin)	36,662,500	35,600,000	4,563,000
3)	Normal Serum Plus Iron to fully saturate the U.I.B.C.*	28,562,500	26,200,000	34,125,000
4)	Leukemic Serum Plus high U.I.B.C.* Serum	37,500	40,400	3,000
5)	Leukemic Serum Plus high U.I.B.C.* serum plus iron to fully saturate the U.I.B.C.*	25,050,000	66,600,000	9,450,000
6)	Leukemic Serum plus Purified Human Transferrin	49,500	21,750	12,000
7)	Leukemic Serum Plus Purified Human Transferrin Plus Iron to Fully saturate the transferrin	31,637,500	78,500,000	16,500,000

* U.I.B.C. = unbound iron binding capacity

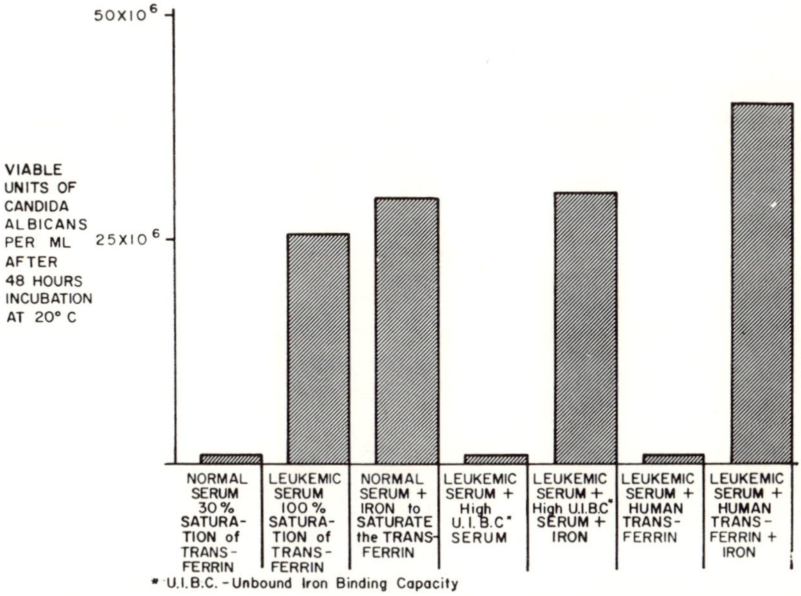

Fig. 1.—Growth of Candida Albicans in serum from normal and leukemic subjects. Mean values of three sets of experiments using sera from three leukemic patients.

Fig. 1). When, however, fully transferrin saturated serum from leukemic patients was combined with a highly transferrin unsaturated serum (obtained from a patient with iron deficiency anemia), candidal growth was inhibited. If to this mixture of serum from leukemic patients and highly transferrin unsaturated serum, sufficient iron was added to fully saturate the unbound iron binding capacity, the protection against candidal growth afforded by the unbound binding capacity was neutralized.

Adding an exogenous source of purified human transferrin to fully transferrin saturated serum from leukemic patients inhibited growth of *Candida albicans.* This inhibition of growth was overcome by the addition of sufficient iron to saturate fully the added transferrin. Leukemic serum whose iron saturation was within normal limits failed to support fungus growth.

Discussion

In 1944 Schade and Caroline[15] described a protein component in raw egg white that was capable of binding iron and inhibiting growth of *Shigella dysenteriae* and other microorganisms. This inhibition of growth could be overcome only by the addition of iron but not by ten vitamins or 30 other elements tested. Two years later, Schade and Caroline[2] demonstrated a bacteriostatic iron binding protein in human plasma and called it siderophilin (now called transferrin or iron-binding globulin). Other antimicrobial substances in human serum have also been described and these include gram negative bactericidins, beta lysins and properdin.[16]

Fresh human serum has also been shown to contain a potent factor which inhibits the growth of certain fungi.[4,5] Serum from normal adults possesses a high capacity to inhibit growth of *Candida albicans*,[6] an effect which can be overcome by the addition of iron.[7,8] This inhibitory activity is greatly diminished in umbilical cord blood and infant blood up to 10 weeks of age.[7] The low resistance of the newborn to candidiasis may be due to the fact that the iron binding capacity of cord blood and newborn blood is nearly fully saturated with iron.[7]

One can postulate a similar mechanism to explain the increased susceptibility of patients with acute leukemia to fungus infections. The high serum iron and/or nearly complete or full saturation of transferrin in the serum of such patients may foster candidal growth. Ionic iron is important in determining whether infectious agents can multiply in mammalian host tissues.[3] Yeasts such as *Candida albicans* can grow in the presence of normal serum or plasma only when sufficient iron is available to saturate fully the transferrin.[7,8] Jackson and Morris[17] have shown that the virulence of *Pasteurella* and other bacteria is enhanced by the addition of iron. Martin, Jandl and Finland[18] demonstrated the enhancement of virulence of *Klebsiella pneumoniae* and *Pseudomonas aeruginosa* in rats and mice when iron salts were administered. Small doses of iron-free human transferrin afforded some degree of protection against acute infections with these organisms. Iron is also essential for the growth of *Clostridium welchii,*[19,20] *Listeria monocytogenes,*[21] *staphylococcus* and *salmonella.*[3] Cations such as magnesium, calcium, cobalt, nickel, copper, zinc and others cannot substitute for iron.[15,17]

Roth and Goldstein[9] have shown that the serum of normal adults possesses marked capacity to inhibit the in vitro reproduction of *Candida albicans* and other species of *Candida*. In patients with acute leukemia, they found the activity or concentration of the inhibitory complex to be greatly diminished. These investigators did not, however, measure serum iron or iron binding capacity in their patients. In a study of eight patients with Hodgkins disease, Cline and Berlin[22] found an increased serum iron concentration in one patient on one occasion and a low value in the same patient on another occasion. The iron binding capacity was fully saturated in another of these patients on one of three occasions. Neither patient is reported to have developed candidal infection.

The hypothesis that the increased frequency of systemic fungal infections, particularly candidiasis, in patients with acute leukemia is causally related to the high iron and/or near complete or full saturation of transferrin in the serum of such patients is supported by clinical observations and in vitro experiments. Twenty-one of thirty-four patients with acute myeloblastic leukemia (64 per cent) and two of six patients with acute lymphoblastic leukemia had elevated serum iron levels and very low or absent unsaturated transferrin levels. Whether the iron binding globulin itself protects an individual by directly inhibiting fungal growth or whether the excess iron in the plasma enhances candidal growth has not yet been determined. These two factors are difficult to study separately because of the high avidity for iron of the unsaturated iron binding capacity of human serum. In this manner, inhibition of multiplication of fungi and bacteria is achieved by depriving these microorganisms of biologically available iron essential for their reproduction.

Leukocytes contain appreciable amounts of iron[23] and the state and physiologic function of this iron has not yet been determined. Leukocytes destroyed by the invading organisms, or leukemic cells destroyed by chemotherapeutic agents may release iron that is biologically available to microorganisms for multiplication. Another possible source of iron in the patient is blood transfusion from which hemolysed erythrocytes release iron into the circulation. However, in the studies here reported several patients had high serum iron levels and low or absent unbound iron binding capacities before any blood had been administered. The possibility that the patient was destroying his own red cells at an accelerated rate with release of excess iron into the blood was not investigated.

Other possible mechanisms may explain the increased incidence of fungus infections in patients with acute leukemia.[11] One proposed explanation is that such patients are usually receiving one or more antibiotics, possibly predisposing them to the development of superinfections. Antibiotics may increase the hazard of candidiasis by changing the intestinal flora, thereby permitting overgrowth of *Candida* in the absence of competing organisms.[24] Other mechanisms may include local tissue damage and increased invasiveness of the *Candida*.[24] In addition, antibiotics inhibit anticandidal antibody synthesis and phagocytic activity,[25] thus reducing host resistance to invasion by *Candida*.

The role of corticosteroids and antileukemic drugs in the sharp increase in mycotic infections in leukemic patients in the last two decades, cannot be minimized.[26,27] Host resistance in leukemic patients with already poor immunologic defenses may be further depressed by corticosteroids and antileukemic drugs. However, in seven of the patients with acute myeloblastic leukemia here reported who had fully saturated iron binding capacities, no specific antileukemic chemotherapy had yet been administered at the time they were studied. Furthermore, preliminary studies in patients with Cooley's anemia who are not receiving such chemotherapeutic agents, reveals enhanced candidal growth in their serum when compared to normal individuals. Patients with Cooley's anemia have low or absent unsaturated transferrin and elevated iron levels in the serum.[28]

Immunologic competence in patients with acute leukemia is not totally lacking in that host defenses against fungi may remain intact. A specific host antibody response to *Candida albicans* is the production of precipitating antibodies specific for a somatic antigen[14] of this fungus in the serum of the patients who develop systemic candidiasis. The specific component in the serum of such patients that reacts with the somatic antigen of *Candida* is presently being studied. Immunoelectrophoretic investigations seem to indicate that this material is distinct from the defined human immunoglobulins.

Further questions remain to be answered. Do patients with iron deficiency anemia who have high levels of unsaturated iron binding capacity develop fewer fungal infections than normal individuals? Would the intravenous administration of purified human transferrin protect patients with acute leukemia against fungal infections? Why do children with Cooley's anemia who have fully saturated transferrin in their plasma not develop systemic candidiasis as do patients with acute leukemia? What is the significance of the reduced levels of iron binding capacity present in patients with acute and chronic bacterial infections? Are these two findings causally related? Do patients with hemochromatosis or other forms of iron overload develop more infections than normal people? What effect, if any, does antifungal chemotherapy (i.e. amphotericin B) have on plasma transferrin levels and per cent saturation?

ACKNOWLEDGMENTS

The authors are indebted to Dr. Arthur L. Schade for helpful advice and encouragement and to Mrs. Claire L. Taschdjian and Mr. Manuel Cuesta for performing the Candida agglutination and precipitin tests. Thanks are due to Mrs. Kay D. Orr for technical assistance and to Miss Gail Wollan for typing the manuscript.

REFERENCES

1. Wintrobe, M. M.: Clinical Hematology (ed. 6). Philadelphia, Lea & Febiger, 1967, p. 133.

2. Schade, A. L. and Caroline, L.: An iron-binding component in human blood plasma. Science 104:340–341, 1946.

3. Weinberg, E. D.: Metallic ions in host-parasite interactions. Bact. Rev. 30:136–144, 1966.

4. Lorincz, A. L., Priestly, J. O., and Jacob, P. H.: Evidence for a humoral mechanism which prevents growth of dermatophytes. J. Invest. Derm. 31:15, 1958.

5. Blank, H., Sagami, S., Boyd, C., and Roth, F. J., Jr.: The pathogenesis of superficial fungous infections in cultured human skin. Arch. Derm. 70:524, 1959.

6. Roth, F. J., Jr., Boyd, C., Sagami, S., and Blank, H.: An evaluation of the fungistatic activity of serum. J. Invest. Derm. 32:549–556, 1959.

7. Caroline, L., Taschdjian, C. L., Kozinn, P. J., and Schade, A. L.: Reversal of serum fungistasis by addition of iron. J. Invest. Derm. 42:415–419, 1964.

8. Esterly, N. B., Brammer, S. R., and Crounse, R. G.: The relationship of transferrin and iron to serum inhibition of *Candida albicans*. J. Invest. Derm. 49:437–442, 1967.

9. Roth, F. J., Jr., and Goldstein, M. I.: Inhibition of growth of pathogenic yeasts by human serum. J. Invest. Derm. 36:383–387, 1961.

10. Esterly, N. B., Brammer, S. R., and Crounse, R. G.: In vitro inhibition of candidal growth by human serum. J. Invest. Derm. 49:246–250, 1967.

11. Schumacher, H. H., Ginns, D. A., and Warren, W. J.: Fungus infection complicating leukemia. Amer. J. Med. Sci. 247:313, 1964.

12. Schade, A. L., Oyama, J., Reinhart, R. W., and Miller, J. R.: Bound iron and unsaturated iron-binding capacity of serum; Rapid and reliable determination. Proc. Soc. Exp. Biol. 87:443, 1954.

13. Thjotta, Y., Jansen, J., and Rasch, S.: Studies on agglutination of fungi. I. Techniques for quantitative determinations. Acta Path. Microbiol. Scand. 33:72, 1953.

14. Taschdjian, C. L., Kozinn, P. J., and Caroline, L.: Immune studies in candidiasis. III. Precipitating antibodies in systemic candidiasis. Sabouraudia 3:312–320, 1964.

15. Schade, A. L., and Caroline, L.: Raw hen egg white and the role of iron in growth inhibition of *Shigella Dysenteriae, Staphylococcus Aureus, Escherichia Coli* and *Saccharomyces cerevisiae*. Science 100: 14–15, 1944.

16. Muschel, A. L.: Serum bactericidal actions. Ann. N. Y. Acad. Sci. 88:1265–1272, 1960.

17. Jackson, S., and Morris, B. C.: Enhancement of growth of *Pasteurella pestis* and other bacteria in serum by the addition of iron. Brit. J. Exp. Path. 42:363–368, 1961.

18. Martin, C. M., Jandl, J. H., and Finland, M.: Enchancement of acute bacterial infections in rats and mice by iron and their inhibition by human transferrin. J. Infect. Dis. 112:158–164, 1963.

19. Rogers, H. J.: Bacteriostatic effects of horse sera and serum fractions on *Clostridium Welchii* type A and the abolition of bacteriostasis by iron salts. Immunology 12: 285–301, 1967.

20. Bullen, J. J., Cushire, G. H., and

Rogers, H. J.: The abolition of the protective effect of *Clostridium Welchii* type A antiserum by ferric iron. Immunology 12: 303–311, 1967.

21. Sword, C. P.: Mechanisms of pathogenesis in *Listeria monocytogenes* infection. I. Influence of Iron. J. Bact. 92:536–542, 1966.

22. Cline, M. J., and Berlin, N. I.: Anemia in Hodgkin's Disease. Cancer 16:526–532, 1963.

23. Laurell, C. B.: Plasma iron and transport of iron in organisms. Pharmacol. Rev. 4:371, 1952.

24. Seelig, M. S.: Mechanisms by which antibiotics increase the incidence and severity of candidiasis and alter the immunological defenses. Bact. Rev. 30:442–457, 1966.

25. Seelig, M. S.: The role of antibiotics in the pathogenesis of candida infections. Amer. J. Med. 40:887–917, 1966.

26. Craig, J. M., and Farber, S.: The development of disseminated visceral mycosis during therapy for acute leukemia. Amer. J. Path. 29:601, 1953.

27. Grubin, J. G., and Samson, J.: Mycotic infections in leukemic patients at autopsy. Cancer 16:61, 1963.

28. Smith, C. H.: Blood Diseases of Infancy and Childhood. St. Louis, C. V. Mosby Co., 1960.

Placental Transfer of Iron in the Rabbit

T. A. Douglas, J. P. Renton and C. Watts

Placental transfer of iron in the rabbit is an active process whereby iron from the maternal circulation is taken up by the placental cells and transferred quickly to the transferrin of the foetal circulation. In this form it is carried to its various depots within the foetus, e.g. foetal marrow and liver (Davies, 1961). It is now known that the transfer of iron from mother to foetal rabbit increases dramatically as gestation advances (Bothwell *et al*, 1958). At the same time as this increase is occurring, alteration in the subcellular architecture of the placenta has also been demonstrated (Enders, 1965).

Although much work has been done on absorption and transport of iron across the intestinal cells, as yet there is no comparable work involving this aspect of placental cells. In order to investigate the mechanism of placental transfer of iron, a study of the uptake of iron by the various subcellular fractions of the placental cells was undertaken.

Since the transfer of iron across the placenta is extremely rapid (Bothwell *et al*, 1958), optimum conditions for the identification of the various forms of iron present within the placental cells must be obtained. Accordingly, preliminary studies of plasma clearance and uptake of iron by the placenta at different stages of gestation were carried out.

MATERIALS AND METHODS

Placental Uptake at Various Stages of Gestation

Pregnant rabbits of known breeding history were injected intravenously with 5 μCi of ^{59}Fe ferric citrate. Two hours later the rabbits were killed by an intracardial injection of pentobarbitone sodium. The total number of foetuses present in each rabbit was noted. All the foetuses and attached placentae were removed without delay. Each placenta was carefully separated from its associated foetus and the surrounding membranes washed in ice-cold 0.15 M saline, blotted dry with filter paper and weighed. The placenta was then finely chopped with scissors, added to 10 ml of 0.25 M sucrose and the mixture homogenized in an ice-cold Potter type perspex-glass homogenizer (Hogeboom *et al*, 1948; Hogeboom & Schneider, 1950). The total ^{59}Fe activity of each of the homogenates was measured, and the results expressed as a percentage of the ^{59}Fe activity injected into the rabbit.

Perfusion of the Rabbit Placenta

The pregnant rabbits were anaesthetized with intravenous nembutal and then intubated. Anaesthesia was continued with halothane; 30000 IU heparin were injected intravenously and the abdomen opened. The pregnant uterus was carefully exteriorized and placed on warm moist sterile swabs. The intestines were drawn to one side and the aorta and the vena cava exposed on the floor of the abdomen. These vessels are very closely allied to one another, the aorta lying underneath and to the left of the vena cava. It was found that it was better to canulate the aorta first since the inflowing saline prevented the thin-walled vena cava from collapsing on sectioning. Pieces of soft twine were passed underneath each vessel. An assistant gently raised the aorta from the abdominal floor by means of the lower piece of twine and the pressure applied in doing this was sufficient to stop the flow of blood from the vessels when it was incised. The aorta was cut with a sharp-pointed pair of scissors and a nylon catheter passed along its length for approximately 2 cm. The canula was now connected to a bottle of ice-cold saline suspended above the operating table and the saline was allowed to flow in freely under gravity. The vena cava was now canulated with a sharp-pointed glass canula. When in position, this was secured by the lower piece of twine and the upper circulation again tied off. The outflowing blood from the vena cava was collected. As soon as the saline was flowing freely into the aorta, the rabbit was sacrificed by intracardiac pentobarbitone sodium.

Plasma Clearance Rates

Plasma clearance rates were studied in both pregnant and non-pregnant rabbits. The pregnant rabbits were all in the last third of gestation. Each rabbit was injected intravenously with either 5 μCi or 30 μCi of ^{59}Fe. Blood samples were withdrawn from an ear vein at approximately 15-min intervals. The first sample was withdrawn 5 min after administration of the ^{59}Fe. The radioactivity of each of the blood samples was measured in a solid scintillation counter. The PCV of each of the samples was also measured. From the two results the ^{59}Fe activity of equal amounts of plasma at the different sampling times was calculated. Since different amounts of ^{59}Fe were injected into the different rabbits studied, the first sample was arbitrarily taken to represent 100% activity and the subsequent samples expressed as a percentage of this activity. In the rabbit in which plasma clearance of ^{59}Fe was studied before conception and at 27 and 30 days of gestation measurements of the ^{59}Fe activity were made on plasma.

Subcellular Fractionation of the Rabbit Placenta

Rabbit placentae were fractionated by the method of Hogeboom *et al* (1948) with modifications by Hogeboom & Schneider (1950), and electron micrographs were prepared of the different subcellular components (Fig 1).

Pregnant rabbits during the last third of gestation were injected intravenously with 5 μCi of ^{59}Fe as ferric citrate in a solution of 1% sodium citrate. Two hours later, the rabbits were killed and all the placentae removed. Each placenta on removal was homogenized in 10 ml 0.25 M sucrose as above and separated into nuclear, mitochondrial, microsomal and non-particulate fractions by centrifugation as shown on the flow sheet. The radioactivity of each of the fractions and of the homogenate was measured in a scintillation counter and the ^{59}Fe activity of each fraction expressed as a percentage of the initial homogenate.

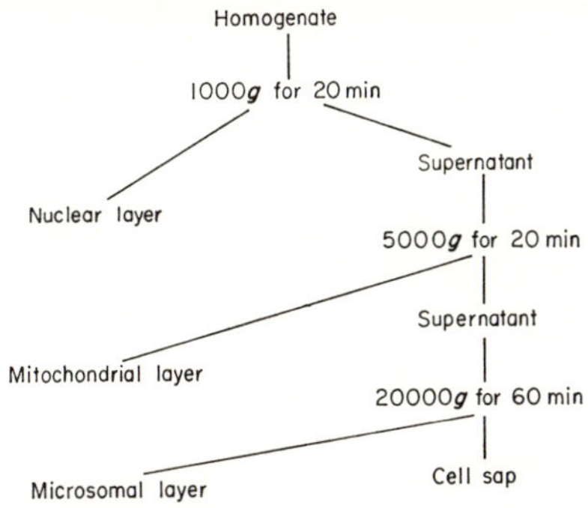

FIG 1. Separation of subcellular fractions of rabbit placenta by differential centrifugation.

Isolation and Identification of Iron-containing Compounds in Placental Cell Sap

The molecular size of the ^{59}Fe-containing compounds was assessed by passing the placental cell sap through columns of G25, G75 and G200 Sephadex prepared as described by Porath & Flodin (1959) and Porath (1959). Further identification of the iron-containing compounds was carried out by starch gel electrophoresis of the cell sap. The method used was that described by Smithies (1955) using the discontinuous system of Poulik (1957) with minor modifications by Ashton (1957). Protein bands were detected by staining with Amido black. Ferritin was stained by treating the gel with a mixture of 2 N-HCl and potassium ferrocyanide. For radioactive measurements, the gel was cut into 0.5 cm strips, digested in nitric acid and counted in a well-type scintillation counter.

Ferritin was prepared by the method of Granick (1943) from livers and spleen of rabbits whose ferritin production had been stimulated by the administration of Imferon (Benger's Laboratories Ltd, England).

RESULTS

Uptake of ^{59}Fe by the Placenta at Different Stages of Gestation

At first sight, it would appear that there is no direct correlation between the stage of gestation and ^{59}Fe uptake by total placental homogenate (Table I). However, when comparisons are made between rabbits carrying the same number of foetuses at different stages of gestation, it is obvious that there is an increase in the ^{59}Fe uptake by the rabbit placenta as gestation advances.

Perfusion of the Rabbit Placenta

It was decided to perfuse the uterus and its contents for no longer than 5 min in order to minimize cellular damage. The results obtained using the described technique resulted in an obvious blanching of the placentae and uterus. However, since foetal blood is not removed by the perfusion technique, a pinkish hue of the uterine contents is still apparent and is due in part to the presence of foetal blood. Comparison, however, of the ^{59}Fe content of the placental homogenate with and without perfusion is shown in Table II. These results indicate a marked reduction in the ^{59}Fe content of the perfused placenta.

TABLE I. Uptake of ^{59}Fe by total rabbit placental tissue at various stages of gestation

Days of gestation	*No. of foetuses*	*Total placental ^{59}Fe-uptake**
11	8	0.13
14	2	0.69
15	5	0.47
16	5	0.73
21	8	3.60
23	5	4.00
23	7	3.30
25	10	6.60
25	6	2.70
27	8	8.10

* The placental activity is expressed as % initial activity injected and is uncorrected for activity due to maternal blood.

TABLE II. Activity of ^{59}Fe in rabbit placentae with and without perfusion

	Perfused	*Unperfused*
	0.55	1.1
	0.4	1.1
	0.35	0.8
	Taken for histology	1.0
	—	1.0
Total	1.3	5.0
Mean	0.4	1.0

Each of the rabbits was 22 days pregnant and all the placentae were removed 2 hr after administration of the radioactive iron.

Placental activity is expressed as % initial amount of ^{59}Fe injected.

Plasma Clearance Rates

Fig 2 shows the mean results of plasma clearance carried out on four non-pregnant, four 27-days' and four 30-days' pregnant rabbits. It will be seen that the plasma clearance rate of ^{59}Fe is faster in the pregnant rabbit compared with the non-pregnant. Moreover the plasma clearance rate increases with gestation. It would seem, therefore, that if at least 30 min were allowed to elapse after administering the radio-iron and before removing the placentae, then the circulating plasma-^{59}Fe of the dam would be markedly reduced.

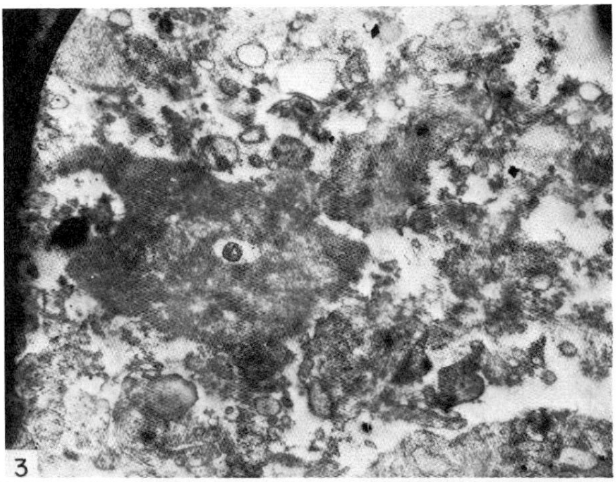

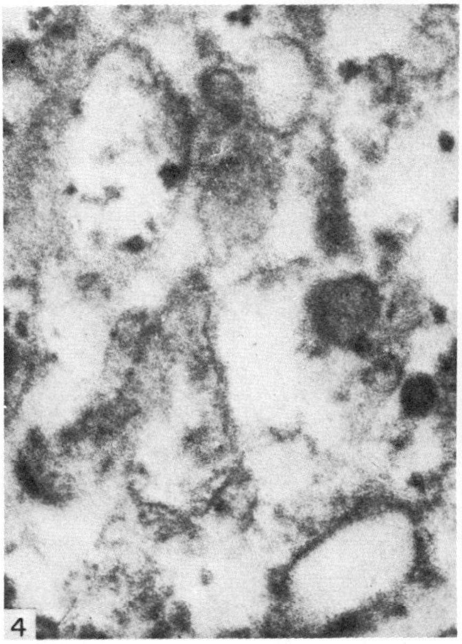

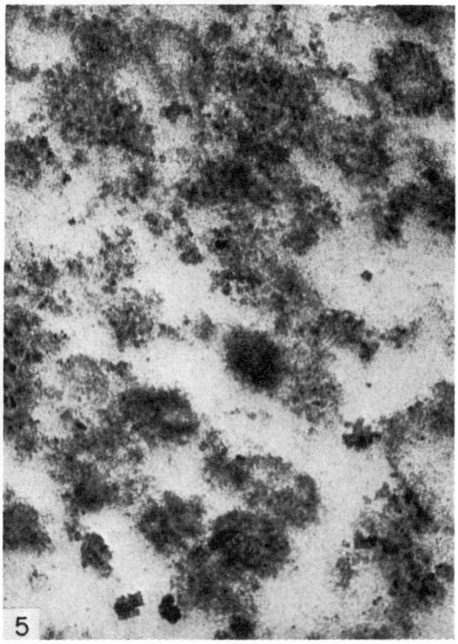

Fig 3. Electron micrograph of nuclear pellet.
Fig 4. Electron micrograph of mitochondrial pellet.
Fig 5. Electron micrograph of microsomal pellet.

Uptake of ^{59}Fe by the Subcellular Fractions of the Rabbit Placenta

The electron micrographs (Figs 3, 4 and 5) demonstrate that the placental tissue was successfully separated into a pellet containing the nuclei of the cells and cell debris (Fig 3), a mitochondrial fraction (Fig 4), and a fraction containing the endoplasmic reticulum of the cell broken down into microsomes (Fig 5), leaving a final supernatant or cell sap.

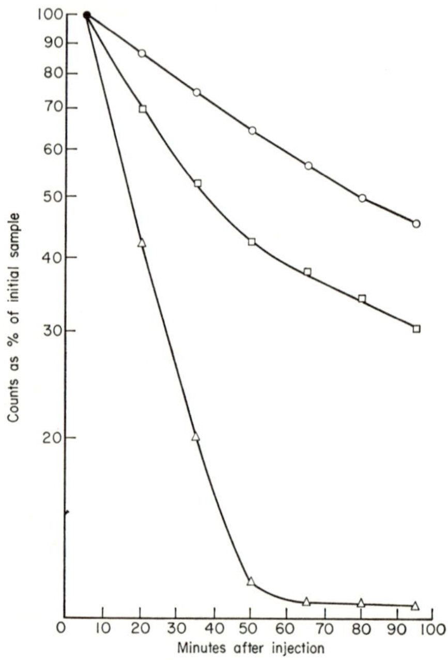

FIG 2. Plasma clearance of ^{59}Fe in rabbits: ○, non-pregnant; □, 27 days pregnant; △, 30 days pregnant.

TABLE III. ^{59}Fe activity in subcellular fractions of rabbit placentae (counts per 100 s) as % total activity

	Nuclear	Mitochondrial	Microsomal	Cell sap	% Recovered
	29	3.8	3.6	51	87
	26	5.3	7.4	55	94
	29	4.3	1.5	57	92
	33	6.6	4.7	49	93
	26	4.6	4.4	60	95
Mean	28.6	4.9	4.3	54.4	92.2
SE ±	1.3	0.5	0.9	2.0	1.4

The above results are on five placentae from a rabbit 22 days pregnant. The placentae were removed 120 min after the injection of ^{59}Fe.

A typical example of the distribution of the ^{59}Fe in the different fractions of the cell is shown in Table III. In most instances the highest concentration of ^{59}Fe is found in the non-particulate part of the cell. On the two occasions when this is not so, the nuclear layer contains the greatest proportions. This layer contains the nuclei of the cells and some unbroken cells. The number of unbroken cells depends on the efficiency of the homogenizing technique. These results, therefore, might be accounted for by insufficient homogenizing.

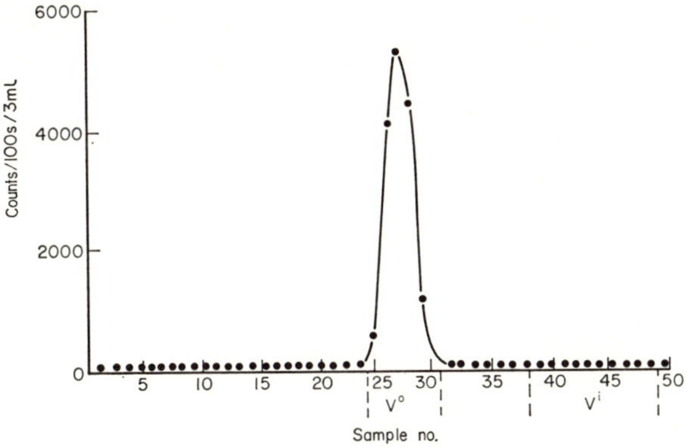

FIG 6. Elution diagram of ^{59}Fe-containing compounds of placental cell sap applied to Sephadex G25. Sample volume, 3 ml; V°, void volume; V^i, inner volume.

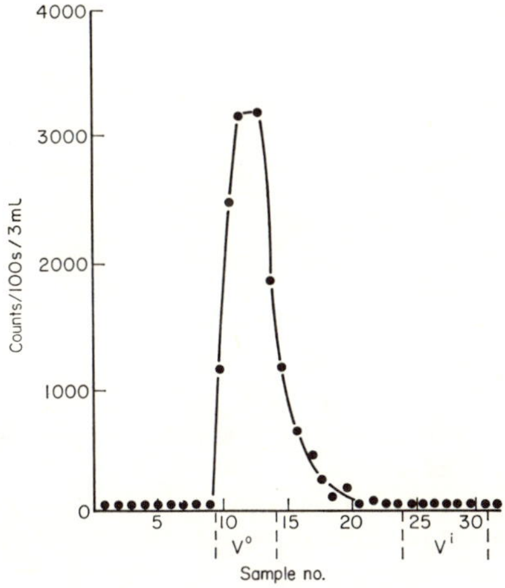

FIG 7. Elution diagram of ^{59}Fe-containing compounds of placental cell sap applied to Sephadex G75. Sample volume, 3 ml; V°, void volume; V^i, inner volume.

Characterization of ^{59}Fe Compounds in the Cell Sap

Aliquots of cell sap, prepared from placentae of rabbits injected intravenously with ^{59}Fe 2 hr prior to killing, were fractionated on columns of G25, G75 and G200 Sephadex. The radioactivity in 3-ml fractions of eluate from each of these columns was measured in the scintillation counter. A single peak of radioactivity was obtained from the G25 column which occurred in the void volume, as is shown in Fig 6. This would suggest that these iron-containing compounds have a molecular weight greater than 5000. When the same cell sap was

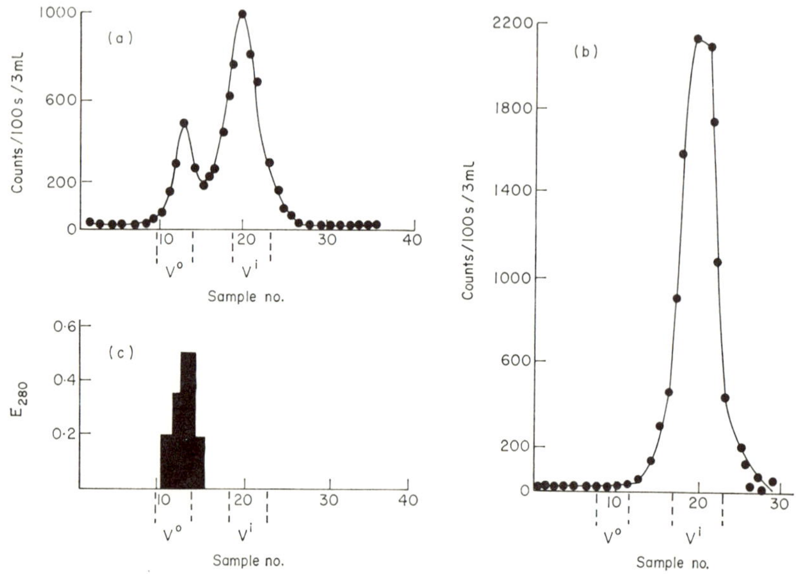

FIG 8. Elution diagram of ^{59}Fe-containing compounds of (a) placental cell sap, (b) maternal serum, and (c) aqueous rabbit ferritin, applied to Sephadex G200. Sample volume, 3 ml; V^o, void volume; V^i, inner volume.

applied to a G75 column, the results indicated that the molecular weight of the iron-containing compounds was greater than 50000 (Fig 7). Two peaks of radioactivity were obtained when the cell sap was passed through a G200 column (Fig 8). The first peak occurred in the inner volume, indicating the presence of compounds of molecular weight between 50000 and 200000. The second peak in the void volume suggested iron-containing compounds with molecular weights greater than 200000.

From these results, it would appear that there were at least two groups of iron-containing compounds present in the cell sap, one having a molecular weight less than 200000 and one greater than 200000. These findings would be consistent with the presence of transferrin, molecular weight 90000 and ferritin with a molecular weight of 400000. It should be remembered that perfusion of the placenta did not remove all the maternal blood nor any of the foetal blood. Therefore, it might be expected that the placental cell sap would contain ^{59}Fe transferrin from these sources. Consequently, plasma from the mother rabbit was applied to the G200 column. As can be seen from Fig 8, the position of the radioactive peak from the maternal plasma corresponded exactly with the peak of radioactivity seen in the inner volume on separation of the placental cell sap. This indicates that one of the ^{59}Fe-containing compounds of the cell sap was probably transferrin which may have originated from residual maternal blood in the placenta. An aqueous solution of pure rabbit ferritin was applied to the G200 column and its presence in the eluate fractions recognized by colour. The radioactive peak found in the placental cell sap in the void volume corresponded to the position of pure ferritin eluted from the same column (Fig 8).

Starch gel electrophoresis of placental cell sap and maternal serum showed that there were two areas of radioactivity in the cell sap, one of which corresponded with the transferrin area found in maternal plasma. In a further experiment, a 27-days' pregnant rabbit was injected intravenously with 50 μCi ^{59}Fe. The supernatant from the placental homogenate was freeze-dried and reconstituted in a small volume of 0.01 M phosphate buffer, pH 7.4, and applied to a G200 Sephadex column. The radioactive fractions in the volume were combined, heated to 80°C and the precipitate removed by centrifugation. This supernatant was concentrated by freeze-drying and applied to the same G200 column. All the radioactivity emerged in a peak coinciding with the elution volume of pure rabbit ferritin.

When pure rabbit ferritin was run along with cell sap on a starch gel and subsequently stained with a mixture of 2 N-HCl and potassium ferrocyanide, a faint blue band was seen in the cell sap which corresponded to one of the bands of pure ferritin. This stained area in the cell sap was radioactive.

DISCUSSION

The transfer of iron across the placenta in the rabbit is unidirectional from mother to foetus (Bothwell *et al*, 1958). The amount of iron transferred from mother to foetal rabbit shows a remarkable increase during the last third of gestation. At day 19 of gestation approximately 4% of the iron leaving the maternal plasma is transferred to the foetus compared with approximately 40% at day 22 of gestation (Davies *et al*, 1959). This increase in the amount of iron transferred by the placenta could be due to the placental cells at this advanced stage being able to transport more iron. At the same time, histological changes in the trophoblastic cells are also taking place. Electron micrographs of placental cells at this stage of gestation have demonstrated the presence of increased amounts of rough endoplasmic reticulum, suggesting greater activity within these cells. It would seem, therefore, that the time to study the mechanism of placental transfer of iron in this species would be during the last third of gestation.

In the rabbit placenta during the last third of gestation there is a relatively large amount of maternal blood and in studying the mechanism of transfer of ^{59}Fe across the placenta, it is desirable to remove as much of the maternal blood as possible. It would also be desirable to remove as much foetal blood as possible from the placenta but technically this is very difficult. By perfusing the placenta *in situ*, a large percentage of the maternal blood can be removed and most of the radioactive iron remaining in the placenta associated with blood will be in the foetal circulation. The result of the plasma clearance studies (Fig 1) would seem to indicate that 2 hr after administration of the radioactive iron, the maternal plasma level of ^{59}Fe is only about 2% of that present immediately after the injection of ^{59}Fe. On the other hand, 2 hr after administering ^{59}Fe intravenously, much of this iron has already crossed the placenta and therefore the chance of finding the ^{59}Fe-containing compounds within placental cells is considerably reduced. However, it would seem desirable to reduce the heavy contamination by the maternal blood at the expense of a possible reduction in the amount of compounds associated with the transfer of iron by the placental cells. Furthermore, the iron taken up by the placenta at this stage of gestation is immediately transferred to the foetus and therefore there is never an accumulation of ^{59}Fe-containing compounds within the placental cells.

Differential centrifugation of various tissues has been employed to separate the subcellular fractions and to study their individual biochemical reactions. The conditions under which satisfactory separation into mitochondrial, microsomal fraction and cell sap have varied from author to author and from tissue to tissue. There is no available information in the conditions applicable to rabbit placenta. Electron micrographs of the various fractions obtained are necessary to establish suitable conditions. The conditions which were employed enabled us to obtain relatively pure mitochondrial and microsomal fractions, leaving a non-particulate supernatant or cell sap. When studying the uptake of ^{59}Fe by the subcellular fractions, it was apparent that most of the iron was in the supernatant cell sap and not associated with either the mitochondrial or the microsomal fractions.

From our studies on the ^{59}Fe-containing compounds in the cell sap, it would appear that all the ^{59}Fe was associated with either transferrin or ferritin. The presence of transferrin in the cell sap could be due to the contamination of the placental homogenates with residual maternal blood and foetal blood. There is no evidence to suggest the occurrence of transferrin within placental cells, and, in fact, it has been demonstrated that iron can cross the placenta unaccompanied by maternal transferrin (Douglas *et al*, 1968).

As, under normal circumstances, ferritin is not found in circulating blood, its presence in the placental cell sap indicates its origin as being from the placental cell. Wöhler (1955) has demonstrated the presence of ferritin in rabbit placentae. In these experiments Wöhler used large quantities of iron. In our experiments we have used only trace amounts of iron and the quantity of ferritin obtained by us has been extremely small. The role which ferritin plays here in the transfer of iron is not known. It has been suggested by Crosby (1963) that ferritin acts as a regulator in the absorption of iron across intestinal cells and its role in the placenta may well be similar. The placenta may be able to store iron in the form of ferritin until this can be taken up by the foetus and in fact there is evidence that if the foetus is removed, iron will be stored in the placental tissue (Bothwell *et al*, 1958).

Identification of ferritin in the placenta using the electron microscope has been inconclusive. Furthermore, immunoelectrophoresis using rabbit liver ferritin antiserum has given negative results for the presence of placental ferritin. Whether there is an antigenic difference in the ferritin from different organs is not known. Most of our evidence is therefore indirect, but it would appear that small amounts of ferritin are present in rabbit placenta under normal circumstances. The form in which the iron crosses the placental cell could be either ionic or bound to some other molecule. In the experiments described here, free iron would be rapidly chelated by the transferrin and the presence of free iron would not be detected under these experimental conditions.

ACKNOWLEDGMENT

This work was supported throughout by a grant from the Agricultural Research Council.

REFERENCES

ASHTON, G.C. (1957) Serum protein differences in cattle by starch gel electrophoresis. *Nature*, **180**, 917.

BOTHWELL, T.H., PRIBILLA, W.F., MEBUST, W. & FINCH, C.A. (1958) Iron metabolism in the pregnant rabbit. Iron transport across the placenta. *American Journal of Physiology*, **193**, 615.

CROSBY, W.H. (1963) Gastro-intestinal tract and iron absorption. *Blood*, **22**, 416.

DAVIES, J. (1961) *Survey of Research in Gestation and Developmental Sciences.* Williams & Williams, Baltimore.

DAVIES, J., BROWN, E.B., JR, STEWART, D., TERRY, C.W. & SISSON, J. (1959) Transfer of radioactive iron via the placenta and accessory fetal membranes in the rabbit. *American Journal of Physiology*, **197**, 87.

DOUGLAS, T.A., RENTON, J.P. & WRIGHT, R. (1968) Role of transferrin in the placental transfer of iron in the rabbit. *American Journal of Obstetrics and Gynecology*, **102**, 1169.

ENDERS, A.C. (1965) A comparative study of the fine structure of the trophoblast in several hemochorial placentas. *American Journal of Anatomy*, **116**, 29.

GRANICK, S. (1943) Ferritin. IV. Occurrence and immunological properties of ferritin. *Journal of Biological Chemistry*, **149**, 157.

HOGEBOOM, G.H. & SCHNEIDER, W.C. (1950) Cytochemical studies of mammalian tissues. III. Isocitric dehyrogenase and triphosphopyridine nucleotide-cytochrome c reductase of mouse liver. *Journal of Biological Chemistry*, **186**, 417.

HOGEBOOM, G.H., SCHNEIDER, W.C. & PALADE, G.E. (1948) Cytochemical studies of mammalian tissue. I. Isolation of intact meitochondria from rat liver: Some biochemical properties of mitochondria and submicroscopic particulate material. *Journal of Biological Chemistry*, **172**, 619.

PORATH, J. (1959) Fractionation of polypeptides and proteins on dextran gels. *Clinica Chimica Acta*, **4**, 776.

PORATH, J. & FLODIN, P. (1959) Gel filtration: A method for desalting and group separation. *Nature*, **183**, 1657.

POULIK, M.D. (1957) Starch gel electrophoresis in a discontinuous system of buffers. *Nature*, **180**, 1477.

SMITHIES, O. (1955) Zone electrophoresis in starch gels: Group variations in the serum proteins of normal human adults. *Biochemical Journal*, **61**, 629.

WÖHLER, F. (1955) Zur Physiologie und Pathologie des Speichereisens; über den intermediären Eisenstoffwechsel der Plazenta. *Deutsche Medizinische Wochenschrift*, **80**, 30.

Maternally Derived Transferrin in Pigeon Squabs

JEFFREY A. FRELINGER

Transferrin is a nonheme iron-binding protein (*1*) that is widely distributed throughout the chordates from lamprey to man (*2*). One of its principal functions is the transport of iron to reticulocytes for incorporation into hemoglobin (*3*). It may be important in nonspecific resistance to disease, as well as for its iron transport function. Transferrin has been found to be polymorphic in most species, the products of different alleles usually differing in electrophoretic mobility (*4*).

Although the development of transferrin has been studied in several mammalian species, including mouse, rabbit, and man (*5*), I am not aware of any reports on developmental studies of transferrin in birds. In mammals, there is very little transport of transferrin to the developing fetus (*6*); in this, transferrin differs from certain immunoglobulins, which are known to be transported intact to the embryo.

Pigeons have been shown to be polymorphic at a transferrin locus, and have only two reported variants, Tf^A and Tf^B (*7*). The alleles are inherited as autosomal codominants, and in populations so far examined they are present in nearly equal frequency. Transferrin is found in the pigeon blood, egg white, egg yolk, crop milk, and probably in the semen. In all these fluids it is under the control of the same gene. In pigeons, which differ in this respect from chickens (*8*), the electrophoretic mobility of transferrin in all these fluids is identical. In this report, therefore, transferrin derived from egg white will not be distinguished by the specific term ovotransferrin, which is often used.

Pigeons (*Columba livia*) were maintained in the laboratory in mating cages (1 pair per cage) or in large fly-pens. Eggs were checked daily and the day of hatching was designated as day 0.

For adults and squabs over 4 days old, when more than 0.5 ml of blood was to be removed, the birds were bled from the brachial vein by syringe and needle. The blood was allowed to clot and the serum was collected. For younger birds, blood was collected directly onto filter paper for electrophoresis. In order to determine whether this would give consistent serum patterns, several squabs were killed by exsanguination and their serums were collected. The results for collection by filter paper and by syringe were identical.

Transferrin typing was carried out on horizontal starch gels by the use of tris–citric acid buffer (*p*H 7.5) in the gel and borate buffer (*p*H 8.7) as electrolyte (*9*). An ice pack was placed on top of the gel to prevent excessive heating; the gels were stained with Coomassie blue.

Antibodies to pigeon transferrin were

prepared in rabbits. Approximately 5 mg of purified pigeon transferrin in Freund's complete adjuvant (Difco) was injected into toe pads. Four weeks later, 2 mg of this transferrin in 1 ml of saline was injected intraperitoneally; and 3 days after that, 3 mg in 1 ml of saline was injected intravenously. The rabbits were bled 1 week after the last injection. When assayed by immunoelectrophoresis against pigeon normal serum, the rabbit antiserum gave a single band in the transferrin position.

For determination of the synthesis of transferrin by newly hatched squabs, the squabs were injected intraperitoneally with [^{3}H]leucine (specific activity, 38.5 c/mmole; New England Nuclear) and allowed 20 minutes to incorporate the isotope. The squabs were killed; their livers were washed in ice-cold phosphate buffered saline (PBS) *(10)* and homogenized in a Waring Blendor for 2 minutes in 15 ml of PBS. The homogenate was centrifuged 1 hour at 30,000*g* and the pellet was discarded. A portion of the supernatant was precipitated with an equal volume of 10 percent trichloroacetic acid (TCA) and counted in a toluene omnifluor scintillation mixture. One-half milliliter of supernatant was reacted with 0.5 ml of antiserum for 1 hour at room temperature, and then for 2 days at 4°C. The pellets were washed four times in cold PBS, precipitated with TCA, filtered, and counted as above.

The following matings were made to test for maternally derived transferrin: Tf^A/Tf^A ♀ × Tf^B/Tf^B ♂; the reciprocal Tf^B/Tf^B ♀ × Tf^A/Tf^A ♂; and Tf^A/Tf^B ♀ × Tf^A/Tf^A ♂. In the AA ♀ × BB ♂ mating the squab is genotypically AB. However, until 8 days after hatching it appears to have only A type transferrin in its serum, as assayed on starch gels. On the eighth day, the squab's own type becomes detectable. A similar result is obtained in BB ♀ × AA ♂ matings, the offspring showing only B type until 8 days. In AB ♀ × BB ♂ matings, although half the squabs are homozygous BB, all show the heterozygous phenotype until they reach 14 to 16 days of age.

Because transferrin is found in crop milk produced by both the male and the female, protein transfer by this route could affect the results. One pair of squabs of AB genotype was separated at hatching; one squab was put with the A parent, the other with the B parent. Both squabs followed the same pattern; that is, the squabs showed the maternal phenotype regardless of the source of crop milk.

These experiments demonstrate the transfer of a maternally derived intact protein through the egg, or as a formal possibility, a portion of the maternal protein-synthesizing machinery. Because the homozygous offspring of matings of AB ♀ × AA ♂ show the heterozygous type even though they do not possess the Tf^B gene, the protein's source can only be maternal.

These observations necessitated a study of active synthesis of transferrin by squabs. We tested squabs at various times after hatching for their ability to incorporate [^{3}H]leucine into protein reacting with monospecific antiserums to transferrin. The results are given in Table 1. Antiserum to human serum, alone and with added human serum, served as coprecipitation controls; these controls are not different from the rabbit normal serum or saline controls. The antiserum to transferrin precipitates about 20 percent of the total labeled protein in the supernatant, while the antiserum to pigeon whole serum precipitates almost all of the counts.

With the use of genetically marked transferrin, this study has shown that, in pigeons, newly hatched squabs derive part of their plasma proteins from their mothers. The transferred protein represents the major portion of the young squab's serum transferrin, even though the young bird is actively synthesizing transferrin during this period. This conclusion is reasonable when the growth rate of a young pigeon is considered. The squab, weighing about 16 g at hatching, doubles its weight in the first 2 days, and by 2 weeks it weighs 150 g *(11)*. This rapid rate of growth involves

Table 1. Active synthesis of transferrin by squab liver. Phosphate buffered saline (0.5 ml) and 0.5 ml of liver homogenate were centrifuged at 30,000*g*. The supernatant and 0.5 ml of the indicated serums were reacted, pellets were washed and precipitated with TCA as described in the text. The values are given in counts per minute per filter and represent the average of duplicate portions of the same homogenate, subjected to the same treatments.

	Squab No. 1 (0 days, 17 g)	Squab No. 2 (0 days, 17 g)	Squab No. 3 (4 days, 70 g)
Saline	74	30	221
Rabbit normal serum	195	105	204
Rabbit antiserum to human serum	95		
Rabbit antiserum to human serum + human serum	87		
Rabbit antiserum to pigeon serum	3721	4483	1919
Rabbit antiserum to pigeon transferrin	1068	1152	884
Supernatant (0.5/ml)	5688	4027	3038

a large increase in mass, and extensive synthesis is required even to maintain a constant concentration of transferrin.

All the observations are consistent with the following model. A large amount of transferrin is absorbed intact by the developing embryo, through the egg white or the yolk, or both. Some time prior to the day of hatching, the squab initiates its own synthesis of transferrin. The failure to detect the squab's own type in genotypically heterozygous squabs is a result of inability to detect low levels of transferrin. Unlike mammals, therefore, pigeons provide the major part of their offspring's transferrin supply by maternal transfer, even though the squab is also engaged in active transferrin synthesis.

References and Notes

1. R. Feeney and S. Komatsu, *Struct. Bonding* **1**, 146 (1966).
2. R. Webster and B. Pollara, *Comp. Biochem. Physiol.* **30**, 509 (1969); E. Giblett, *Progr. Med. Genet.* **2**, 34 (1962).
3. E. Baker and E. Morgan, *Biochemistry* **8**, 1133 (1969); J. Fletcher, *Clin. Sci.* **37**, 273 (1969); S. Kornfeld, *Biochim. Biophys. Acta* **194**, 25 (1969).
4. C. Baker, *Comp. Biochem. Physiol.* **20**, 949 (1967); J. Clark, D. Osuga, R. Feeney, *J. Biol. Chem.* **283**, 3621 (1963); E. Ezekiel, L. Lai, E. Kaldor, *Comp. Biochem. Physiol.* **10**, 69 (1963); E. Giblett, C. Hickman, O. Smithies, *Nature* **183**, 1589 (1959).
5. D. Shreffler, *Proc. Nat. Acad. Sci. U.S.* **46**, 1378 (1960); E. Morgan, *Aust. J. Exp. Biol. Med. Sci.* **47**, 361 (1969); D. Gilten and A. Biasucci, *J. Clin. Invest.* **48**, 1433 (1969); P. Tojvanen, T. Rossi, T. Hirvonen, *Scand. J. Haematol.* **6**, 113 (1969).
6. E. Baker and E. Morgan, *Quart. J. Exp. Physiol. Cog. Med. Sci.* **54**, 173 (1969).
7. J. Mueller, O. Smithies, M. Irwin, *Genetics* **47**, 1385 (1962); R. Brown and H. Sharp, *Anim. Blood Groups Biochem. Genet.* **1**, 11? (1970).
8. A. Ogden, J. Morton, D. Gilmour, E. McDermid, *Nature* **195**, 1026 (1962); A. Stratil, *Comp. Biochem. Physiol.* **24**, 13 (1968); C. Baker, *Genetics* **58**, 211 (1968).
9. F. Kristjansson, *Genetics* **48**, 1059 (1963).
10. 0.075*M* phosphate and 0.075*M* NaCl (*p*H 7.2).
11. W. Levi, *The Pigeon* (Levi, Sumter, S.C., ed. 3, 1957), pp. 269–271; and personal observation.

12. I thank Dr. Ray Owen for valuable discussion, support, and criticism. Supported by AEC contract AT 04376706 FP and PHS grant GM 00086.

Immunity, Transferrin, and Survival in Kwashiorkor

H. McFARLANE, PH.D., M.R.C.PATH. ;
S. REDDY, M.B., B.S., M.R.C.P.ED. ;
K. J. ADCOCK, M.B., B.S., D.R.C.O.G.
H. ADESHINA, A.M.I.L.T. :
A. R. COOKE, M.B., B.S., D.T.M. & H. ; J. AKENE

Summary: In a study of 40 children with kwashiorkor, serum albumin, transferrin, and immunoglobulin levels were measured. Treatment included chloroquine, pyrimethamine, multivitamins, folic acid, iron compounds, and a high-protein diet. After two weeks the mean serum transferrin values in the children who survived and those who died were 1·30 mg./ml. and 0·33 mg./ml., respectively. Many of the children died immediately after treatment started, and it is suggested that in children with severe kwashiorkor and low serum transferrin levels any increase in free-circulating iron may result in overwhelming infection and death. Thus the appropriate time for instituting iron therapy in such patients should be reconsidered.

Introduction

In kwashiorkor assessment of the degree of malnutrition or its prognosis on clinical grounds alone is universally accepted as being difficult. Hence several attempts have been made to find suitable biochemical tests to fulfil this need (Waterlow *et al.*, 1960). The low serum transferrin levels found in kwashiorkor may be significant (Antia *et al.*, 1968) and of several biochemical tests McFarlane *et al.* (1969) found the serum transferrin to be the most accurate index for assessing kwashiorkor.

Infection is more prevalent in this disease than in the rest of the population (Scrimshaw *et al.*, 1960), and there is evidence of an immune deficiency state in kwashiorkor. Brown and Katz (1965), in Uganda, noted that the serum immunoglobulin concentration in kwashiorkor was severely depressed, whereas Najjar *et al.* (1969) observed high serum IgG, IgA, and IgM in marasmic infants with no clinical evidence of kwashiorkor. On the other hand, mean levels of serum immunoglobulin values in both severe and moderate kwashiorkor did not show much difference (McFarlane *et al.*, 1970), though some individual kwashiorkor children had reduced serum immunoglobulin values. We report here the results of the Heaf test and a sequential study of albumin, transferrin, and immunoglobulins in children with kwashiorkor.

Patients and Methods

Of the 40 children studied with kwashiorkor, who were attending the general outpatient clinic of University College Hospital, Ibadan, 21 were girls and 19 boys aged 1½ to 5 years. Of these seven had hepatomegaly, one of whom also had splenomegaly; only one child was jaundiced; and almost all had varying degrees of diarrhoea, two having malaria. Ascaris ova were found in the stools of two children. Clinical evidence of bacterial infection was found in four children—two had otitis media, one had conjunctivitis and one had furunculosis.

The Heaf test was done with the standard technique and was negative in all cases. No abnormality was detected on routine chest *x*-ray examination. Twenty-nine were haemaglobin genotype AA. All the children were treated initially with chloroquine and thereafter with weekly doses of pyrimethamine; a multivitamin mixture plus 5 mg. of folic acid was given daily. The children were given a high-protein diet in the form of milk powder that was known to have a high-protein content. Sulphadimidine and potassium chloride were prescribed for those with diarrhoea, and the bacterial infections noted above were treated with antibiotics as indicated. Oral ferrous sulphate was prescribed for most of those who had low packed cell volume after the diarrhoea had subsided. When oral iron was not available intramuscular iron was given. Most of the children were followed up for six weeks or more, though many died or dropped out of the study. All were seen every other day during the first two weeks and thereafter once or twice a week, depending on the severity of the illness.

Serum proteins were estimated by the method of Gornall *et al.* (1949), serum uric acid by the method of Feichtmeir and Wrenn (1955), and serum transferrin and immunoglobulins by the Hyland immunoplate method.

Results

Serum Albumin and Serum Transferrin

The time course sequence of albumin and transferrin concentration in the children with kwashiorkor who survived and in those who died is shown in Fig. 1. The mean albumin values are plotted on the same semilogarithmic scale as the transferrin values for ease of comparison. The serum albumin patterns were similar when plotted on linear paper. Before treatment began the mean serum albumin values of children who survived was similar to that of those who died, whereas there was a pronounced initial difference in the mean serum transferrin value between these two groups (Fig. 1).

The initial mean serum transferrin value in those who survived was twice as high as in those who were lost to follow-up and three times as high as in those who subsequently died. After treatment the difference between the groups became even greater, and at the end of two weeks the mean serum transferrin value in those who survived (1·3 mg./ml.) was about four times higher than in those who eventually died (0·33 mg./ml.). In comparison the mean serum albumin concentration in those who died was 1·6 g./100 ml. and in those who recovered 2·2 g./100 ml.

Most patients who were responding to treatment showed an appreciable rise in the serum transferrin level even as early as the second day after treatment and a twofold to fourfold increase by the fourth day. Most probably the rise in the serum transferrin concentration on the second day was not more pronounced because of the redistribution of body fluids caused by the loss of oedema. In fact in some patients the serum transferrin values fell noticeably by the second day but in those who survived the values usually promptly increased again by the third to the fourth day of treatment.

The pattern of the transferrin results in four children who initially had low serum transferrin values is shown in Fig. 2. Immediately after treatment had started (phase 1) the serum transferrin value fell significantly, which seemed to last for about 24 to 48 hours. This was followed by phase 2, starting on the third day, when a very sharp rise occurred, reaching a peak between the sixth and eighth day. During the second week of treatment (phase 3) there was a pronounced fluctuation in the levels. This was followed by phase 4, which continued after the third week with values showing less fluctuation. The serum albumin in these four children did not show such pronounced changes. The serum transferrin values were mostly in the upper limit of the normal range, whereas for the corresponding period the serum concentrations of albumin were in the lower limit of the normal range.

Patients Who Died.—Only 2 of the 13 patients who died had serum transferrin values above 0·4 mg./ml. before treatment. The percentage increase after treatment was negligible

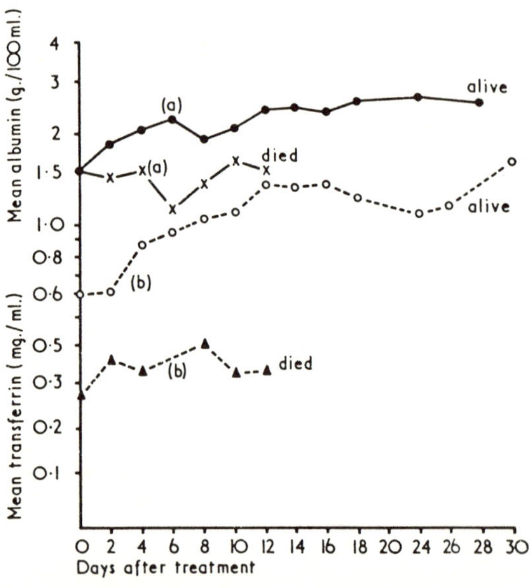

FIG. 1.—Difference between serum albumin (a) and transferrin (b) in kwashiorkor children who survived and in those who died. Note the pronounced difference in the transferrin values.

in most of those who eventually died. Just before death, most of them had values of less than 0·33 mg./ml. Two who died by the second day after they were first seen had values of 0·32 and 0·22 mg./ml. and two others who died on the fourth day had values of 0·21 and 0·3 mg./ml.

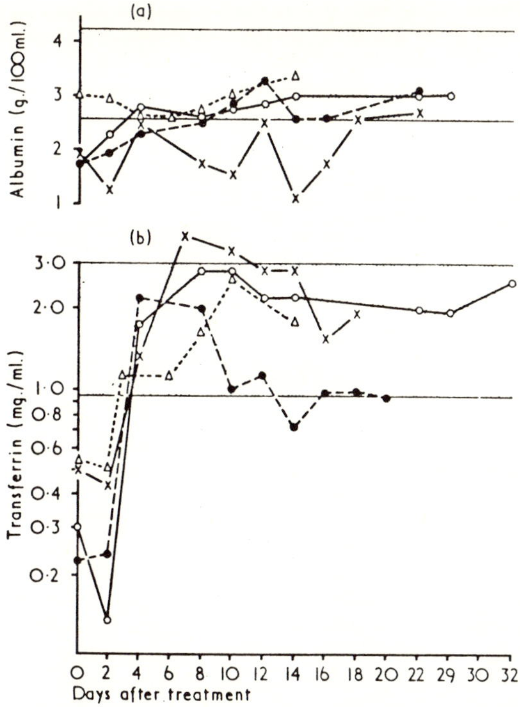

FIG. 2.—Comparison of values of serum albumin (a) and transferrin (b) in 4 children who survived. The shaded areas represent the normal range.

Children Lost to Follow-up.—Of the 11 children who were lost to follow-up by the end of the second week of the study all but one had initial serum transferrin values of less than 0·4 mg./ml. Nine had initial values ranging from 0·038 to 0·38 mg./ml., and none had appreciably increased transferrin values after four days of treatment. The prognosis was generally unfavourable if the serum transferrin still remained less than 0·45 mg./ml. after four to seven days of treatment. Thus the most probable reason for their dropping out was death.

Serum Immunoglobulins

The serum immunoglobulin patterns showed pronounced variations. The IgG concentrations ranged from 10 to 40 mg./ml., IgA from 0·8 to 4 mg./ml., and IgM from 0·6 to 2 mg./ml. As in our previous studies (McFarlane *et al.,* 1970), a few children had low serum immunoglobulin levels and a few high levels, but most of the values were similar to those in age-matched controls. One child, who had diarrhoea and otitis media and eventually died, had a low serum IgG throughout.

Serum Uric Acid

Serum uric acid was in no way related to the nutritional state, and the patterns were similar in those who survived and those who died.

Discussion

The serum albumin results did not give any guide to the subsequent progress of the child with kwashiorkor. The mean values of those who died and of those who survived were not significantly different. Interestingly all three serum immunoglobulin (IgG, IgA, and IgM) levels were not generally affected by lack of protein intake. Mean values were mostly similar in those who died and in those who survived. Some patients showed an increase in concentration of these immunoglobulins after corrective treatment but this was not the rule. In three children the serum IgG concentration rose immediately before death, and in an unpublished study (McFarlane *et al.*, 1967) about 10 to 20% of children with kwashiorkor had IgG values above 30 mg./ml. The reason for this is not clear, but the high serum IgG may be related to infection. Cohen and Hansen (1962) showed that four children with kwashiorkor with signs of infection also had high rates of γ-globulin synthesis. Four children had reduced levels of IgA throughout, but this appeared to be related to their ages rather than to any abnormality in synthesis or catabolism. Most children had normal serum IgM during the six weeks or more of treatment, though occasionally the IgM was slightly reduced in a few. Watson and Freesemann (1970) suggested that the high initial levels of immunoglobulins in kwashiorkor may be a response to infection. Diarrhoea in almost all the children may also be an indication of infection, which is known to be prevalent in malnutrition.

The negative Heaf test in all the children could be regarded as evidence of impairment of the cell-mediated immune response which is known to exist in kwashiorkor. In Ibadan, J. A. Idowu (personal communication, 1970) stated that 5 to 15% of normal children under 5 years usually show a positive Heaf test. Lloyd (1968) noticed a depression of the

Heaf test in children with malnutrition, and Watts (1969) declared that the atrophied thymus of the kwashiorkor child is the most likely cause of the impaired cell-mediated immune response. Hutt (1969) stated that in malnourished children not only are the Heaf and Mantoux reactions depressed but also the conversion rate after B.C.G. vaccination. Studying the serum immunoglobulins in pulmonary tuberculosis in Nigeria, Malomo *et al.* (1970) found that most of the Mantoux-negative subjects were undernourished children.

Plasma uric acid levels did not show any constant abnormal patterns. A few children initially had high values which quickly reverted to normal on treatment. In some children the serum uric acid concentration increased after treatment had begun but later returned to pretreatment values.

Of the serum proteins measured the transferrin showed the most remarkable changes. Those children who had a poor prognosis had considerably lower mean transferrin values before, during, and after initiating treatment than those who subsequently did well. On the first day the children were seen those with a good prognosis had mean serum transferrin levels of 0·76 mg./ml., whereas those with a grave prognosis had a mean value of 0·29 mg./ml. By the end of the second week this difference had risen about fivefold.

Serum transferrin is responsible for the transport of iron in the body and under normal conditions only negligible concentrations of iron are found free in the circulation. An estimation of the mean total intravascular transferrin mass in four kwashiorkor children who responded well showed that in the early recovery phase the synthetic rate of serum transferrin was extremely high and that after four days of treatment the intravascular transferrin mass increased from about 175 to 1,000 mg. At this time, however, the mean serum transferrin concentration of 2 mg./ml. in these children can bind an equivalent of about 3·4 μg. of iron, which far exceeds the concentration of iron found in their serum. On the other hand, the transferrin levels of those who did not respond to treatment was about 0·32 mg./ml. This could bind only about 0·55 μg. of iron and may leave an appreciable concentration of free iron in the plasma since the serum iron in these children ranged from 0·48 to 0·80 μg./ml. Edozien and Udeozo (1960) observed that in kwashiorkor the percentage saturation of the total iron-binding capacity was generally above the normal range. Using an in-vitro technique, Schade (1963, 1966) showed that serum transferrin has a bacteriostatic action and that iron-requiring pathogenic bacteria like *Staphylococcus aureus, Shigella paradysenteriae,* and *Pseudomonas aeruginosa* will grow more readily in sera which contain an excess of free iron caused by oversaturation of the available transferrin than in sera which contain all the iron bound to transferrin.

At death children with kwashiorkor have acute bacterial infections, and Soltys and Brody (1970) remarked that the occurrence of Gram-negative sepsis in certain conditions in which the concentration of free transferrin is diminished implies that this iron-binding protein may be a component of an auxiliary antibody-globulin system. Barber (1961) suggested that iron-free transferrin prevents the formation of lipid peroxides, which are known to be toxic to several biological systems.

Interestingly a high percentage of the children with kwashiorkor died immediately after treatment had started. The only constant finding among them was the greatly reduced transferrin. Unfortunately it was not possible to determine the exact cause of death of these children as necropsies were not done. Conceivably in children with severe kwashiorkor and low serum transferrin any increase of the serum iron, particularly during the first week of treatment, from whatever source, may encourage bacterial infections since all the available serum transferrin is of the bound type. The free iron would then be available to promote bacterial growth (Rogers, 1967), resulting in overwhelming infection and finally death. Further studies are in progress to elucidate this mechanism, but it may be therapeutically sound to reconsider the appropriate time at which iron therapy is instituted in these patients. The haemosiderosis which is so often seen in kwashiorkor at necropsy may be the result of the low serum transferrin and increased free circulating iron.

We should like to thank the University of Ibadan for a Senate Research Grant to conduct these studies.

References

Antia, A. U., McFarlane, H., and Soothill, J. F. (1968). *Archives of Disease in Childhood*, **43**, 459.

Barber, A. A. (1961). *Archives of Biochemistry and Biophysics*, **92**, 38.

Brown, R. E., and Katz, M. (1965). *East African Medical Journal*, **42**, 221.

Cohen, S., and Hansen, J. D. L. (1962). *Clinical Science*, **23**, 351.

Edozien, J. C., and Udeozo, I. O. K. (1960). *Journal of Tropical Pediatrics and African Child Health*, **6**, 60.

Feichtmeir, T. V., and Wrenn, H. T. (1955). *American Journal of Clinical Pathology*, **25**, 833.

Gornall, A. G., Bardawill, C. J., and David, M. M. (1949). *Journal of Biological Chemistry*, **177**, 751.

Hutt, M. S. R. (1969). *Journal of Tropical Pediatrics*, **15**, 153.

Lloyd, A. V. C. (1968). *British Medical Journal*, **3**, 529.

McFarlane, H., *et al.* (1969). *Lancet*, **1**, 392.

McFarlane, H., *et al.* (1970). *Tropical and Geographical Medicine*, **22**, 61.

Malomo, I. M., McFarlane, H., and Idowu, J. A. (1970). *Transactions of the Royal Society of Tropical Medicine and Hygiene*, **64**. In press.

Najjar, S. S., Stephan, M., and Asfour, R. Y. (1969). *Archives of Disease in Childhood*, **44**, 120.

Rogers, H. J. (1967). *Immunology*, **12**, 285.

Schade, A. L. (1963). *Biochemische Zeitschrift*, **338**, 140.

Schade, A. L. (1966). In *Proceedings of the Colloquium on the Protides of the Biological Fluids*, ed. H. Peeters, vol. 14, p. 13. Amsterdam, Elsevier.

Scrimshaw, N. S., Wilson, D., and Bressani, R. (1960). *Journal of Tropical Pediatrics and African Child Health*, **6**, 37.

Soltys, H. D., and Brody, J. I. (1970). *Journal of Laboratory and Clinical Medicine*, **75**, 250.

Waterlow, J. C., Cravioto, J., and Stephen, J. M. L. (1960). *Advances in Protein Chemistry*, **15**, 131.

Watson, C. E., and Freesemann, C. (1970). *Archives of Disease in Childhood*, **45**, 282.

Watts, T. (1969). *Journal of Tropical Pediatrics*, **15**, 155.

TRANSFERRIN AND ALBUMIN DISTRIBUTION AND TURNOVER IN THE RABBIT

by E. H. MORGAN

INTRODUCTION.

The metabolism of albumin and, less frequently, transferrin has been studied separately in man and laboratory animals by many workers. The results, in general, indicate that the two proteins occupy similar plasma spaces and have similar relative distributions between the intravascular and interstitial body fluid compartments. However, the relative turnover rate of transferrin is greater than that of albumin (Gitlin, Janeway and Farr, 1956; Awai and Brown, 1963; Cohen, Freeman and McFarlane, 1961; Freeman, 1961; Jarnum and Lassen, 1961; Katz, 1961; Gordon, 1963; Masuya and Kozuru, 1963). Another difference between transferrin and albumin is that transferrin, *in vitro* at least, is reversibly bound to the surface of reticulocytes (Jandl and Katz, 1963; Morgan and Laurell, 1963). The amount of transferrin so bound is relatively small; but no measurements have been made of transferrin bound to other cells of the erythropoietic tissue or to other tissues with the exception of placenta (Laurell and Morgan, 1964). Furthermore, the amount of transferrin bound to cells in the living animal has not been estimated, although it has been postulated that under certain circumstances a relatively large fraction of plasma transferrin may become sequestrated at cellular sites (Mitchell, Halden, Jones, Bryan, Stirman and Muirhead, 1960).

The aim of the present work was to study the distribution and turnover of albumin and transferrin simultaneously in the same rabbits by use of purified homologous proteins labelled with ^{131}I and ^{125}I. The initial dilution of the two proteins in the plasma was used to measure the amount of transferrin bound at tissue sites both in normal rabbits and rabbits with accelerated erythropoiesis.

Materials and Methods

Animals.

Mature New Zealand rabbits of both sexes were used. They were housed in individual metabolism cages.

Purification and labelling of proteins.

Rabbit albumin and transferrin were purified as described previously (Morgan and Laurell, 1963). They were iodinated with ^{131}I or ^{125}I (Radiochemical Centre, Amersham, England) by the method of McFarlane (1958) to an average extent of 0·5-1·0 iodine atoms per protein molecule (assuming molecular weights of 70,000 and 75,000 for albumin and transferrin respectively). Precipitation with a final concentration of 10% trichloroacetic acid showed that more than 99% of the radioactivity was protein bound. The labelled proteins were injected into the recipient animals within 2 hrs. of labelling.

Experimental procedure.

The solutions of albumin and transferrin, each protein labelled with a different isotope, were mixed, samples were taken for the preparation of standards and 1 ml. aliquots were injected into rabbits by a marginal ear vein. The amount of protein injected into each rabbit was 8 mg. albumin and 3 mg. transferrin. In the first experiment this contained approx. 400,000 counts/min. of each isotope and in the second experiment 4,000,000 counts/min. Blood samples were collected from the other ear to the one injected by incision of a marginal vein. The first sample (3 ml.) was obtained 10 min. after the injection and the other samples (0·5 ml.) at various time intervals thereafter for up to 14 days. The first sample was used to obtain haematocrit, reticulocyte count, serum radioactivity and serum albumin and transferrin concentrations. Serum radioactivity only was measured in the later blood samples. Faeces and urine were collected each day. They were homogenized in a Waring blender, using about 1 ml. octyl alcohol to prevent frothing, the volume was measured and aliquots were counted for radioactivity. For 2 days before injection of the labelled proteins, and on each day of the experiments, the rabbits were injected subcutaneously with 20 mg. potassium iodide dissolved in physiological saline.

Two experiments were performed. In the first experiment 4 untreated normal rabbits and 4 with haemorrhagic anaemia were injected with albumin labelled with ^{125}I and transferrin labelled with ^{131}I. Six blood samples were taken during the first 70 min. after the injection and thereafter daily samples were collected. The haemorrhagic anaemia was produced by bleeding

TABLE 1

Haematological values and initial distribution volumes (plasma volumes) and rates of transcapillary passage (slopes) of radioactive iodine-labelled transferrin and albumin in 4 normal rabbits and 4 rabbits with haemorrhagic anaemia. Each value is the mean ± standard deviation.

Rabbit	Body weight (Kg.)	Haema-tocrit (%)	Reticu-locytes (%)	Transferrin		Albumin	
				Plasma volume (ml.)	Slope ($hr.^{-1}$)	Plasma volume (ml.)	Slope ($hr.^{-1}$)
Normal	2·81 ±0·53	31·5 ± 2·6	0·50 ±0·25	105 ± 13	0·26 ±0·02	104 ±11	0·27 ±0·02
Anaemic	2·16 ±0·09	18·8 ± 3·4	15·2 ± 1·3	108 ± 10	0·27 ±0·014	106 ± 9·2	0·27 ±0·04

the rabbits 3 times during the week preceding the protein injections, 25-30 ml. blood being removed on each occasion. At the time of injection the haematocrits of the bled rabbits were decreased and relative reticulocyte counts were increased relative to the corresponding values for the untreated animals (Table 1).

In the second experiment 4 normal rabbits were given albumin-^{131}I and transferrin-^{125}I. A blood sample was taken 10 min. later and thereafter samples were collected daily. The albumin and transferrin used in this experiment were from different preparations than those used in the first experiment.

Analytical methods.

Paper electrophoresis was performed according to Laurell, Laurell and Skoog (1956). Total serum protein concentration was measured by a biuret method (Kingsley, 1942) and serum albumin concentration by paper electrophoresis and elution of the bromphenol blue from the albumin zone and from the other protein zones combined. Transferrin concentration was determined from the serum total iron binding capacity (Morgan and Carter, 1960) and an assumed molecular weight of 75,000. The relative reticulocyte counts were made on blood smears stained with new methylene blue. Haematocrits were determined by centrifugation of the blood in Wintrobe tubes for 1 hr. at a force of 1,500 *g*.

Radioactivity was counted in a well type scintillation detector. Iodine-^{131} and ^{125}I were differentiated by the use of a pulse-height analyser and by counting standards of the pure isotopes. The efficiency of counting was approx. 20% for ^{131}I and 45% for ^{125}I. All samples and standard solutions were made up to the same volume and, for each experiment, were all counted on the same day.

Analysis of results.

The method of least squares was used to obtain the regression lines of the serum radioactivity due to the two isotopes in the first hour after injection in the first experiment. The slopes of these regression lines were used as a measure of the rate of transcapillary passage of the proteins from vascular to extravascular spaces. Plasma volume was calculated from the injected dose and the plasma activity found by extrapolation of the regression lines to zero time. In the second experiment plasma volume was estimated from the dose, the serum radioactivity in the 10 min. blood sample and the mean rate of disappearance of the labelled proteins from the plasma as determined in the first experiment.

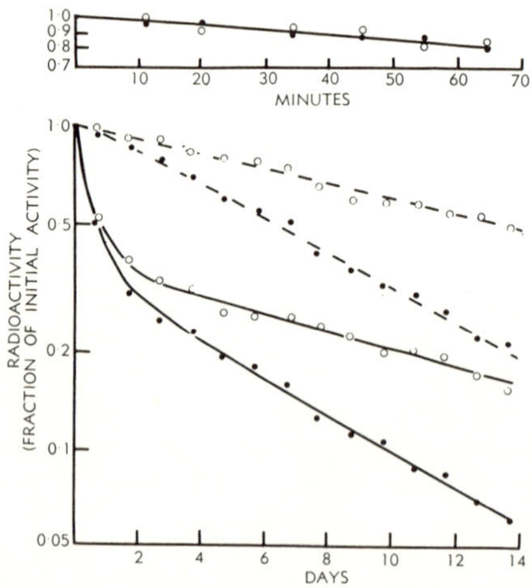

Fig. 1. Changes in plasma (————) and whole body (— — — — —) radioactivity after the intravenous injection of radioactive iodine-labelled transferrin (•) and albumin (o) in a normal rabbit.

The final distribution of the proteins between the intravascular and extravascular spaces, and their fractional and absolute turnover rates, were calculated from the serum and excreted radioactivity data by the method of Nosslin, as described by Anderson (1964). Since these analyses require that the animals are in a steady state with regard to the proteins being studied, they were applied only to the normal rabbits, not to those which had been bled. The changes in serum and whole-body radioactivity found in one of the normal rabbits are illustrated in Fig. 1.

RESULTS

Initial distribution volumes.

No significant difference was found between the plasma volumes determined in each rabbit from the serum radioactivity due to albumin and transferrin in the 8 normal rabbits or in the 4 with haemorrhagic anaemia (Tables 1 and 2).

TABLE 2

Distribution and turnover of radioactive iodine-labelled transferrin and albumin in 8 rabbits. Each value is the mean ± standard deviation.

	Body weight (Kg.)	Plasma volume (ml.)	Serum concentration (g./100 ml.)	Plasma pool (g.)	Total pool (g.)	Pools ratio	Fractional turnover rate (plasma pools/day)	Absolute turnover rate (g./day)
Transferrin	3·20 ±0·56	124 ± 23	0·22 ±0·02	0·28 ±0·06	0·60 ±0·13	2·16 ±0·17	0·31 ±0·03	0·086 ±0·018
Albumin	3·20 ±0·56	122 ± 22	4·62 ±0·44	5·81 ±1·38	13·15 ±3·60	2·24 ±0·19	0·17 ±0·03	0·93 ±0·12

Rate of transcapillary passage.

The slopes of the regression lines of serum albumin and transferrin radioactivity during the first hour after the injections were almost identical in both the normal and bled rabbits. There was no significant difference between the means for the two proteins, nor between the values for each protein in the normal and the bled animals (Table 1).

Final distribution and turnover.

The plasma and whole body pools and turnover rates of the two proteins in the 8 normal rabbits are given in Table 2. The relative distribution of albumin and transferrin between intravascular and extravascular spaces were very similar in all 8 rabbits and the mean values were not significantly different. Approx. 45% of the total body content of each protein was situated in the intravascular space, and 55% was extravascular. The fractional turnover rate, which is a measure of the rate of catabolism of the proteins, was approx. twice as great for transferrin as for albumin. No correlation was found between the fractional turnover rates of albumin with those of transferrin, nor between the fractional turnover rates of albumin or transferrin with their serum concentrations. The absolute turnover rates, which may be used as a measure of the rates of synthesis of the proteins, were approx. 10 times as great for albumin as for transferrin.

DISCUSSION.

When rabbit transferrin labelled with ^{131}I is incubated *in vitro* with rabbit reticulocytes, transferrin is rapidly bound by the cells to reach maximum value within 10 min. (Morgan and Laurell, 1963). If all types of primitive erythroid cells of the rabbit bind *in vivo* as much transferrin as do reticulocytes *in vitro*, the transferrin bound to cells would represent 0·5-1·0% of the plasma transferrin. In the present experiments it may be assumed that mixing with plasma and maximal uptake of labelled transferrin by erythropoietic tissue would have occurred within 10 min. of the injections. At this time, however, there was no difference between the distribution volumes of labelled transferrin and albumin. Hence, the amount of transferrin bound to cells in excess of any albumin bound was too small to be measured, even though in 4 of the animals erythropoiesis had been stimulated by haemorrhage. The results therefore suggest that cells of the erythropoietic tissue more primitive than reticulocytes do not bind *in vivo* significantly more transferrin than do reticulocytes *in vitro*. Nor is there any evidence that tissues other than the erythropoietic tissue bind circulating plasma transferrin to any degree.

No differences were found between the rates at which albumin and transferrin left the plasma in the first hour after the injection nor in their relative distributions between intravascular and extravascular spaces. This is probably due to the similarity of molecular size of albumin and transferrin. The molecular weight of rabbit albumin is 68,000 (Charlwood, 1959) and that of transferrin has been determined at 70,000 to 77,000 (Greene and Feeney, 1968; Baker, Shaw and Morgan, 1968). The similarity in intravascular : extravascular pools ratios of the two proteins is further evidence for the fact that only small amounts of transferrin are bound at cell surfaces since, if large amounts were bound, the ratio of plasma to total pools of transferrin as measured in these experiments would be reduced.

The rate of catabolism of transferrin was approx. twice as great as that of albumin. An almost identical relationship to this has been found in humans (Jarnum and Lassen, 1961), but in the rat the relative turnover rate of albumin is almost as great as that of transferrin (Morgan, 1966). The greater catabolic rate of transferrin could possibly be related to its function of donating iron to erythropoietic and other acceptor tissues. However, it has been shown that transferrin is not destroyed during the process of iron donation to reticulocytes (Paoletti and Durand, 1958), nor is its catabolism increased when the rate of erythropoiesis is accelerated (Awai and Brown, 1963; Morgan, 1966). Hence, it seems unlikely that transferrin catabolism is related to its iron-carrying function.

Acknowledgements. The writer is indebted to Dr. B. Nosslin for assistance with the mathematical analyses. The work was supported in part by a grant from the National Health and Medical Research Council.

REFERENCES.

ANDERSON, S. B. (1964): "Metabolism of Human Gamma Globulin (γSS-Globulin)", p. 115. Blackwell, Oxford.

AWAI, M., and BROWN, E. B. (1963): 'Studies of the metabolism of I^{131}-labeled human transferrin'. *J. Lab. Clin. Med.*, **61**, 363.

BAKER, E., SHAW, D. C., and MORGAN, E. H. (1968): 'Isolation and characterization of rabbit serum and milk transferrins. Evidence for difference in sialic acid content only'. *Biochemistry*, **7**, 1371.

CHARLWOOD, P. A. (1959): 'Molecular weights of rat, rabbit and guinea-pig serum albumins'. *Biochem. Biophys. Acta*, **32**, 283.

COHEN, S., FREEMAN, T., and MCFARLANE, A. S. (1961): 'Metabolism of ^{131}I-labelled human albumin.' *Clin. Sci.*, **20**, 161.

FREEMAN, T. (1961): '^{131}I-transferrin metabolism in the human subject.' In "Protides of the Biological Fluids, IX Colloquium", p. 213. Ed. H. Peeters. Elsevier: Amsterdam.

GITLIN, D., JANEWAY, C. A., and FARR, L. E. (1956): 'Studies on the metabolism of plasma proteins in the nephrotic syndrome. I. Albumin, γ-globulin, and iron-binding globulin.' *J. Clin. Invest.*, **35**, 44.

GORDON, A. H. (1963): 'The rates of catabolism of rat transferrin *in vivo* and by the perfused rat liver.' In "Protides of the Biological Fluids, X Colloquium", p. 71. Ed. H. Peeters. Elsevier: Amsterdam.

GREENE, F. C., and FEENEY, R. E. (1968): 'Physical evidence for transferrins as single polypeptide chains.' *Biochemistry*, **7**, 1366.

JANDL, J. H., and KATZ, J. H. (1963): 'The plasma-to-cell cycle of transferrin.' *J. Clin. Invest.*, **42**, 314.

JARNUM, S., and LASSEN, N. A. (1961): 'Albumin and transferrin metabolism in infectious and toxic diseases.' *Scandinav, J. Clin. Lab. Invest.*, **13**, 357.

KATZ, J. H. (1961): 'Iron and protein kinetics studied by means of doubly labeled human crystalline transferrin.' *J. Clin. Invest.*, **40**, 2143.

KINGSLEY, G. R. (1942): 'Direct biuret method for the determination of serum proteins as applied to photoelectric and visual colorimetry.' *J. Lab. Clin. Med.*, **27**, 840.

LAURELL, C.-B., LAURELL, S., and SKOOG, N. (1956): 'Buffer composition in paper electrophoresis.' *Clin. Chem.*, **2**, 99.

LAURELL, C.-B., and MORGAN, E. H. (1964): 'Iron exchange between transferrin and the placenta in the rat.' *Acta Physiol. Scand.*, **62**, 271.

MCFARLANE, A. S. (1958): 'Efficient trace labelling of proteins with iodine.' *Nature*, **182**, 53.

MASUYA, T., and KOZURU, M. (1963): 'Clinical and experimental studies on the metabolism of transferrin. II. Turnover studies with iodine-labelled human transferrin.' *Kyushu J. Med. Sci.*, **14**, 233.

MITCHELL, J., HALDEN, E. R., JONES, F., BRYAN, S., STIRMAN, J. A., and MUIRHEAD, E. E. (1960): 'Lowering of transferrin during iron absorption in iron deficiency.' *J. Lab. Clin. Med.*, **56**, 555.

MORGAN, E. H. (1966): 'Transferrin and albumin distribution and turnover in the rat.' *Amer. J. Physiol.*, **211**, 1486.

MORGAN, E. H., and CARTER, G. (1960): 'Plasma iron and iron-binding capacity levels in health and disease: with an improved method for the estimation of plasma iron concentration and total iron-binding capacity.' *Aust. Ann. Med.*, **9**, 209.

MORGAN, E. H., and LAURELL, C.-B. (1963): 'Studies on the exchange of iron between transferrin and reticulocytes.' *Brit. J. Haematol.*, **9**, 471.

PAOLETTI, C., and DURAND, M. (1958): 'Absence de consommation de la sidérophiline au cours de la synthèse de l'hemoglobine *in vitro*.' *Rev. Franç ét Clin. Biol.*, **3**, 259.

A STUDY OF IRON TRANSFER FROM RABBIT TRANSFERRIN TO RETICULOCYTES USING SYNTHETIC CHELATING AGENTS

E. H. MORGAN

INTRODUCTION

Reticulocytes are able to take up iron from the plasma iron-binding protein, transferrin and utilize it for haem synthesis[1]. This process involves uptake of the iron–transferrin complex by the cells and release of the iron from transferrin before its incorporation into haemoglobin[2,3]. The mechanism by which iron is released from its strong complex with transferrin and its subsequent metabolic path are still poorly understood despite investigations by many workers[4–9]. One method of studying this problem has been to use synthetic iron chelating agents, either for comparisons with transferrin as iron donors, or to block the utilization of transferrin-bound iron. It has been shown that several such agents can act as iron donors for reticulocytes, while others are ineffective in this regard[10–12]. Similarly some chelators such as 2,2'-bipyridine and 1,10-phenanthroline block iron uptake by reticulocytes from transferrin[5,13,14] while EDTA has little effect except at relatively high concentrations[4].

The present investigation used both of the above approaches in an effort to obtain more information on the mechanism of iron release from transferrin and its subsequent metabolic path. The initial experiments confirmed that bipyridine and 1,10-phenanthroline were very effective inhibitors of reticulocyte iron uptake from transferrin, and showed that in the presence of actively metabolizing reticulocytes iron was rapidly transferred from transferrin to the synthetic chelators. Experiments were also performed using synthetic chelators as the iron donor for comparison with the natural iron carrier, transferrin. The results showed both similarities and differences between transferrin and the other chelators as sources of iron for reticulocytes.

MATERIALS AND METHODS

Chemicals

Sulphonated bathophenanthroline, 1,10-phenanthroline and 2,2'-bipyridine were obtained from the G. Frederick Smith Chemical Co., Columbus, Ohio, U.S.A. Sodium citrate, EDTA, nitrilotriacetic acid and *N*-β-hydroxyethyliminodiacetic acid, *plus* the metabolic inhibitors and metabolites used in the experiments were purchased from the Sigma Chemical Co., St. Louis, Mo., U.S.A. Desferroxamine was kindly provided by Ciba Ltd., Basle, Switzerland. Iron-59 ($FeCl_3$, 10–20 $\mu C/\mu g$) and iodine-125 (NaI, carrier free) were purchased from the Radiochemical Centre, Amersham, England.

Reticulocytes and rabbit tissues

Reticulocytes were obtained from bled rabbits and washed prior to use as previously described[9]. Rabbit tissues were obtained from animals killed by a blow on the head. The tissues were quickly removed, and placed in ice-cold 0.15 M NaCl, and slices 0.5 mm thick were cut by hand[15], washed in cold saline, blotted with filter paper, weighed and then suspended in incubation medium. Bone marrow was obtained from the femora and tibiae, suspended in cold saline, dispersed by repeated passage through a needle and syringe and centrifuged to remove fat. Placental tissue was obtained from rabbits on the 28th or 29th days after mating.

Transferrin and albumin purification and labelling

Transferrin and albumin were prepared from rabbit serum and labelled with ^{125}I and in the case of transferrin with ^{59}Fe as previously described[9,16]. The amount of iron added to label purified transferrin or transferrin in serum was sufficient to raise its iron concentration only to 30–50% of its iron-binding capacity.

Chelator solutions

The chelators were dissolved in 0.15 M NaCl, the pH of the solution adjusted to 7.4 with NaOH or HCl and the concentration made to 10 mM. The solutions were then diluted with phosphate-buffered saline (0.15 M NaCl, 0.01 M sodium phosphate, pH 7.4) to the desired final concentration. Iron-59 chelate solutions were prepared by adding $^{59}FeCl_3$ to the chelate solution and adjusting the pH to 7.4 with NaOH.

Iron uptake by reticulocytes

The procedure used for incubating reticulocytes with labelled transferrin and for washing and counting the cells was the same as used in earlier experiments[9,16]. Reticulocytes were incubated with the other ^{59}Fe–chelate solutions in a similar way.

Dialysis experiments

Washed reticulocytes, bone marrow cells or tissue slices were placed in bags of 16/32″ Visking dialysis tubing together with 1.5 ml of a solution containing iron–transferrin or iron–chelate *plus* another synthetic iron chelator in the iron-free form, dissolved in phosphate buffered saline. The volume of cell suspension used was 0.25 to 0.5 ml, and the weight of tissue slices 0.25 to 0.5 g. The dialysis sac was closed, quickly rinsed with cold 0.15 M NaCl, dried with filter paper and placed in a 20 ml conical flask containing 10 ml of a solution of the same synthetic chelators which were added to the dialysis sac dissolved in phosphate-buffered saline. The concentration of transferrin was 0.04 mM (assuming a molecular weight of 75000[17]) and of the synthetic chelator was 0.1 to 10 mM as specified below. The same concentrations of synthetic chelators were used inside and outside of the sac. The flask was then incubated with shaking at a rate of 60 oscillations/min and a temperature of 37°, unless otherwise stated. Samples of the solution surrounding the sac were removed after 1 min and at further intervals of 15–30 min for periods of 1 to 4 h. In those experiments in which ^{59}Fe was used radioactivity was measured in these samples and in standards prepared from the initial labelled transferrin solution. In other experiments employing non-radioactive iron the accumulation of iron outside of the sac was determined from the absorbance of the solution at the wavelength of maximal light absorption of the iron–chelate complex oustide of the sac. In control experiments the cells, tissues or synthetic chelators were omitted from the sac, or the rate of diffusion of iron–bipyridine from inside to outside of the sac was measured using ^{59}Fe–bipyridine in the presence of unlabelled bipyridine without transferrin, and with or without reticulocytes.

Analytical methods

Iron concentration and total iron-binding capacity of transferrin containing solutions were measured using sulphonated bathophenanthroline[18]. Protein was determined by a biuret procedure[19]. Radioactivity was measured in a dual-channel well type scintillation counter. Reticulocytes were counted on dry smears after staining with new methylene blue. Haem iron was extracted from erythrocytes by the method of Thunell[20].

RESULTS

Effect of chelators on reticulocytes iron uptake from transferrin

Reticulocytes were incubated with transferrin labelled with ^{59}Fe and ^{125}I in the presence of several different synthetic iron chelating agents (Fig. 1). The concentrations of transferrin and other chelators were 0.04 mM and 1 mM, respectively. None of the chelators affected transferrin uptake by cells as measured by their uptake of ^{125}I. This showed rapid uptake to reach a plateau level within about 15 min as has been described previously[2,3]. The effect of chelator on iron uptake varied with the chelator. Several (citrate, nitrilotriacetic acid, *N*-β-hydroxyethyliminodiacetic acid and desferroxamine) had no effect, while bipyridine and 1,10-phenanthroline resulted in almost complete inhibition of iron uptake. Sulphonated bathophenanthroline produced an intermediate degree of inhibition and EDTA had a small inhibiting effect. In other experiments it was found that nitrilotriacetic acid, *N*-β-hydroxyethyliminodiacetic acid and desferroxamine did not reduce the rate of iron uptake when used at 5 mM concentration, while the effect of EDTA increased with a rise in concentration. Bipyridine was found to produce negligible inhibition of iron uptake when used at a concentration of 0.05 mM, but produced approximately 15 % inhibition at 0.1 M and 65 % inhibition at 0.25 mM. Similar effects on iron uptake were observed whether the ^{59}Fe was bound to purified transferrin or to transferrin present in whole serum.

Iron exchange between transferrin and synthetic chelators

The fact that bipyridine and 1,10-phenanthroline inhibited iron uptake without affecting transferrin uptake indicated that they act subsequently to the processes involved in transferrin uptake[9,16], either at the time of, or after, removal of the iron from transferrin. They could act by blocking the intracellular metabolic pathway of iron possibly by inhibiting one or more enzymatic process, or simply by chelating the newly assimilated iron and making it unavailable for haem synthesis and possibly removing it from the cell[14,21]. In the latter case radioactive iron would be expected

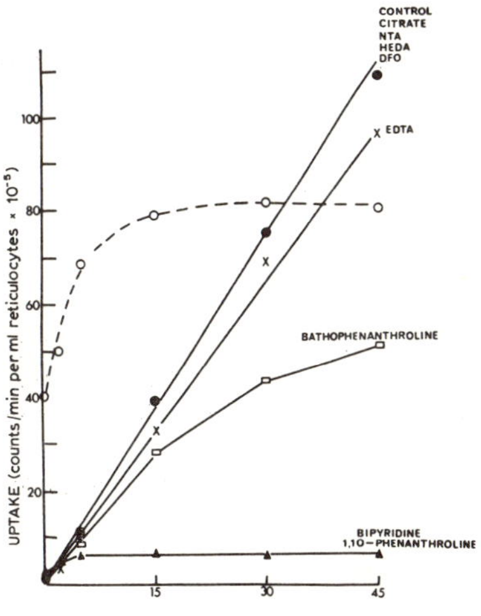

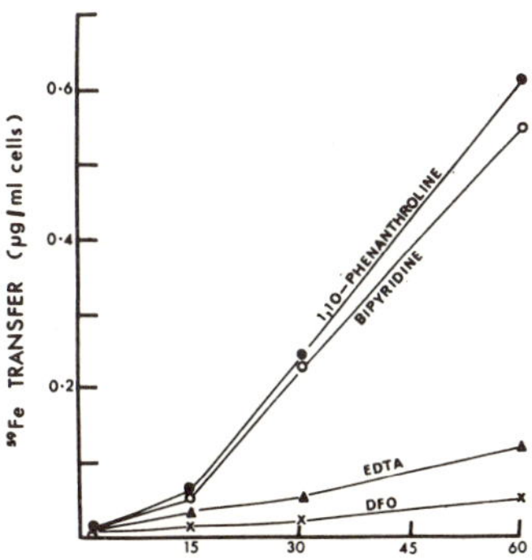

Fig. 1. Effect of iron chelators on reticulocyte uptake of transferrin (-----) and transferrin-bound iron (———). None of the chelators affected transferrin uptake, hence only one curve is shown for transferrin. The concentrations used were: iron, 0.03 mM; transferrin, 0.04 mM; synthetic chelators, 1 mM; reticulocytes, 22 %. NTA, nitrilotriacetic acid; HEDA, *N*-β-hydroxyethyliminodiacetic acid; DFO, desferroxamine.

Fig. 2. Exchange of iron between transferrin and different iron chelators in the presence of reticulocyte-rich blood cells. The concentrations used were: iron, 0.03 mM; transferrin, 0.04 mM; synthetic chelators, 1 mM; reticulocytes, 19 %. DFO, desferroxamine.

to accumulate on the chelate in the incubation medium. The dialysis experiments were performed to investigate this possibility.

Reticulocytes were incubated with transferrin-bound ^{59}Fe in dialysis sacs in the presence of several chelators at 1 mM concentration. It was found that essentially no transfer of ^{59}Fe from the inside to the outside of the dialysis sac occurred in the absence of a chelator, or in the presence of those chelators which did not affect iron uptake by reticulocytes. On the other hand, rapid radioiron transfer occurred in the presence of bipyridine or 1,10-phenanthroline, and slower transfer when EDTA was used (Fig. 2). Iodine-125 did not pass to the external solution, indicating that there was no leakage of transferrin through the dialysis membrane. At the end of the ex-

TABLE 1

IRON EXCHANGE BETWEEN TRANSFERRIN AND BIPYRIDINE IN THE PRESENCE OF CELLS OR TISSUE SLICES

The cells and tissue slices were incubated with transferrin–^{59}Fe while being dialysed against 2 mM 2,2′-bipyridine.

Cell or tissue	*Iron exchange (μg/ml cells (or g tissue) per h)*
Reticulocyte	3.35
Bone marrow	5.25
Liver	0.069
Spleen	0.49
Kidney	0.056
Heart muscle	0.046
Placenta	0.091
Nil	0.049

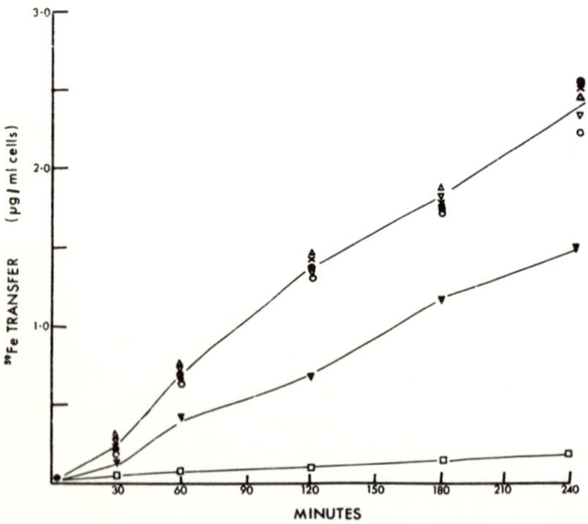

Fig. 3. Effect of 2,2′-bipyridine concentration on iron exchange between transferrin and bipyridine in the presence of reticulocyte-rich blood cells (26% reticulocytes). Bipyridine concentration: □, 0.1 mM; ▼, 0.5 mM; ▽, 1.0 mM; △, 2.0 mM; ×, 3.0 mM; ●, 5.0 mM; ○, 10 mM. Other conditions were as in Fig. 2.

periments the outside solutions containing bipyridine or 1,10-phenanthroline showed the pink colours characteristic of the combination of ferrous iron with the chelators. If the reticulocytes were omitted from the sac or were heated at 90° for 10 min prior to the experiment no ^{59}Fe transfer occurred even in the presence of bipyridine or 1,10-phenanthroline. Similar results for ^{59}Fe transfer were obtained whether the ^{59}Fe was bound to purified transferrin or to that present in serum.

Dialysis experiments were also performed using bone marrow cells or slices of rabbit liver, spleen, kidney, heart muscle or placental tissue. As shown in Table I only bone marrow, in addition to reticulocytes, had the capacity of mediating iron transfer from transferrin to bipyridine.

The effect of bipyridine concentration on the iron transfer process was investigated using a constant amount of reticulocytes but varying the chelator concentration from 0.1 to 10 mM. Iron transfer increased to a maximal rate as the concentration was

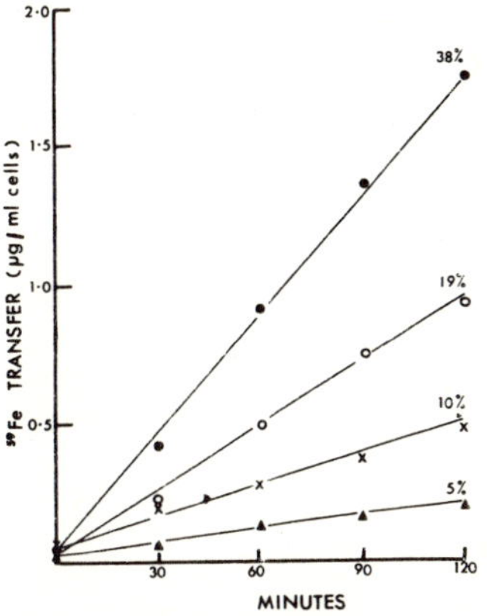

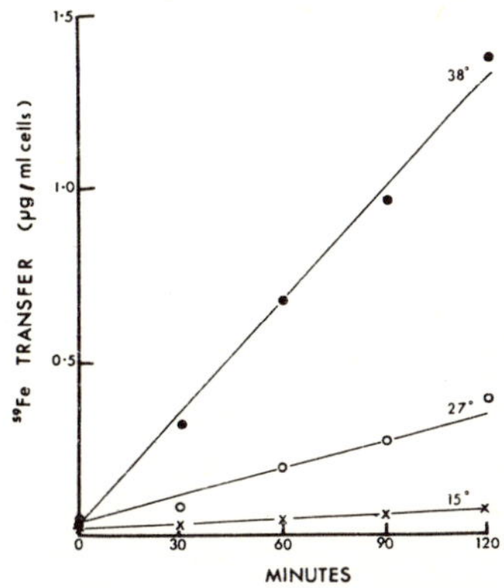

Fig. 4. Effect of reticulocyte concentration on iron exchange between transferrin and 2,2′-bipyridine. The reticulocyte concentrations varied from 5 to 38%; other conditions were as in Fig. 2.

Fig. 5. Effect of incubation temperature on iron exchange between transferrin and 2,2′-bipyridine in the presence of reticulocyte-rich blood cells (25% reticulocytes). Other conditions were as in Fig. 2.

TABLE II

COMPARISON OF UPTAKE OF TRANSFERRIN-BOUND IRON BY RETICULOCYTES AND EXCHANGE OF IRON BETWEEN TRANSFERRIN AND BIPYRIDINE IN THE PRESENCE OF RETICULOCYTES

Rabbit erythrocytes (28% reticulocytes) were incubated with transferrin–^{59}Fe either alone (iron uptake) or with dialysis against 2 mM 2,2′-bipyridine (iron transfer to bipyridine).

Volume of cells (ml)	*Iron uptake (µg/h)*	*Iron transfer to bipyridine (µg/h)*
0.05	0.050	0.043
0.1	0.12	0.090
0.2	0.22	0.16
0.4	0.34	0.29
0.6	0.47	0.35

raised from 0.1 to 1 mM but showed no increase when the bipyridine concentration was raised further (Fig. 3). In a similar way the effect of reticulocyte concentration was studied using 2 mM bipyridine but varying the reticulocyte percentage of the cells used from 5 to 38% by mixing cells from an unbled and from a bled rabbit. As shown in Fig. 4 the rate of iron transfer was proportional to the reticulocyte concentration.

The rate of iron exchange between transferrin and bipyridine in the presence of reticulocytes was markedly affected by temperature (Fig. 5). It was extremely slow at temperatures below 15° and increased as the temperature was raised to 38°. A 10° temperature rise produced an approximately 4-fold increase in iron transfer. In contrast, a 10° temperature increase raised the rate of diffusion of ^{59}Fe–bipyridine across the dialysis membrane by a factor of only 1.5.

TABLE III

EFFECT OF METABOLIC INHIBITORS ON IRON EXCHANGE BETWEEN TRANSFERRIN AND BIPYRIDINE IN THE PRESENCE OF RETICULOCYTES

Reticulocytes were incubated with transferrin–^{59}Fe in the presence of metabolic inhibitors and with dialysis against 2 mM 2,2′-bipyridine.

Inhibitor	*Concentration (mM)*	*Iron exchange (μg/h per ml reticulocytes)*
Control	—	2.8
Sodium arsenite	10	0.10
Iodoacetamide	10	0.23
N-Ethylmaleimide	5	0.14
p-Chloromercuribenzoate	1	0.50
NaCN	10	0.37
2,4-Dinitrophenol	10	0.13
Rotenone	0.001	0.27
NaN_3	10	0.83
NaF	10	1.2

TABLE IV

IRON EXCHANGE FROM TRANSFERRIN TO BIPYRIDINE IN THE PRESENCE OF RETICULOCYTE GHOSTS AND VARIOUS METABOLITES

Reticulocyte ghosts were incubated with transferrin–^{59}Fe in the presence of different metabolites and with dialysis against 2 mM 2,2′-bipyridine. The rates of iron exchange are given as percentages of the exchange observed in the presence of the same volume (0.25 ml) of intact reticulocytes (control).

Additions	*Iron exchange (% control)*
Nil	1.4
ATP (4 mM)	1.6
Ascorbic acid (2 mM)	2.9
ATP (4 mM), ascorbic acid (2 mM)	2.6
Sodium citrate (5 mM)	3.7
NADH (5 mM)	1.3
Sodium citrate (5 mM), NADH (5 mM)	3.9
Glutathione (5 mM)	2.9
Sodium citrate (5 mM), glutathione (5 mM)	3.7
No ghosts or cells	1.6

The rate of iron exchange between transferrin and bipyridine in dialysis experiments was compared with the rate of iron uptake from transferrin by reticulocytes using the same transferrin and reticulocyte concentrations but in the absence of bipyridine. As shown in Table II these two rates were similar but uptake by reticulocytes in the absence of bipyridine was slightly greater than transfer to bipyridine at all reticulocyte concentrations used.

Several metabolic inhibitors have been shown to affect iron uptake by reticulocytes[9]. When they were used in dialysis experiments similar effects were found on transfer from transferrin to bipyridine (Table III). Marked inhibition of iron transfer occurred when sulphydryl reagents (sodium arsenite, iodoacetamide, *N*-ethylmaleimide, *p*-chloromercuribenzoate) or inhibitors of oxidative metabolism (sodium cyanide, dinitrophenol, rotenone, sodium azide) were used. Fluoride produced 57 % inhibition. The inhibitory effects of iodoacetamide, *N*-ethylmaleimide and *p*-chloromercuribenzoate, but not of sodium arsenite were largely overcome by including cysteine in the incubation solution at 5 times the molar concentration of the inhibitors.

Dialysis experiments with reticulocyte ghosts

Washed reticulocytes were haemolysed and then restored by the method of VIVADER[22] using 0.138 M KCl in the restoring solution. Dialysis experiments were performed using the ghosts instead of intact erythrocytes, with and without the metabolites listed in Table IV. Ghosts alone or after the addition of ATP, sodium citrate, ascorbic acid, NADH or glutathione were unable to mediate iron exchange between transferrin and bipyridine. In order to determine whether the loss of this iron-transferring capacity was the result only of disruption of the cells, or was due to loss of essential intracellular constituents, further experiments were performed in which the entire cell lysate was included in the dialysis sac with the cells disrupted by osmotic shock, freezing and thawing or ultrasonification. In all cases the disrupted cells were found to be unable to mediate the iron-transfer process.

Reticulocyte iron uptake from synthetic chelators

When reticulocytes were incubated with ^{59}Fe bound to citrate, nitrilotriacetic acid or *N*-β-hydroxyethyliminodiacetic acid, iron was taken up by the cells and was incorporated into haem, whereas little uptake and incorporation occurred from EDTA as the ^{59}Fe donor, and none from desferroxamine, bipyridine or 1,10-phenanthroline. The mechanism of iron uptake from citrate, nitrilotriacetic acid and *N*-β-hydroxyethyliminodiacetic acid was then compared with that from transferrin, using reticulocyte-rich and reticulocyte-poor blood, incubation at 4° and at 37°, and certain metabolic inhibitors. Table V summarizes the results obtained with citrate and nitrilotriacetic acid, with or without sodium arsenite and rotenone. Similar results were obtained with *N*-β-hydroxyethyliminodiacetic acid. Iron uptake from all of the iron-binding substances was similar in several respects. It was much greater with reticulocyte-rich blood than with blood of low reticulocyte count and was inhibited by low temperature, sodium arsenite (10 mM) or rotenone (2.5 μM). After 45 min incubation at 37° more than 75 % of the radioiron taken up by the reticulocytes was incorporated into haem. Other experiments showed that *N*-ethylmaleimide (5 mM) and antimycin A (0.05 mM) also inhibited iron uptake from these chelators.

Dialysis experiments using synthetic chelators as the iron source

Reticulocytes were placed in dialysis sacs with non-radioactive iron (0.1 mM) bound to various chelators (0.5 mM) *plus* iron-free bipyridine (1 mM). The sacs were incubated in phosphate-buffered saline containing the same concentrations of chelators and iron as in the sacs. The rate of iron transfer from its initial complex to that with bipyridine was measured by determining the absorbance at 520 mμ of the fluid outside of the sac after different periods of incubation. Control dialyses were performed in which reticulocytes were omitted from the sac, so that the exchange due to the presence of reticulocytes could be determined. It was found that there was a rapid reticulocyte mediated exchange when citrate, nitrilotriacetic acid or *N*-β-hydroxyethyliminodiacetic acid were used as the iron donors, a very slow exchange when EDTA was used, and none from desferroxamine (Fig. 6). However, several differences were observed between iron transfer from synthetic chelators to bipyridine and that from transferrin to bipyridine. Using citrate, nitrilotriacetic acid or *N*-β-hydroxyethyliminodiacetic acid the exchange was mediated just as well by mature erythrocytes as by reticulocytes, and was more rapid if haemolysed cells were used instead of intact cells. The supernatant from osmotically lysed erythrocytes was as effective as the total haemolysate, but the cell stroma showed little ability to mediate the iron-exchange process (Fig. 7). Liver, spleen, kidney and heart muscle tissue slices and bone marrow cells were also effective, producing iron transfer from the synthetic chelators to bipyridine at rates 60–130 % as great as that achieved with reticulocytes.

TABLE V

IRON UPTAKE BY RETICULOCYTES AND MATURE ERYTHROCYTES FROM TRANSFERRIN, SODIUM CITRATE AND NITRILOTRIACETIC ACID

Reticulocyte-rich blood cells (24 % reticulocytes) and reticulocyte-poor blood cells (4 % reticulocytes) were incubated at 4° or 37° with ^{59}Fe (iron concentration 0.02 mM) bound to transferrin (0.04 mM), citrate (0.2 mM) or nitrilotriacetic acid (0.2 mM) with or without the addition of sodium arsenite (10 mM) or rotenone (0.0125 mM).

Iron donor	*Cells*	*Incubation temp.*	*Inhibitor*	*Iron uptake (μg/h per ml cells)*	*% ^{59}Fe incorporated into haem after 60 min*
Transferrin	Reticulocytes	37°	—	0.62	92
		4°	—	0.015	94
		37°	Arsenite	0.009	0
		37°	Rotenone	0.011	0
	Erythrocytes	37°	—	0.022	28
Citrate	Reticulocytes	37°	—	0.41	76
		4°	—	0.022	36
		37°	Arsenite	0.022	5
		37°	Rotenone	0.020	4
	Erythrocytes	37°	—	0.008	27
Nitrilotriacetic acid	Reticulocytes	37°	—	0.36	80
		4°	—	0.049	66
		37°	Arsenite	0.068	3
		37°	Rotenone	0.12	4
	Erythrocytes	37°	—	0.021	20

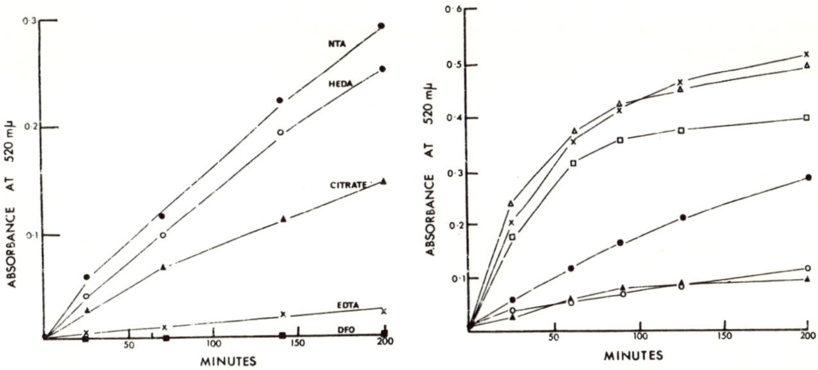

Fig. 6. Iron exchange between sodium citrate, nitrilotriacetic acid (NTA), *N*-*β*-hydroxyethyliminodiacetic acid (HEDA), EDTA or desferroxamine (DFO) and 2,2′-bipyridine in the presence of reticulocyte-rich blood cells. The concentrations used were: iron, 0.1 mM; bipyridine, 1 mM; other chelators, 0.5 mM; reticulocytes, 29%.

Fig. 7. Iron exchange between nitrilotriacetic acid and 2,2′-bipyridine at 37° in the presence of intact reticulocytes (●) or mature erythrocytes (□), osmotically haemolysed reticulocytes (×), or the supernatant (△) or stroma (▲) from osmotically haemolysed reticulocytes. Also shown is the exchange at 4° in the presence of intact reticulocytes (○). The reticulocyte concentration in the reticulocytes was 34% and in the mature erythrocytes, 3%; other incubation conditions as in Fig. 6. The absorbance values shown have been corrected for the changes which occurred in control incubations in the absence of cells or the products of their lysis.

Sodium arsenite (10 mM), dinitrophenol (10 mM), rotenone (0.05 mM) and antimycin A (0.05 mM) had no effect on iron transfer in the presence of reticulocytes. The reducing agents glutathione (0.5 mM) and hydroxylamine chloride (0.5 mM) caused rapid iron exchange between citrate, nitrilotriacetic acid or *N*-*β*-hydroxyethyliminodiacetic acid, and bipyridine in the absence of reticulocytes, but they did not produce measurable iron exchange between transferrin and bipyridine when incubations were performed for up to 4 h.

Permeability of reticulocytes to synthetic iron chelators

An attempt was made to determine the permeability of reticulocytes to chelators by incubating the cells for 1 min or 15 min at 4° and for 15 min at 37° with a solution containing rabbit albumin (5 mg/ml) labelled with ^{125}I and several different iron chelators (1 mM) labelled with ^{59}Fe. The cell suspensions were then centrifuged at 4° for 5 min at 2000 × *g*. Radioactivity was determined in the cells and in an aliquot of the supernatant solution as well as in aliquots of the original incubation solutions. The ^{125}I values were used to determine the degree of trapping of incubation solution in the cell layer. Iron-59 in the cells in addition to that attributable to trapped incubation solution was presumably either bound to the cell surface or had entered the cells. When the incubations were performed at 4° significant ^{59}Fe uptake by the cells occurred when bipyridine, 1,10-phenanthroline, sodium citrate, nitrilotriacetic acid and *N*-*β*-hydroxyethyliminodiacetic acid were used but not with EDTA or desferroxamine (Table VI). Incubation at 37° produced a great increase in ^{59}Fe uptake from citrate, nitrilotriacetic acid and *N*-*β*-hydroxyethyliminodiacetic acid compared with uptake at 4°, but uptake from bipyridine and 1,10-phenanthroline increased very little.

TABLE VI

RETICULOCYTE UPTAKE OF RADIOIRON FROM SYNTHETIC CHELATORS AT 4° AND 37°

0.25 ml cells (35% reticulocytes) were incubated with 0.25 ml of a solution of chelator–^{59}Fe and albumin–^{125}I for 1 and 15 min at 4° or 15 min at 37°, centrifuged and radioactivity determined in the cell layer.

Chelator	*Radioiron uptake (% total radioiron)*		
	1 min at 4°	*15 min at 4°*	*15 min at 37°*
2,2′-Bipyridine	3.1	3.7	5.3
1,10-Phenanthroline	3.5	4.2	6.8
Sodium citrate	1.2	1.5	33
Nitrilotriacetic acid	0.60	0.82	25
N-*β*-Hydroxyiminodiacetic acid	3.3	4.5	29
EDTA	0.03	—0.05	1.0
Desferroxamine	—0.35	0.02	0.44

DISCUSSION

The different effects of the various chelators used on reticulocyte iron uptake from transferrin could be due to differences in their binding affinity for iron or in their ability to penetrate the cell membrane. The fact that many of the chelators, even in concentrations as high as 5 mM, had no effect on iron uptake indicates, as pointed out by JANDL *et al.*[4], that at no time is the iron present in a free ionized form outside of the cell. The recent demonstration that transferrin actually passes into the interior of reticulocytes[23] and there probably donates its iron to the cell indicates why this would be so. The two chelators most effective in blocking iron uptake were bipyridine and 1,10-phenanthroline, both of which have a much higher affinity for ferrous than for ferric iron, while the ineffective chelators bind ferric iron more strongly than ferrous iron. It is therefore possible that in the reticulocyte iron is reduced at the same time as, or immediately after, it is removed from transferrin, and that only ferrous iron chelators can then effectively compete for the iron with the normal intracellular acceptor. Possibly reduction of the iron while still bound to transferrin is necessary for its removal from the protein. It is also likely that reticulocytes are more permeable to bipyridine and 1,10-phenanthroline than to the ferric-iron chelators. This would be expected from the structure of these molecules, and appears to be confirmed for all of the chelates except *N*-*β*-hydroxyethyliminodiacetic acid by the experiment in which an attempt was made to compare these permeabilities (Table VI). Of course, this experiment cannot distinguish between surface binding of the chelator or penetration into the interior of the cells. In addition, it is possible that the ^{59}Fe dissociated from the chelators and was then taken up by the cells. The latter explanation seems unlikely with the incubations performed at 4°, but no doubt explains the increase in ^{59}Fe uptake from citrate, nitrilotriacetic acid and *N*-*β*-hydroxyethyliminodiacetic acid found when the incubations were performed at 37°. Further evidence that ability to penetrate the cell membrane may be necessary for a chelator to block iron uptake from transferrin is provided by the fact that sulphonated bathophenanthroline was less effective an inhibitor than bipyridine or 1,10-phenanthroline. Although sulphonated bathophenanthroline is a ferrous-iron chelator it is more water soluble than the other two chelators and probably penetrates cell membranes less effectively.

The results of the dialysis experiments indicate that the mechanism of action of bipyridine and 1,10-phenanthroline is to enter the reticulocyte, act as an iron acceptor after the iron has dissociated from transferrin, and then leave the cell carrying the iron out also. The chelator thus competes with the normal intracellular iron acceptor for the newly released iron. The effect on rate of iron uptake or iron transfer to chelator of changing the chelator concentration from 0.05 to 1.0 mM is probably due to competition between the chelator and the normal acceptor for this iron. However, the fact that iron transfer did not increase when chelator concentration was raised above 1.0 mM, *plus* the effects of reticulocyte concentration, temperature, metabolic inhibitors and prior heating of the cells to 90° indicate that removal of the iron from transferrin was a function of the reticulocytes, not the chelator, and that it depended on reticulocyte metabolism. In addition the rate of iron transfer from transferrin to bipyridine was only 15–30% less than that of iron uptake by reticulocytes in the absence of bipyridine (Table II). Hence it is probable that bipyridine does not disturb the normal mechanism of iron removal from transferrin, and that the initial steps in iron uptake by reticulocytes (transferrin uptake and removal of iron from transferrin) are the rate-limiting steps in iron accumulation by rabbit reticulocytes.

It has been shown that reticulocyte ghosts have very little capacity for taking up iron from transferrin[3–5]. It was thought that this may have been due to loss of an iron acceptor during the process of hemolysis even though the capacity to remove iron was retained by the ghosts, possibly by the action of a membrane-bound enzyme. If so, bipyridine could possibly replace the acceptor and restore this function to the ghosts. The use of reticulocyte ghosts in dialysis experiments would thus have provided a useful system for studying the mechanism of iron release from transferrin. However, restoration of the iron–transferrin capacity to ghosts was not achieved even though ATP, ascorbic acid, NADH, citrate and glutathione, all of which may have been necessary[5,24–26], were added to the system. In addition the complete mixture of disrupted cells *plus* their contents was also unable to produce iron exchange between transferrin and bipyridine. It is therefore likely that disruption of cell integrity deprives the reticulocyte of its ability to remove iron from transferrin.

The results of the experiments on reticulocyte iron uptake from synthetic chelating agents confirms previous work in which it was shown that several chelators are able to donate iron to reticulocytes[11]. Several similarities and also some differences were found between transferrin and the other chelators as iron donors. Uptake from citrate, nitrilotriacetic acid and *N*-β-hydroxyethyliminodiacetic acid was affected by temperature, reticulocyte concentration and metabolic inhibitors in a manner similar to that from transferrin, and the iron was utilized for haem synthesis. However, transfer from the chelators to bipyridine was not affected by reticulocyte concentration or metabolic inhibitors, and seemed to depend only on reduction of the iron to the ferrous form, a process which could be achieved by the reducing systems present in erythrocyte cell sap. The difference between reticulocyte uptake of iron from transferrin and from the other chelators must lie in the steps which occur before the iron can be bound by bipyridine. These steps are uptake and then dissociation of the transferrin–iron or the chelate–iron complex. The uptake of transferrin probably occurs by pinocytosis[23, 27] and is inhibited by sulphydryl reagents[9]. Uptake of the synthetic chelators probably occurs by diffusion and is unaffected by such reagents. Dissociation of the iron–transferrin complex requires more than simple reduction of the iron since the reducing agents used (glutathione and hydroxylamine chloride) did not cause iron exchange between transferrin and bipyridine although they were effective with the other iron–chelates. Possibly the additional process involves proton donation to the transferrin by a mechanism dependent on mitochondrial function[9].

The mechanism of iron uptake by bone marrow cells is probably similar to that by reticulocytes, as shown by similar behaviour of the two types of cells in the dialysis experiments. However, there are differences between these two cell-types and the other tissues studied in the present work. One must conclude that either the tissues studied had little ability to remove iron from transferrin, or that the iron was removed in such a way that it could not be chelated by bipyridine. The first explanation may well apply to all of the tissues except placenta, which in late pregnancy in the rabbit, can remove iron from plasma transferrin and transfer it to the foetuses more effectively than it is taken up by the bone marrow[28, 29]. Moreover, iron uptake by placental tissues involves transferrin uptake[29, 30] as does that by erythropoietic tissue. It, therefore, seems likely that the mechanism of iron uptake by placenta from transferrin is different to that by erythropoietic tissue, and the same conclusion may also apply to liver, spleen, kidney and heart.

ACKNOWLEDGEMENTS

The writer is indebted to Miss M. Struthers for valuable technical assistance. The work was supported by a grant from the Australian Research Grants Committee.

REFERENCES

1 R. J. Walsh, E. D. Thomas, S. K. Chow, R. G. Fluharty and C. A. Finch, *Science*, 110 (1949) 396.
2 J. H. Jandl and J. H. Katz, *J. Clin. Invest.*, 42 (1963) 314.
3 E. H. Morgan and C.-B. Laurell, *Brit. J. Haematol.*, 9 (1963) 471.
4 J. H. Jandl, J. K. Inman, R. L. Simmons and D. W. Allen, *J. Clin. Invest.*, 38 (1959) 161.
5 A. Mazur and A. Carleton, *J. Biol. Chem.*, 238 (1963) 1817.
6 S. S. Zail, R. W. Charlton, J. D. Torrance and T. H. Bothwell, *J. Clin. Invest.*, 43 (1963) 670.
7 W. B. Greenough, T. Peters, Jr. and E. D. Thomas, *J. Clin. Invest.*, 41 (1962) 1116.
8 D. Allen and J. H. Jandl, *Blood*, 15 (1960) 71.
9 E. H. Morgan and E. Baker, *Biochim. Biophys. Acta*, 184 (1969) 442.
10 F. Cleton, A. Turnbull and C. A. Finch, *J. Clin. Invest.*, 42 (1963) 327.
11 J. V. Princiotto, M. Rubin, G. C. Shashaty and E. J. Zapolski, *J. Clin. Invest.*, 43 (1964) 825.
12 M. D. Gerlanc, E. J. Zapolski, M. Rubin and J. V. Princiotto, *Blood*, 35 (1970) 493.
13 P. Clark and R. J. Walsh, *Australian J. Exptl. Biol.*, 38 (1960) 135.
14 J. V. Primosigh and E. D. Thomas, *J. Clin. Invest.*, 47 (1968) 1473.
15 F. J. Ballard and I. T. Oliver, *Biochem. J.*, 90 (1964) 261.
16 E. Baker and E. H. Morgan, *Biochemistry*, 8 (1969) 1133.
17 E. Baker, D. C. Shaw and E. H. Morgan, *Biochemistry*, 7 (1968) 1371.
18 E. H. Morgan and G. Carter, *Australian Ann. Med.*, 9 (1960) 209.
19 G. R. Kingsley, *J. Lab. Clin. Med.*, 27 (1942) 840.

20 S. Thunell, *Clin. Chim. Acta*, 11 (1965) 321.
21 L. Felicetti, B. Colombo and C. Baglioni, *Biochim. Biophys. Acta*, 129 (1966) 380.
22 G. A. Vivader, *Biochemistry*, 3 (1964) 795.
23 E. H. Morgan and T. C. Appleton, *Nature*, 223 (1969) 1731.
24 M. Gutman, R. Margalit and A. Schejter, *Biochemistry*, 7 (1968) 2778.
25 P. Aisen and A. Leibman, *Biochem. Biophys. Res. Commun.*, 32 (1968) 220.
26 P. Saltman, *J. Chem. Education*, 42 (1965) 682.
27 T. C. Appleton, E. H. Morgan and E. Baker, *Proc. of the Symposium Erythropoieticum Prague, 1970*, in the press.
28 T. H. Bothwell, W. F. Pribilla, W. Mebust and C. A. Finch, *Am. J. Physiol.*, 193 (1958) 615.
29 E. Baker and E. H. Morgan, *Quart. J. Exptl. Physiol.*, 54 (1969) 173.
30 C.-B. Laurell and E. H. Morgan, *Acta Physiol. Scand.*, 62 (1964) 271.

THE EFFECT OF METABOLIC INHIBITORS ON TRANSFERRIN AND IRON UPTAKE AND TRANSFERRIN RELEASE FROM RETICULOCYTES

E. H. MORGAN AND ERICA BAKER

INTRODUCTION

The mechanisms whereby plasma iron bound to its carrying protein, transferrin, is taken up by immature erythropoietic cells and is incorporated into heme are poorly understood. It has been shown that one of the initial reactions in this process is the binding of the transferrin molecule to the cell, and that this step and the subsequent release of iron from transferrin and its uptake by the cell is a temperature-sensitive process, and one which can be inhibited by certain metabolic inhibitors[1–4]. On the basis of this evidence it has been assumed that both steps are dependent on cellular metabolism, but the mechanism linking metabolism to transferrin and iron uptake is uncertain. The aim of the present work was to investigate this problem by studying

Abbreviations: PCMB, *p*-chloromercuribenzoate; PCMBS, *p*-chloromercuribenzenesulfonate.

the effects of various inhibitors of different metabolic functions on transferrin and iron uptake by rabbit reticulocytes, and also on the release of transferrin from the cells.

MATERIALS AND METHODS

Reticulocytes

Reticulocytosis was produced in adult hybrid rabbits of either sex by repeated bleeding. The rabbits were bled from a marginal ear vein, 10–15 ml blood per kg body wt. being removed 3 times in 1 week, and the reticulocyte-rich blood for the experiments collected during the following week. Heparin was used as an anticoagulant. The blood was immediately centrifuged, the plasma removed and the cells washed 3 times with ice-cold 0.15 M NaCl. All centrifugation was performed at 4°. The reticulocyte count in the blood samples used in the experiments varied from 20 to 35 %. No attempt was made to separate reticulocytes from mature erythrocytes. It has been demonstrated previously[1–3], and confirmed during the present work, that the amount of iron and transferrin uptake by reticulocyte-rich blood is directly proportional to the reticulocyte count and is absent in blood containing no reticulocytes. Therefore, the only blood cells taking up significant amount of transferrin and iron are reticulocytes, and, for brevity, the cells of reticulocyte-rich blood will be referred to as reticulocytes.

Transferrin and albumin

Rabbit transferrin and albumin were purified as previously described[5,6].

Inhibitors

The inhibitors used were purchased from Sigma Chemical Co., St. Louis. With the exceptions noted below they were dissolved in 0.15 M NaCl solution and the pH adjusted to 7.4 with 0.1 M NaOH or 0.1 M HCl. Rotenone and oligomycin were dissolved at high concentration in 95 % ethanol, and then diluted to the final concentration with 0.15 M NaCl. The rotenone was then in the form of an emulsion. *p*-Chloromercuribenzoate (PCMB) and *p*-chloromercuribenzene sulfonate (PCMBS) were dissolved in 0.025 M glycylglycine buffer in NaCl.

Radioactive isotopes

^{59}Fe was obtained as $FeCl_3$ of specific activity 5–12 μC/μg, and ^{131}I and ^{125}I as NaI, carrier-free, from The Radiochemical Centre, Amersham, England.

Isotope labeling of proteins

Transferrin (in the form of its iron complex) and albumin were labeled by the iodine monochloride method[7], to an average maximum of one iodine atom per protein molecule. Non protein-bound radioiodine was removed from the protein solutions by passage of the solutions through a column of the cation-exchange resin, IRA 410, followed by dialysis overnight against Hanks' solution[8]. For many experiments transferrin was also labeled with ^{59}Fe by first removing iron from transferrin, adding ^{59}Fe as ferric citrate, adjusting the pH to 7.4 with $NaHCO_3$ and incubating at 37° for 30 min, followed by overnight dialysis against Hanks' solution. Care was taken that the amount of iron added did not exceed 60% of the iron-binding capacity of the transferrin.

Transferrin and iron-uptake experiments

The reticulocytes (usually 0.5 ml) were incubated with shaking at 37° for 15 min with 0.5 ml of the inhibitor solutions at twice their final concentrations, or with 0.5 ml of the media in which the inhibitors were dissolved. The cell suspensions were then cooled in an ice bath for 5 min followed by the addition of 0.5 ml of an ice-cold solution of transferrin labeled with ^{59}Fe and ^{125}I. After mixing, a 0.2-ml aliquot was removed from each tube and transferred to 10 ml 0.15 M NaCl in another ice bath, and the reticulocytes were then incubated with shaking at 37°. Additional 0.2-ml aliquots were removed at different time intervals, usually after 2, 5, 10, 15 and 30 min incubation, and transferred to 10 ml ice-cold 0.15 M NaCl. The reticulocyte aliquots were washed 3 times with 10 ml saline by centrifugation at 2000 $\times$ g for 10 min, removal of the supernatant and resuspension in saline. After washing, the cells were hemolyzed with 2.0 ml water, and the radioactivity was measured.

Transferrin-release experiments

Only transferrin release from reticulocytes was studied because it has been shown that almost all of the iron taken up by reticulocytes is retained by the cells[9], while the transferrin is released into the surrounding medium after its iron has been taken up by the cells[2,3]. ^{125}I-labeled transferrin (2–4 mg transferrin per ml) was incubated with reticulocytes for 30 min. The cells were then washed 4 times with cold saline, 0.5 ml ice-cold inhibitor (twice final concn.) or its solution medium was added, mixed and allowed to stand in an ice-bath for 10 min. After this 0.5 ml rabbit plasma was added, the tubes mixed and a 0.2-ml aliquot transferred to 2.0 ml cold saline. The remainder of the reticulocyte suspension was incubated at 37° with shaking and additional 0.2-ml aliquots were transferred to 2.0 ml cold saline after 2, 5, 10 and 30 min incubation. The aliquots were centrifuged at 2000 $\times$ g for 10 min, and the radioactivity was counted in the cells and supernatant solutions. The rate of release of transferrin from the reticulocytes was calculated from these results.

Analytical methods

Protein was measured by a biuret method[10], and iron concentration and total iron-binding capacity by the use of sulfonated bathophenanthroline[11]. Reticulocytes were measured by counting dried smears after staining with new methylene blue, and hematocrit by the microhematocrit method. Heme iron was extracted from reticulocytes by the method of THUNELL[12]. Radioactivity was measured using a well-type scintillation counter equipped with a two-channel γ-spectrometer which enabled simultaneous determination of two isotopes present in the one sample.

RESULTS

Effect of inhibitors on iron and transferrin uptake by reticulocytes

When reticulocytes were incubated with transferrin labeled with ^{125}I and ^{59}Fe in the absence of inhibitors the two isotopes were taken up by the cells in different manners (Fig. 1). Iron uptake commenced from near zero in the sample taken on mixing in the cold before commencing incubation at 37° and was linear for the 30 min time of incubation at 37°. The rate of iron uptake was measured from the slope of the line obtained by plotting uptake of ^{59}Fe against time. In contrast to iron uptake, transferrin uptake by reticulocytes, as measured with ^{125}I, occurred in three distinct

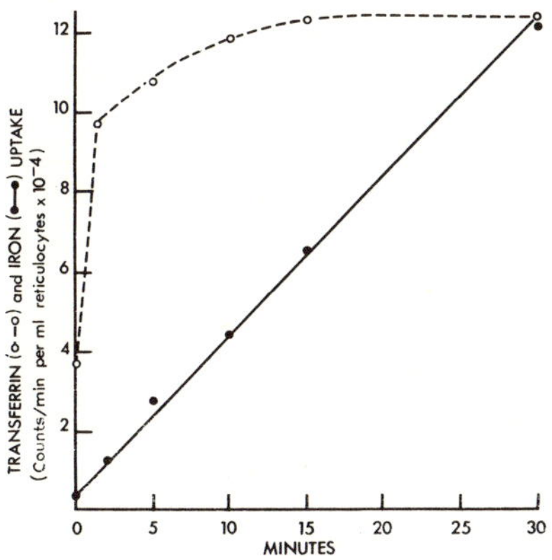

Fig. 1. Transferrin and iron uptake by rabbit reticulocytes. After 30 min incubation transferrin uptake was 0.0052 μM per ml reticulocytes and iron uptake was 0.024 μM per ml reticulocytes.

phases, *viz.* (1) an initial binding on mixing in the cold which represented 20–40% of the maximum uptake obtained on subsequent incubation—the adsorption reaction[13]; (2) a progressive uptake during the first 10–15 min incubation at 37° which was most rapid at first and then gradually slowed—the association reaction[13]; and (3) a plateau or constant level of transferrin bound to the cells after about 15 min incubation. Three measurements of transferrin uptake were made: (1) the amount of adsorbed transferrin, (2) the initial rate of the association reaction determined from the slope of the line joining the ^{125}I values at 0 and 2 min incubation, and (3) the amount of transferrin taken up during the association reaction, obtained by subtracting the 0-min ^{125}I value from the plateau level. None of the inhibitors used affected the amount of transferrin bound during the adsorption phase. Hence this value will not be reported.

The effects of the inhibitors used may be divided into 3 groups, *viz.* (1) no effect on either iron or transferrin uptake, (2) decreased iron uptake but much less effect on transferrin uptake, and (3) approximately the same degree of inhibition of both transferrin and iron uptake.

The inhibitors with no effect on transferrin or iron uptake were sodium malonate in the concentration range 0.25–50 mM and ouabain, 0.05–5 mM (Table I). Further experiments were performed in conjunction with the ouabain experiments to determine whether Na^+ was necessary in the incubation medium to allow transferrin or iron uptake by reticulocytes. Transferrin labeled with ^{125}I and ^{59}Fe dissolved in isotonic NaCl, KCl or LiCl was incubated with reticulocytes washed 3 times with the same solutions. The uptake of iron and transferrin were identical with all three media.

Several inhibitors caused a much greater decrease of iron uptake than of trans-

TABLE I

ACTION OF METABOLIC INHIBITORS WHICH HAD NO EFFECT ON TRANSFERRIN AND IRON UPTAKE BY RETICULOCYTES

Inhibitor	*Final concn. (mM)*	*Uptake (% control value)*		
		Iron	*Transferrin*	
		Rate	*Rate*	*Amount*
Sodium malonate	0.25	99	100	98
	2.5	97	100	97
	25	100	100	110
	50	98	100	100
Ouabain	0.05	99	100	98
	0.5	108	100	97
	1.5	100	98	105
	5.0	101	98	97

TABLE II

ACTION OF METABOLIC INHIBITORS WHICH AFFECTED IRON UPTAKE BY RETICULOCYTES TO A GREATER EXTENT THAN TRANSFERRIN UPTAKE

Inhibitor	*Concentration (mM)*	*Uptake (% control value)*		
		^{59}Fe	*Transferrin*	
		Rate	*Rate*	*Amount*
Rotenone	0.00005	86	98	101
	0.0005	30	98	96
	0.005	14	94	94
	0.01	3	67	80
2,4-Dinitrophenol	0.5	41	90	103
	1.25	31	100	101
	2.5	18	90	75
	5	8	95	72
Oligomycin	0.0125	45	95	90
	0.0250	43	99	92
	0.0625	48	100	95
NaCN	5	61	100	99
	10	30	95	85
	25	20	90	72
	50	16	88	85
NaN_3	5	61	90	100
	10	38	88	100
	25	10	71	46
	50	9	72	51
NaF	5	102	97	105
	10	91	100	98
	25	41	102	101
Cycloheximide	0.5	43	98	105

TABLE III

EFFECT OF INHIBITORS WHICH BLOCKED BOTH TRANSFERRIN AND IRON UPTAKE BY RETICULOCYTES

Inhibitor	*Concentration (mM)*	*Uptake (% control value)*		
		Iron	*Transferrin*	
		Rate	*Rate*	*Amount*
Sodium arsenite	0.1	89	86	97
	0.5	21	37	74
	1.0	18	18	51
	5.0	2	12	17
Iodoacetamide	0.25	100	105	95
	0.5	73	63	101
	1.0	65	75	91
	5.0	2	11	12
N-Ethylmaleimide	0.1	101	94	98
	0.5	89	98	97
	1.0	85	74	94
	2.0	5	2	1
	5.0	0	0	0
PCMB	0.005	100	100	105
	0.05	85	85	95
	0.25	69	81	81
	0.5	55	68	75
	1.0	5	17	22
PCMBS	0.005	105	103	99
	0.05	18	47	48
	0.1	4	5	15
	0.4	3	3	4
Lead acetate	0.05	98	97	101
	0.1	98	95	103
	0.25	91	94	102
	0.5	64	51	56

ferrin uptake (Table II). The most effective was rotenone which partially inhibited iron uptake at a concentration of 50 nM, and almost completely inhibited it at 10 μM, at which concentration there was only a 30 % reduction of transferrin uptake. NaF, NaCN, NaN_3, and 2,4-dinitrophenol at relatively high concentrations produced 60–90 % inhibition of iron uptake, but 0–30 % inhibition of transferrin uptake. The other inhibitors in this group were oligomycin and cycloheximide which both produced about 50 % inhibition of iron uptake without affecting transferrin uptake.

The inhibitors which decreased iron and transferrin uptake to approximately the same degree were sodium arsenite, iodoacetamide, *N*-ethylmaleimide, PCMB, PCMBS and lead acetate (Table III). The first five of these reagents, which are all recognized as sulfhydryl reagents, almost completely inhibited the uptake of transferrin and iron at concentrations of 0.5–5 mM. Lead acetate was tested only at lower concentrations, up to 0.5 mM. When used at concentrations of 0.025 and 0.05 mM iron and transferrin uptake were unaffected but incorporation of ^{59}Fe into heme after 30 min incubation was reduced to 72 and 51 % of the control value, respectively.

TABLE IV

EFFECT OF PRIOR ADDITION OF CYSTEINE OR GLUTATHIONE ON THE INHIBITORY EFFECT OF SULFHYDRYL REAGENTS ON TRANSFERRIN AND IRON UPTAKE BY RETICULOCYTES

Inhibitor	*Concentration (mM)*	*Cysteine concn. (mM)*	*Uptake (% control value)*		
			Iron	*Transferrin*	
			Rate	*Rate*	*Amount*
Iodoacetamide	5	—	4	10	6
	5	5	48	50	81
	5	10	87	96	98
N-Ethylmaleimide	2	—	3	5	6
	2	4	57	58	83
	2	8	92	102	99
PCMB	1	—	5	17	22
	1	2	64	72	55
	1	10	76	81	93
PCMBS	0.4	—	5	12	17
	0.4	2	77	59	95
	0.4	8	89	85	98
Sodium arsenite	5	—	8	8	20
	5	10	6	5	21
	5	20	3	7	18
	5	20*	46	80	87

* Glutathione.

At 0.5 mM iron and transferrin uptake were only reduced by about 40 % but incorporation into heme was reduced by 90 % to 10 % of the control value.

In order to determine whether the inhibitory effects of the sulfhydryl reagents listed above were specific for the binding of transferrin, reticulocytes were incubated with [^{125}I]transferrin and [^{131}I]albumin with and without the inhibitors. The amount of albumin bound by the control cell samples was 5–7 % of the amount of transferrin bound; but whereas the inhibitors blocked the binding of transferrin, they had no effect on the amount of albumin left on the cells after three saline washes.

The effects of iodoacetamide, *N*-ethylmaleimide, PCMB and PCMBS on both iron and transferrin uptake were largely prevented by the prior addition of cysteine in 1–4 times the molar concentration of the inhibitor (Table IV), but not by addition of cysteine after the inhibitors. Inhibition due to sodium arsenite was not reversed by cysteine even when it was used in 20 times the molar concentration of arsenite. However, reduced glutathione in 5 times the molar concentration of arsenite largely reversed its inhibitory effect.

Rate of onset of inhibition by sulfhydryl reagents

The rate at which sulfhydryl reagents produced inhibition was investigated in two ways. In the first, ^{125}I- and ^{59}Fe-labeled transferrin were mixed with PCMB (1 mM), PCMBS (1 mM), sodium arsenite (10 mM), *N*-ethylmaleimide (10 mM) or iodoacetamide (10 mM) and added simultaneously to reticulocytes immediately prior to commencing incubation. Cell samples were removed, washed and counted after 0.5 and 1.0 min incubation and then at 1-min intervals for 20 min. The onset of inhibition was immediate with all of the agents used, so that transferrin and iron uptake were almost completely blocked.

The second method used was to incubate reticulocytes with ^{125}I- and ^{59}Fe-labeled transferrin for 15 min at 37°, then to add the inhibitor and take further cell samples during the succeeding 25 min. The inhibitors used were sodium arsenite (10 mM), iodoacetamide (10 mM) and *N*-ethylmaleimide (5 mM), added with or without cysteine in a concentration of 40 mM. As can be seen from Fig. 2, the addition of the inhibitors alone resulted in the immediate and complete blockage of further iron uptake, but had no effect on the amount of transferrin bound. When cysteine was added with iodoacetamide or *N*-ethylmaleimide, it prevented the inhibition of iron uptake; but cysteine did not affect the inhibition due to sodium arsenite.

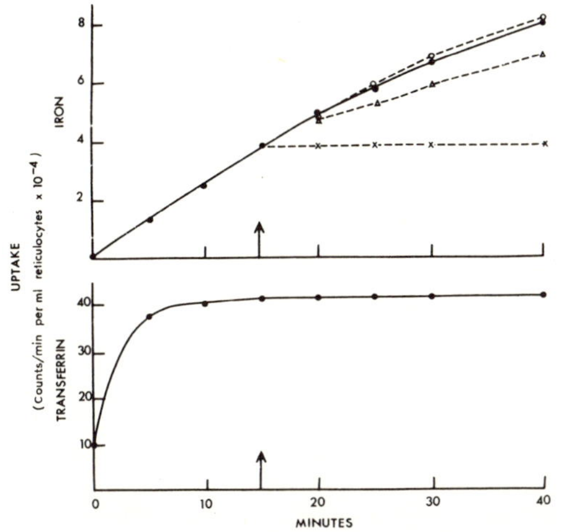

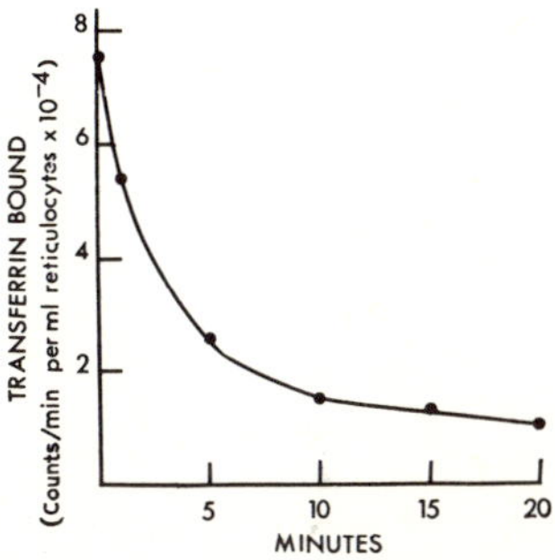

Fig. 2. Effect of metabolic inhibitors on transferrin and iron uptake by rabbit reticulocytes. The inhibitors or inhibitors *plus* cysteine were added at the time shown by the arrows. ●—●, control; ×---×, sodium arsenite (10 mM), iodoacetamide (10 mM), *N*-ethylmaleimide (5 mM); △---△, iodoacetamide (10 mM) *plus* cysteine (40 mM); ○---○, *N*-ethylmaleimide (5 mM) *plus* cysteine (40 mM). None of the inhibitors with or without cysteine affected the amount of transferrin bound, and the results for transferrin uptake with all treatments were the same as the control.

Fig. 3. Transferrin release from rabbit reticulocytes. Reticulocytes containing [^{125}I]transferrin were washed in the cold, then reincubated for different times in rabbit plasma and the amount of [^{125}I]transferrin remaining on the cells was measured.

Effect of inhibitors on transferrin release from reticulocytes

When reticulocytes were incubated with [^{125}I]transferrin, washed and reincubated in rabbit plasma the bound transferrin was released into the incubation medium, at first quickly and then more slowly (Fig. 3). Two measurements of the release process were made, (1) the initial rate of release calculated from the difference between

TABLE V

EFFECT OF METABOLIC INHIBITORS WITH OR WITHOUT THE PRIOR ADDITION OF CYSTEINE ON THE RELEASE OF TRANSFERRIN FROM RETICULOCYTES

Inhibitor	*Concentration (mM)*	*Cysteine concn. (mM)*	*Transferrin release (% control value)*	
			Initial	*Amount after 20 min*
Sodium arsenite	4	—	4	13
	10	—	5	10
	10	40	99	97
Iodoacetamide	4	—	65	71
	10	—	29	61
	10	40	85	105
N-Ethylmaleimide	2	—	4	10
	5	—	3	6
	5	20	125	139
NaCN	20	—	91	87
NaF	10	—	100	104
	20	—	86	99
NaN_3	20	—	85	92
2,4-Dinitrophenol	5	—	85	87
	10	—	74	73
Rotenone	0.0005	—	107	104
	0.005	—	99	104
	0.01	—	103	103

the amount of [^{125}I]transferrin free from the cells at 0 and at 2 min incubation, and (2) the amount of transferrin released after 20 min incubation, the difference between the 0- and the 20-min values for cell-free transferrin. The effects of several inhibitors on these two measurements of the release process are summarized in Table V. Sodium arsenite (10 mM), *N*-ethylmaleimide (5 mM) and, to a lesser extent, iodoacetamide (10 mM) inhibited transferrin release from the reticulocytes; but this effect was reversed by the addition of cysteine in 4 times the molar concentration of the inhibitor. Indeed the addition of cysteine along with *N*-ethylmaleimide led to a more rapid and greater release of transferrin than in the control where no inhibitor or *N*-ethylmaleimide was used. NaCN, NaF, NaN_3 and rotenone had very little effect on transferrin release, while 2,4-dinitrophenol had only a relatively small effect.

The effect of cysteine on transferrin release from reticulocytes was investigated by incubating reticulocytes with [^{125}I]transferrin for 30 min, washing them 4 times and then reincubating in Hanks' solution or Hanks' solution containing 0.1, 1 and 10 mM cysteine. The rate of release of transferrin from the reticulocytes was the same with all mixtures, whether or not cysteine was present.

DISCUSSION

The inhibitors which affected iron and/or transferrin uptake may be broadly classified into two groups, (1) those which inhibited iron uptake much more than transferrin uptake (Table II), and (2) those which inhibited iron and transferrin uptake to approximately the same degree (Table III). All of the inhibitors of the first group, with the exception of cycloheximide and NaF act mainly on oxidative metabolism. Cycloheximide and NaF inhibit protein synthesis in reticulocytes[14]. At concentrations of rotenone up to 0.005 mM; 2,4-dinitrophenol, 1.25 mM; CN^- and N_3^-, 10 mM; F^-, 25 mM and oligomycin 0.0625 mM there was inhibition of iron uptake with little or no effect on transferrin uptake. Hence the reduced rate of iron uptake was not a consequence of a primary effect on transferrin uptake, but was due to a decreased rate of release of iron from transferrin and its uptake by the cell. The mechanism of this latter process is not known, but on the basis of the effect of the inhibitors of Table II, it appears likely that it depends on the activity of the mitochondrial electron transfer chain.

The inhibitor effective at lowest concentration was rotenone which blocks electron transfer between NADH and cytochrome *b* but does not affect electron transfer from succinate to cytochrome *b* (ref. 15). Rotenone has been shown to block O_2 consumption of liver slices and liver mitochondria at approx. 0.001 mM (ref. 16), a concentration at which it was effective against iron uptake by reticulocytes.

Oligomycin, like rotenone, inhibits NADH-linked oxidation much more effectively than succinate oxidation[17]. In contrast to the above two substances, malonate, which inhibits succinate dehydrogenase, had no effect on iron uptake at concentrations as high as 50 mM. Such concentrations have been shown to block rabbit reticulocyte succinate dehydrogenase[18]. Hence it appears likely that iron uptake by reticulocytes is in some way dependent on NADH-linked electron transfer, but is independent of succinate-linked electron transfer.

Iron uptake ceases as reticulocytes change to mature erythrocytes. One of the changes which occurs during this process is the loss of mitochondria[19] and of oxidative metabolism which occurs in mitochondria[18]. Dependence of iron uptake on mitochondrial function, as suggested above, would explain this loss of the capacity to take up iron as reticulocytes mature. The mechanism whereby mitochondrial function is linked to iron uptake is uncertain. For several reasons it seems highly unlikely, however, that the mitochondria serve only as a source of available energy in the form of high energy compounds such as ATP. Firstly, several of the inhibitors of Table II almost completely blocked iron uptake after preincubation with reticulocytes for only 15 min, in which time little depletion of cellular ATP would have occurred. Secondly, the evidence for NADH-linked but not succinate-linked oxidation as the source of the energy for iron uptake suggests a greater specificity than would be found if ATP or a similar compound were the only requirement for iron uptake. Thirdly, mature cells, although they have a somewhat lower concentration of ATP than reticulocytes, do have a ready source of ATP in glycolysis, yet they do not take up iron; and iron uptake by reticulocytes was not inhibited by concentrations of F^- which block glycolysis[20]. Hence it appears likely that iron uptake by reticulocytes is closely linked to the mitochondrial respiratory chain and is not simply dependent on respiration for a supply of ATP.

All of the inhibitors which blocked transferrin uptake to a similar degree to that of iron uptake, except lead acetate, are sulfhydryl reagents. Since transferrin uptake must occur prior to iron uptake by reticulocytes the effects of these substances on iron uptake can probably be explained by the blocking of transferrin uptake. The sulfhydryl reagents can also inhibit respiration[21], so the possibility that some of their effect on iron uptake may be due to such a cause cannot be excluded. Sulfhydryl reagents have been shown to react with the erythrocyte membrane, and thereby to affect glucose and cation transfer[22, 23]. Their effect on transferrin uptake is probably also produced at the cell membrane. This is likely because of the relative impermeability of the erythrocyte cell membrane to PCMB and more especially to PCMBS to which it is almost impermeable[22]. These two reagents had an effect similar to that of the other sulfhydryl reagents, and produced their effect just as quickly, as shown by the inhibition of transferrin uptake when the reagents were added to the reticulocytes simultaneously with the transferrin.

The most obvious explanation of the inhibition of transferrin uptake by sulfhydryl reagents is that membrane sulfhydryl groups are involved in the binding of transferrin by the cells. The reversal of the effect of the sulfhydryl reagents with cysteine and glutathione could be taken as evidence to support this. However, if such were the case it would be expected that the addition of the reagents to reticulocytes which had previously taken up transferrin would cause the release of the bound transferrin. However, the opposite effect was found: transferrin release was inhibited. It may also be considered that transferrin binding by reticulocytes involved sulfhydryl–disulfide interchange, as has been postulated for the binding of vasopressin to toad bladder cells[24], and that sulfhydryl reagents act by stabilizing the resulting bonds between transferrin and the cell membrane. However, the bonds should be split by cysteine, leading to an increase in the rate of transferrin release. Such an effect was not observed when cysteine was added to the reincubation solution. It therefore seems more likely that the sulfhydryl reagents act by producing a change in the structure of the reticulocyte membrane which in turn reduces transferrin (and iron) uptake and release.

A possibility which must be considered is that during the process of transferrin uptake and release by reticulocytes the transferrin molecule actually passes deeply into or through the cell membrane. The movement of the transferrin molecules would probably be due simply to diffusion. There is no conclusive evidence that transferrin uptake or release is dependent on cellular metabolism, since the reagents of Table II had little effect on transferrin uptake at concentrations which almost certainly largely or completely blocked both glycolysis and oxidative metabolism. The activation energy of transferrin uptake by rabbit reticulocytes, 12 kcal/mole (ref. 13), is of a level which would be expected for a process of restricted diffusion. The action of the sulfhydryl reagents could be simply to produce an alteration of the reticulocyte membrane which reduces its permeability to transferrin either from outside to inside (uptake) or inside to outside (release). Other facts which appear to be more in keeping with passage of transferrin molecules through the membrane rather than binding to receptors on its surface are the relatively long mean residence time of transferrin molecules on the rabbit reticulocyte (10 min) (unpublished results) and the fact that the rate of release of transferrin from the cell is independent of the presence or concentration of transferrin in the surrounding medium[13].

On the basis of the above discussion a useful working hypothesis for the uptake of transferrin and iron by rabbit reticulocytes may be as follows. Transferrin molecules diffuse well into or through the reticulocyte plasma membrane carrying iron to the surface of the mitochondria. Here the transferrin is bound to the mitochondria; and due to the proton pumping activity of mitochondria[25], which is dependent on an intact respiratory chain, protons are donated to transferrin causing release of its iron. The iron then passes into the mitochondria, possibly as a complex with ATP and ascorbic acid[26], or with NADH[27]. Either complex would lead to reduction of the iron to the ferrous state, in which it is incorporated into protoporphyrin to form heme under the action of the enzyme iron chelatase which is found in mitochondria[28]. Transferrin molecules are released from the mitochondria after donating their iron and diffuse out of the reticulocyte in the iron-free form.

The effects of three inhibitors (ouabain, cycloheximide and lead acetate) require special comment. Firstly ouabain, although used up to very high concentrations, was found to have no effect on transferrin or iron uptake. This suggests that the ouabain-sensitive membrane ATPase is not involved in iron uptake. However, the present results are contrary to those of WISE AND ARCHDEACON[29] who found a partial inhibition of iron uptake by rabbit reticulocytes with 1 and 100 μM ouabain. The reason for this difference is unknown. The mechanism of the action of cycloheximide on iron uptake is uncertain. It has been shown, however, that cycloheximide inhibits heme as well as globin synthesis by rabbit reticulocytes[30]. Possibly the effect on iron uptake is related to, or is a consequence of inhibition of heme synthesis. The latter of these two possibilities seems unlikely, however, when considered in relation to the effects of lead acetate. This also inhibits heme synthesis[31], but had little effect on iron uptake until very high concentrations were used. At these concentrations transferrin uptake was also reduced. It is possible that at the higher concentration the lead reacted with the reticulocyte membrane to produce changes which led to reduction of transferrin and consequently of iron uptake.

ACKNOWLEDGEMENTS

This work was supported by grants from the Australian Research Grants Committee and the National Institutes of Health (5 R05 TW-00212-02), and was performed during tenure of a CSIRO senior postgraduate studentship by E.B.

REFERENCES

1 J. H. JANDL, J. K. INMAN, R. L. SIMMONS AND D. W. ALLEN, *J. Clin. Invest.*, 38 (1959) 161.
2 J. H. JANDL AND J. H. KATZ, *J. Clin. Invest.*, 42 (1963) 314.
3 E. H. MORGAN AND C.-B. LAURELL, *Brit. J. Haematol.*, 9 (1963) 471.
4 E. H. MORGAN, *Brit. J. Haematol.*, 10 (1964) 442.
5 E. H. MORGAN, *J. Physiol. London*, 171 (1964) 26.
6 E. BAKER, D. C. SHAW AND E. H. MORGAN, *Biochemistry*, 7 (1968) 1371.
7 A. S. MCFARLANE, *J. Clin. Invest.*, 42 (1963) 346.
8 J. H. HANKS AND R. E. WALLACE, *Proc. Soc. Exptl. Biol. Med.*, 71 (1949) 196.
9 E. H. MORGAN, E. R. HUEHNS AND C. A. FINCH, *Am. J. Physiol.*, 210 (1966) 579.
10 G. R. KINGSLEY, *J. Lab. Clin. Med.*, 27 (1942) 840.
11 E. H. MORGAN AND G. CARTER, *Australasian Ann. Med.*, 9 (1960) 209.
12 S. THUNELL, *Clin. Chim. Acta*, 11 (1965) 321.
13 E. BAKER AND E. H. MORGAN, *Biochemistry*, in the press.

14 S.-Y. Lin, R. D. Mosteller and B. Hardesty, *J. Mol. Biol.*, 21 (1966) 51.
15 M. E. Pullman and G. Schatz, *Ann. Rev. Biochem.*, 36 (1967) 539.
16 P. E. Lindahl and K. E. Oberg, *Exptl. Cell Res.*, 23 (1961) 228.
17 H. A. Lardy, D. Johnson and W. C. McMurray, *Arch. Biochem. Biophys.*, 78 (1958) 587.
18 D. Rubenstein, P. Ottolenghi and O. F. Denstedt, *Can. J. Biochem. Physiol.*, 34 (1956) 222.
19 C. F. Simpson and J. M. Kling, *J. Cell Biol.*, 36 (1968) 103.
20 M. Maizels, *J. Physiol. London*, 112 (1951) 59.
21 J. H. Quastel, in R. M. Hochster and J. H. Quastel, *Metabolic Inhibitors*, Vol. 2, Academic Press, New York, 1963, p. 473.
22 J. Vansteveninck, R. I. Weed and A. Rothstein, *J. Gen. Physiol.*, 48 (1965) 617.
23 A. F. Rega, A. Rothstein and R. I. Weed, *J. Cellular Comp. Physiol.*, 70 (1967) 45.
24 I. L. Schwartz, H. Rasmussen, M. A. Schoessler, L. Silver and C. T. O. Fong, *Proc. Natl. Acad. Sci. U.S.*, 46 (1960) 1288.
25 P. Mitchell and J. Moyle, *Nature*, 208 (1965) 147.
26 A. Mazur, S. Green and A. Carleton, *J. Biol. Chem.*, 235 (1960) 595.
27 M. Gutman, R. Margalit and A. Schejter, *Biochemistry*, 7 (1968) 2778.
28 M. S. Jones and O. T. G. Jones, *Biochem. Biophys. Res. Commun.*, 31 (1968) 977.
29 W. C. Wise and J. W. Archdeacon, *Proc. Soc. Exptl. Biol. Med.*, 118 (1965) 653.
30 A. I. Grayzel, J. E. Fuhr and I. M. London, *Biochem. Biophys. Res. Commun.*, 28 (1967) 705.
31 M. Gajdos-Torok, *Compt. Rend. Soc. Biol.*, 154 (1960) 508.

Factors Affecting the Synthesis of Transferrin by Rat Tissue Slices*

E. H. MORGAN

The concentration of transferrin in the plasma varies in highly predictable ways in humans at different stages of the life cycle and in certain diseases (1) and in laboratory animals under different experimental conditions. In the rat and rabbit, for instance, hemolytic and iron deficiency anemias, cobalt or thyroxine administration, and exposure to reduced atmospheric pressure are accompanied by a rise in plasma transferrin level, while transfusional polycythemia, fasting, or treatment with propylthiouracil are associated with a fall in this level (2–5). It is probable that the changes in transferrin concentration are the result of alterations in the rate of synthesis of the protein, but direct experimental evidence on this is lacking. There is evidence for transferrin synthesis by liver, spleen, bone marrow, lymph nodes, thymus, and peritoneal macrophages in the rat (6, 7) and by some of these tissues in addition to the liver in mouse, rabbit, guinea pig, monkey, and humans (7–11). However, the rate of transferrin synthesis in tissues other than the liver has not been measured. Hence, the relative importance

* This work was supported by a grant from the Australian Research Grants Committee and by Grant 5 R05 TW00212 from the National Institutes of Health.

of the other tissues for transferrin synthesis when compared with the liver is uncertain.

This work aims to determine the major sites of transferrin synthesis in the rat and then to study the effect of various factors, known to influence plasma transferrin concentration, on transferrin synthesis *in vitro* by tissue slices from the more important organs.

MATERIALS AND METHODS

Animals—Male rats of an inbred Wistar strain, 3 months old, weighing 180 to 220 g, were used. Except where indicated, they were fed a high protein laboratory rat diet and water *ad libitum*, and were not fasted prior to the experiments.

Chemicals—L-^{14}C-Leucine with a specific activity of 34 μCi per mmole was purchased from the Radiochemical Centre (Amersham, England). Cycloheximide was obtained from Sigma. Actinomycin D was a gift from Merck. Human transferrin was from Behringwerke (Marburg-Lahn, Germany).

Purification of Rat Proteins and Preparation of Antisera—Rat albumin, transferrin, and γG-globulin were purified by ammonium sulfate precipitation, ion exchange chromatography, and zone electrophoresis as previously described (12) except that the chromatography step was performed with DEAE-Sephadex and a gradient from 0.01 M Tris buffer (pH 8.5) to 0.1 M Tris buffer (pH 7.5). Rabbits were immunized against these proteins and against human transferrin by the intramuscular injection of 3 or 4 doses each of 10 mg of protein dissolved in 1.0 ml of complete Freund's adjuvant, given at 3- to 4-week intervals. Antisera were obtained by bleeding the rabbits from a marginal ear vein. When examined by immunoelectrophoresis against rat serum the antisera each showed only one arc against rat albumin, transferrin, and γG and human transferrin, respectively. The antisera were standardized by quantitative immunoprecipitation (13). No cross-reaction was demonstrable by double diffusion in agar between rat transferrin and anti-human transferrin or between human transferrin and anti-rat transferrin.

Incorporation Studies in Vivo—^{14}C-Leucine, 8 μCi, was injected under ether anesthesia into the femoral vein exposed by a small incision on the inner side of the thigh. The rats were then allowed to recover from the anesthetic. Twenty minutes after the injections, they were reanesthetized with ether and perfused with chilled calcium-free Locke-citrate solution. The liver, spleen, kidneys, small intestine, and lungs were then removed and placed in ice-cold calcium-free Locke-citrate. The femurs were also removed, their ends were cut off, and the bone marrow was blown into 0.25 M sucrose. The organs were quickly dried with filter paper, weighed, and homogenized in

3.0 times their weight of 0.25 M sucrose with a Potter-Elvehjem homogenizer. The suspension was centrifuged at 18,000 × *g* for 10 min. The supernatant was recentrifuged at 105,000 × *g* for 45 min to obtain a microsome pellet. This pellet was washed once with 0.25 M sucrose and was then suspended with homogenization in 0.6% sodium deoxycholate in 0.05 M Tris buffer, pH 8.0 (1 ml per g of original tissue weight). After standing at 4° for 4 hours, the suspension was centrifuged at 105,000 × *g* for 2 hours. The supernatant solution was then "cleared" (14) by the addition of 0.05 ml of human serum followed by 1.0 ml of anti-human transferrin, mixing and incubation at 37° for 1 hour, refrigeration overnight, and centrifugation at 4,000 × *g* for 20 min. Aliquots of the cleared supernatant were then precipitated in the same way with 1.0-ml volumes of anti-rat albumin, transferrin, and γG-globulin. The precipitates were washed three times with ice-cold 0.15 M NaCl solution, and the radioactivity was counted.

Incorporation Studies in Vitro With Tissue Slices—Rats were killed by a blow on the head. Their liver, and other organs when required (spleen, femoral bone marrow, kidney, small intestine), were quickly removed and placed in ice-cold Krebs-Henseleit bicarbonate buffer (15) containing glucose (2 mg per ml) but from which the KH_2PO_4 was omitted. The organs were blotted and weighed, and slices 0.5 mm thick were cut by hand (16). The slices were washed in the Krebs-Henseleit buffer and blotted with filter paper; approximately 300-mg quantities were then weighed and placed in 25-ml conical flasks, to which 3 ml of the Krebs-Henseleit buffer containing L-amino

TABLE I

Incorporation of ^{14}C into proteins extracted from microsome fractions of rat tissues 20 min after intravenous administration of ^{14}C-leucine

Each value is the mean from 5 animals ± standard error of the mean.

Tissue	^{14}C incorporation		
	Albumin	Transferrin	γG-Globulin
	cpm/organ		
Liver	25,100 ± 5,200	4,600 ± 1,400	1,825 ± 480
Spleen	57 ± 14	139 ± 25	1,828 ± 540
Kidney	140 ± 62	90 ± 11	64 ± 6.3
Intestine	88 ± 22	67 ± 7.6	4,580 ± 260
Lung	23 ± 5.4	69 ± 11	970 ± 320
Bone marrow	20 ± 5.8	45 ± 5.1	460 ± 110

acids and ^{14}C-leucine, approximately 0.5 Ci per flask, were added. The millimolar concentrations of amino acids were alanine, 0.40; arginine, 0.15; aspartic acid, 0.20; asparagine, 0.30; cysteine, 0.10; cystine, 0.05; glutamic acid, 0.20; glutamine, 0.20; glycine, 0.40; hydroxyproline, 0.20; histidine, 0.10; isoleucine, 0.10; leucine, 0.20; lysine, 0.35; methionine, 0.05; phenylalanine, 0.10; proline, 0.15; serine, 0.25; threonine, 0.20; tryptophan, 0.15; tyrosine, 0.10; valine, 0.15. The flasks were gassed with 95% O_2-5% CO_2, stoppered, and incubated at 37° with shaking at 120 oscillations per min in a water bath. Unless otherwise specified, incubation was performed for 2 hours. The slices were then homogenized in a Potter-Elvehjem homogenizer together with their incubation solution and 1.0 ml of leucine solution (0.5 g per liter) in 0.15 M NaCl solution containing 1 mM merthiolate. The suspension was treated by ultrasonic dispersion for 1 min and centrifuged at 20,000 × g for 30 min. The supernatant solution was cleared as before with human serum and anti-human transferrin. Aliquots of the cleared solution were then precipitated with anti-rat albumin, transferrin or γG-globulin as described above; the precipitates were washed three times with 0.15 M NaCl solution and counted.

Measurement of Radioactivity—The immunoprecipitates were dissolved in 0.2 ml of Hyamine hydroxide, transferred to counting vials with 10 ml of scintillation solution (17), and counted in a Nuclear-Chicago liquid scintillation counter. Quenching correction was made by the channels ratio method.

Analytical Methods—Protein was determined by a biuret method (18). Serum iron concentration and total iron-binding capacity, which was used to measure transferrin concentration, and tissue non-heme iron were measured by published methods (19, 20). The hematocrit was measured by the microhematocrit procedure and hemoglobin as oxyhemoglobin.

RESULTS

Incorporation in Vivo of ^{14}C-Leucine into Microsomes of Different Organs—The incorporation of ^{14}C-leucine into the albumin, transferrin, and γG-globulin immunoprecipitates from the extracts of the microsome fractions of several organs removed from five rats 20 min after the intravenous injection of the labeled amino acid is shown in Table I. Large incorporation into the albumin and transferrin precipitates occurred only in the liver. Compared with incorporation by liver, the incorporation of ^{14}C into the transferrin precipitates of spleen, lung, and bone marrow were very low but they were significantly higher ($p > 0.05$) than the incorporation into the albumin precipitates of these organs. No significant difference ($p < 0.05$) was found between the incorporation into albumin and transferrin precipitates of kidney and small intestine. The ^{14}C-leucine was incorporated into γG-globulin precipitates of liver, spleen, intestine, bone marrow, and lung, but not of kidney. Microsome fractions were also isolated from testes and heart of two of the rats. Less than 50 cpm of ^{14}C were found in both organs of both rats for the immunoprecipitates of the three proteins.

Incorporation of ^{14}C-Leucine into Transferrin by Slices from Different Rat Tissues—Slices of liver, spleen, kidney, and small intestine, and suspensions of femoral bone marrow from four rats were incubated with ^{14}C-leucine for 2 hours. Incorporation into the albumin precipitates from the liver slices was 40 to 120 times as great as with the other tissues (Table II). In the case of transferrin, however, relatively high incorporations per g of tissue were found with spleen and bone marrow as well as liver,

TABLE II

Incorporation of ^{14}C into albumin, transferrin, and γG-globulin by rat tissue slices during 2 hours of incubation with ^{14}C-leucine

Each value is the mean from 4 animals ± standard error of the mean.

Tissue	Incorporation		
	Albumin	Transferrin	γG-Globulin
	cpm/g		
Liver	15,500 ± 1,700	1,920 ± 260	820 ± 360
Spleen	230 ± 14	2,130 ± 440	24,800 ± 2,400
Kidney	260 ± 45	61 ± 20	79 ± 21
Intestine	250 ± 43	100 ± 22	18,400 ± 4,500
Bone marrow	370 ± 34	2,200 ± 740	21,300 ± 2,600

but very low values were obtained with kidney and small intestine. Incorporations into the γG-globulin precipitates were greatest with spleen, intestine, and bone marrow; intermediate with liver; and very low with kidney tissue.

Investigation of Incorporation Method in Vitro with Liver, Spleen, and Bone Marrow—The above mentioned experiments indicated that incorporation of ^{14}C-leucine into transferrin occurred in spleen, bone marrow, and possibly also lung, as well as liver; but that in the living rat the liver was probably the most important organ for transferrin synthesis. Further experiments were then performed with liver and spleen slices to determine whether incorporation of ^{41}C-leucine into transferrin could be used as a measure of transferrin synthesis. Incorporation into albumin by liver, and into γG-globulin by spleen were also measured for comparison with the transferrin results.

The effect of incubation time on incorporation of ^{14}C-leucine was investigated by suspending liver and spleen slices in incubation solution at 4° and then homogenizing the mixture either without incubation or after 1, 2, or 3 hours of incubation at 37°. There was a progressive increase of incorporation into transferrin as well as into albumin and γG-globulin during the period of incubation (Fig. 1).

The incorporation of ^{14}C-leucine into transferrin and albumin by liver slices and into transferrin and γG-globulin by spleen slices was reduced to less than 22% of the control values by including potassium cyanide (5 mM), 2,4-dinitrophenol (5 mM), sodium arsenite (5 mM), or cycloheximide (125 μg per ml) in the incubation medium. Actinomycin D, on the other hand, in a concentration of 2.5 μg per ml had no effect on ^{14}C-leucine incorporation.

The effect of leucine concentration in the incubation solution on ^{14}C-leucine incorporation into the proteins was investigated by incubating liver and spleen slices in the incubation medium containing the standard concentrations of all the amino acids except leucine, and with increasing concentrations of leucine.

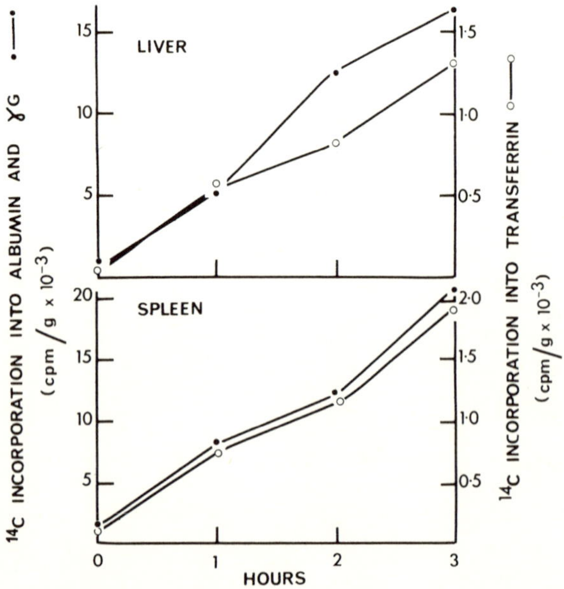

FIG. 1. Effect of duration of incubation on incorporation of ^{14}C-leucine into albumin and transferrin by liver slices and into transferrin and γG-globulin by spleen slices.

Incorporation of radioactivity decreased as the leucine concentration of the incubation solution was raised but the ratio of the counts incorporated into transferrin and albumin by liver, and into transferrin and γG-globulin by spleen, remained constant (Fig. 2).

Effect of Anemia, Polycythemia, and Level of Iron Stores on Incorporation of *^{14}C-Leucine into Transferrin*—Acute hemolytic anemia was produced by the intraperitoneal injection of 20 mg of phenylhydrazine hydrochloride in 0.9% NaCl solution, neutralized with NaOH, into rats 5 days before they were killed. Chronic hemolytic anemia was produced by the intra-

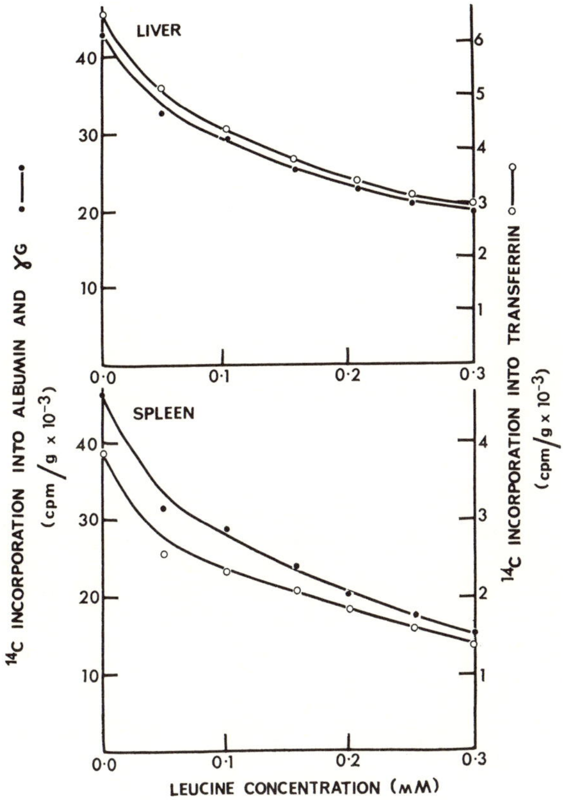

FIG. 2. Effect of leucine concentration of incubation solution on ^{14}C-leucine incorporation into albumin and transferrin by liver slices and into transferrin and γG-globulin by spleen slices. The concentration of ^{14}C-leucine was maintained constant.

TABLE III

Incorporation of ^{14}C-leucine into plasma proteins by liver and spleen slices from rats given various prior treatments

Each value is the mean from 4 animals expressed as percentages of corresponding mean values from 4 untreated control rats ± standard error of the mean. See text for details of treatments.

Treatment	Weight		Incorporation			
			Liver		Spleen	
	Liver	Spleen	Albumin	Transferrin	Transferrin	γG-Globulin
	% control		% control		% control	
Phenylhydrazine	113 ± 4	254[a] ± 10	102 ± 4	103 ± 33	89 ± 9	85 ± 11
Methyl cellulose	140[a] ± 3	490[a] ± 23	99 ± 6	113 ± 27	138 ± 24	118 ± 18
Bleeding	73[a] ± 2	174[a] ± 6	131 ± 16	263[a] ± 48	153[a] ± 10	91 ± 9
Iron-dextran	115 ± 8	140 ± 19	79 ± 11	110 ± 7	93 ± 4	88 ± 10
Transfusion	116 ± 10	171[a] ± 12	122 ± 16	59[a] ± 8	112 ± 4	86 ± 8
Thyroxine	102 ± 6	143[a] ± 14	252[a] ± 13	166[a] ± 6	143 ± 25	82 ± 18
Propylthiouracil	86 ± 7	69[a] ± 9	59[a] ± 2	43[a] ± 2	138 ± 33	120 ± 12

[a] Significant difference from mean control value ($p < 0.05$).

peritoneal injection of 2.5 ml of 2.5% methyl cellulose in 0.9% NaCl solution three times per week for 4 weeks. The incorporation of ^{14}C-leucine into albumin, transferrin, and γG-globulin per unit weight of tissue from the anemic rats showed no significant difference from the controls (Table III). The liver weights were moderately increased and the weights of the spleens greatly increased in both forms of anemia. There was no difference in mean body weights between treated and control animals. Hence, the total capacity for ^{14}C-leucine incorporation into transferrin may have been enhanced due to the increase in size of the organs.

Iron deficiency anemia was produced by twice weekly bleeding of 2 to 3 ml of blood by cardiac puncture of rats fed an iron-deficient milk diet (2) for 2 months prior to the incorporation studies. Control rats were fed the same diet supplemented with iron and were not bled. When the rats were killed for the preparation of liver and spleen slices, the bled rats were anemic (mean hematocrit 15% compared with 42% for the controls), with decreased mean corpuscular hemoglobin concentrations (means, 26% and 35%) and elevated plasma total iron-binding capacity levels (means, 790 μg/100 ml and 415 μg/100 ml). The mean non-heme iron concentrations of the anemic and control rats were 14 and 56 μg per g, wet weight, for liver and 26 and 225 for spleen. The incorporation of ^{14}C-leucine into transferrin by liver slices was greatly increased, and that into albumin was increased to a lesser extent in the anemic rats. Incorporation into transferrin by spleen slices was also increased, but that into γG-globulin showed no change (Table III).

Marked iron overload was produced by injection of iron-dextran intramuscularly into rats in a daily dose of 20 mg of iron for 10 consecutive days. The last injection was given 2 months before the incorporation experiments. Control rats were given intramuscular injections of 0.9% sodium chloride solution. At the time of death, the iron-overloaded rats had similar hemoglobin and total iron-binding capacity levels to the controls, but the mean liver non-heme iron concentrations for treated and control rats were 4670 and 42 μg per g, wet weight, and the spleen values were 3000 and 155 μg per g, wet weight, respectively. However, there was no significant difference in the incorporation of ^{14}C-leucine into transferrin and albumin or γG-globulin by liver and spleen slices from the treated and control rats (Table III).

Polycythemia was induced by the single intraperitoneal injection of 16 ml of washed and freshly obtained rat erythrocytes suspended in 0.9% NaCl solution (hematocrit 40%). Controls received 16 ml of 0.9% NaCl solution intraperitoneally. It has been shown that erythrocytes are rapidly absorbed from the peritoneum in the rat and then survive normally in the circulating blood (21, 22). Incorporation studies were performed with liver and spleen slices 4 days after the injections. Administration of the cells caused a rise in the mean hematocrit value from 43% (controls) to 71% and depression of incorporation of ^{14}C into transferrin but not into albumin or γG-globulin by liver or spleen slices (Table III).

Effect of Thyroid Activity on ^{14}C-Leucine Incorporation into Transferrin—Rats were given daily subcutaneous injections of 0.1 mg of L-thyroxine dissolved in 0.9% NaCl-0.05 N NaOH for 4 weeks or daily doses of 200 mg of propylthiouracil suspended in 0.25 ml of olive oil by stomach tube for the same period of time. These doses have been shown to produce marked changes in oxygen consumption and in plasma total iron-binding capacity in the rat (4). Control rats received no treatment. Treatment with thyroxine resulted in increased incorporation of ^{14}C into transferrin and albumin by liver slices but no significant change in incorporation by spleen slices. Propylthiouracil produced decreased incorporation by liver slices and again no significant change with spleen slices (Table III).

Effect of Fasting—Groups of 4 rats were fasted for 1, 2, 3, and 4 days but were given free access to water. Control animals were fed the normal diet plus water freely. ^{14}C-Leucine incorporation measurements were made with liver slices only. Fasting was associated with a progressive loss of body weight of approximately 10 g per day, and also a loss of liver weight from a mean of 4.6% body weight in the controls to 3.3 to 3.4% of body weight in the fasted animals. Incorporation of ^{14}C-leucine into albumin and transferrin per g of liver slices also fell during the first 2 to 3 days of fasting. On the third and fourth days, this fall was greater for incorporation into albumin than into transferrin (Table IV).

Effect of Exposure to Reduced Atmospheric Pressure—Groups of rats were exposed in a decompression chamber to an atmospheric pressure of 380 mm of Hg for times varying from 1 to 14 days while receiving normal diet and drinking water. The animals showed a small loss of body weight and a proportionate loss of liver weight during the first few days of exposure. Incorporation of ^{14}C-leucine into transferrin by liver slices showed a significant increase relative to control values after 24-hour exposure to reduced pressure, but there was no further increase thereafter. On the other hand, incorporation into albumin showed a significant decrease after 3 days of low pressure and decreased even more with further decompression (Table V). The capacity of spleen slices from the treated rats to incorporate the ^{14}C-leucine into γG and transferrin did not differ significantly from that of the controls.

In a second experiment, groups of rats were again exposed to an atmospheric pressure of 380 mm of Hg for 1 to 4 days and were given drinking water but no food. Control animals maintained at ambient pressure were similarly fasted. Body weight loss was very similar in the rats exposed to low pressure and the controls, but liver weight decreased less during the first 3 days of exposure to reduced pressure than it did in the control animals. The incorporation of ^{14}C-leucine into transferrin by liver slices of rats in the low pressure group relative to the controls increased progressively with the duration of treatment and after 4 days was approximately twice as great as in the control rats. In contrast, incorporation into albumin was not significantly different in the rats exposed to reduced pressure from that in the fasted control animals (Table VI).

The mechanism of the effect of exposure to reduced atmospheric pressure on ^{14}C incorporation into transferrin was investigated by the use of actinomycin D. Four groups of 12 rats each were used. The first group was given actinomycin D dissolved in 0.9% NaCl solution intraperitoneally in two doses of 50 μg/100 g of body weight, one 2 hours before and the second immediately before placing the animals in the decompression chamber for 24 hours. The second group of animals was subjected to decompression without prior treatment with actinomycin. Group 3 was kept at ambient pressure for 24 hours after receiving the same doses of actinomycin as Group 1; and Group 4 was kept at ambient pressure without being given actinomycin. All of the rats were fasted during the experiment. It was found that actinomycin had no effect on the incorporation of ^{14}C into albumin or transferrin by slices

TABLE IV

Effect of fasting on body and liver weights and incorporation of ^{14}C-leucine into albumin and transferrin by liver slices

Each value is the mean from 4 animals expressed as a percentage of the mean from 4 nonfasted control rats ± standard error of the mean.

Duration of fasting	Body weight	Weight loss	Liver weight	Incorporation	
				Albumin	Transferrin
days	*g*		*% body wt.*	*% control*	
1	182 ± 5.1	14.4 ± 0.75	3.4 ± 0.07	74[a] ± 10	73[a] ± 8.9
2	172 ± 7.5	25.7 ± 2.6	3.4 ± 0.22	70[a] ± 15	59[a] ± 13
3	159 ± 6.7	32.5 ± 2.0	3.3 ± 0.11	31[a] ± 4.2	45[a] ± 5.2
4	153 ± 6.7	43.3 ± 3.4	3.3 ± 0.04	31[a] ± 6.0	58[a] ± 7.8

[a] Significant difference from mean control value ($p < 0.05$).

TABLE V

Effect of exposure to a pressure of 380 mm of Hg on incorporation of ^{14}C-leucine into plasma proteins by liver slices

The rats were fed the standard diet. Each incorporation value is the mean from 4 animals expressed as a percentage of the corresponding mean value obtained from 4 rats maintained at ambient pressure ± standard error of the mean.

Duration of exposure	Body weight	Weight loss	Incorporation into liver	
			Albumin	Transferrin
days	*g*		*% control*	
1	185 ± 12	6.7 ± 0.9	111 ± 7.1	136[a] ± 11
2	169 ± 8	18 ± 3.4	96 ± 2.5	124[a] ± 2.6
3	197 ± 15	16 ± 3.0	79[a] ± 8.6	135[a] ± 13
7	186 ± 7	34 ± 6.5	71[a] ± 9.4	139[a] ± 14
14	214 ± 6	8.5 ± 2.3	52[a] ± 4.6	152[a] ± 17

[a] Significant difference from mean control value ($p < 0.05$).

TABLE VI

Effect of exposure to a pressure of 380 mm of Hg while fasting on incorporation of ^{14}C-leucine into albumin and transferrin by liver slices

Each liver weight and incorporation value is the mean from 4 animals expressed as a percentage of the corresponding value from 4 rats maintained at ambient pressure but fasted ± standard error of the mean.

Duration of exposure	Body weight	Liver weight	Incorporation	
			Albumin	Transferrin
days	*g*	*% control*	*% control*	
1	175 ± 2.8	132[a] ± 6.2	105 ± 7.9	131[a] ± 5.8
2	167 ± 3.6	129[a] ± 4.5	103 ± 10	189[a] ± 14
3	160 ± 6.3	112[a] ± 3.9	109 ± 22	198[a] ± 19
4	155 ± 8.8	100 ± 2.7	108 ± 16	211[a] ± 21

[a] Significant difference from mean control value ($p < 0.05$).

from the livers of the animals maintained at normal pressure. In addition, it had no significant effect on the increase of incorporation into transferrin which followed exposure to reduced pressure. Attempts were made to see whether a larger dose of actinomycin would alter the response to reduced pressure by repeating this experiment with double the dose of actinomycin, but all of the rats exposed to the reduced pressure died during the exposure.

DISCUSSION

There is good evidence that the incorporation of ^{14}C-labeled amino acids into albumin by liver slices is due to synthesis of albumin and can be used to measure this synthesis (14, 23). This is supported in the present work by the progressive incorporation of ^{14}C-leucine into albumin by liver slices during 3 hours of incubation, and the inhibition of incorporation by several general metabolic inhibitors, and by cycloheximide which inhibits protein synthesis in rat liver (24, 25) and in other tissues. The effects of incubation time and of the inhibitors on ^{14}C-leucine incorporation into transferrin by liver and spleen slices and into γG-globulin by spleen indicate that the incorporation into these proteins was also due to synthesis. Although incorporation into transferrin per g of tissue was approximately the same for spleen and bone marrow as for liver, the far greater total weight of liver than the other tissues indicates that the liver is much more important than either spleen or marrow for transferrin synthesis. The results of the experiments *in vivo* emphasize the dominance of the liver in transferrin synthesis and suggest that this may in fact be considerably greater than indicated by the experiments *in vitro*.

The main purpose of this investigation was to study the effects of several factors, known to influence plasma transferrin concentration, on transferrin synthesis, with the use of the incorporation of ^{14}C-leucine into transferrin by tissue slices as a measure of synthesis. For this method to be valid, it is necessary either to know the specific activity of the precursor amino acid in the incubation system or at least to know that the specific activity was the same with slices from different animals. An attempt was made to reduce the effect of variations in intracellular leucine pools between animals by using much more leucine in the incubation medium than is present in rat liver (26, 27). The use of a second protein as well as transferrin with both liver and spleen slices made it possible to determine whether a change of incorporation of leucine into transferrin after a certain treatment was due to a general effect on the incorporation of the labeled amino acid into protein, such as from a change of the intracellular amino acid pool, or to a specific change in rate of transferrin synthesis. The results of the experiments in which the leucine concentration of the incubation solution was altered (Fig. 2) showed that the effect of leucine concentration on ^{14}C incorporation was the same into transferrin and albumin by liver, or into transferrin and γG-globulin by spleen. Hence, it appears that the two proteins of each pair utilize leucine from the same pool in both liver and spleen, and a change in leucine concentration or specific activity would affect incorporation into both proteins proportionately.

An increase in the incorporation of ^{14}C-leucine into transferrin by liver slices was found in the rats with hemorrhagic iron deficiency anemia and in those treated with thyroxine or by exposure to reduced atmospheric pressure. Only in the thyroxine-treated rats was there also a similar increase of incorporation into albumin. Hence, hemorrhagic anemia and reduced pressure probably lead to a specific increase in transferrin synthesis, whereas thyroxine stimulates protein synthesis by the liver more generally, as has been previously established (28, 29). A significant depression of ^{14}C-leucine incorporation into transferrin was found with liver slices from the polycythemic rats and from the rats given propylthiouracil or from which food was withheld. The effect of polycythemia was specific for transferrin, but propylthiouracil and fasting also affected incorporation into albumin. The effect of polythiouracil was probably the result of reversal of the general effect of thyroxine on protein synthesis by liver cells. These results indicate that the increased plasma transferrin level found in iron deficiency anemia and after the administration of thyroxine (5) or exposure to reduced atmospheric pressure are the result of increased synthesis by the liver. The decreased transferrin levels found in transfusional polycythemia (30), propylthiouracil treatment (5), or fasting (4), on the other hand, are the result of decreased synthesis by the liver. Possibly, the major underlying cause of these changes in transferrin synthesis is the relative balance between oxygen supply and requirement (3), acting directly on the liver parenchymal cell, or indirectly through a humoral agent produced in a tissue other than the liver. The failure of treatment with iron-dextran to produce any evidence of a change in transferrin synthesis indicates that an increase of tissue non-heme iron does not inhibit transferrin synthesis in the rat, which is in keeping with the failure of iron-dextran and other causes of iron overload in the absence of anemia or polycythemia to affect plasma transferrin concentration in the rat (3, 30, 31).

Exposure to reduced atmospheric pressure produced a significant increase in the incorporation of ^{14}C-leucine into transferrin by liver slices, which was apparent within one day and which lasted for at least two weeks. Incorporation into albumin, on the other hand, was depressed by the third day of exposure (Table V). This treatment led to body weight loss, probably due to loss of body water (32) and to decreased food intake. Therefore, in order to determine the influence of food intake on the results with low pressure, experiments were performed with fasted rats both at ambient pressure and reduced pressure. Fasting at ambient pressure caused an approximately equal inhibition of incorporation of ^{14}C into both transferrin and albumin (Table IV), probably as the result of decreased ribosomal RNA synthesis (33). However, when the fasted rats were exposed to reduced atmospheric pressure, there was no significant difference in the incorporation of ^{14}C-leucine into albumin when compared with fasted rats at normal pressure, although incorporation into transferrin was markedly enhanced (Table VI). It therefore appears that exposure to reduced atmospheric pressure resulted in decreased food intake, while transferrin synthesis was stimulated despite the tendency of decreased food intake to a lower rate of transferrin synthesis. The biochemical mechanism whereby decreased atmospheric pressure, or the other causes of increased transferrin synthesis, produced their effect is uncertain. The results of the experiments in which actinomycin D was used suggest that the mechanism may not involve increased formation of the messenger RNA for transferrin synthesis. The dose of actinomycin used has been shown to inhibit the induction or stimulation of enzyme activity in rat liver (34, 35) and also to inhibit the incorporation of ^{14}C-adenine into rat liver RNA (36). It is possible, however, that a larger dose is required to inhibit transferrin messenger RNA synthesis, but attempts to use a larger dose resulted in death of the rats during exposure to the reduced pressure.

Acknowledgment—I am indebted to Mr. A. Leslie for performing the tissue non-heme measurements.

REFERENCES

1. BOTHWELL, T. H., AND FINCH, C. A., *Iron metabolism*, J. and H. Churchill Ltd., London, 1962.
2. MORGAN, E. H., *Aust. J. Exp. Biol. Med. Sci.*, **39**, 371 (1961).
3. MORGAN, E. H., *Quart. J. Exp. Physiol. Cog. Med. Sci.*, **47**, 57 (1962).
4. MORGAN, E. H., *Quart. J. Exp. Physiol. Cog. Med. Sci.*, **48**, 181 (1963).
5. MORGAN, E. H., *Quart. J. Exp. Physiol. Cog. Med. Sci.*, **48**, 176 (1963).
6. PHILLIPS, M. E., AND THORBECKE, G. J., *Int. Arch. Allergy Appl. Immunol.*, **29**, 553 (1966).
7. STECHER, V. J., AND THORBECKE, G. J., *J. Immunol.*, **99**, 643 (1967).
8. ASOFSKY, R., AND THORBECKE, G. J., *J. Exp. Med.*, **14**, 471 (1961).
9. PRUNIER, J. H., BEARN, A. G., AND CLEVE, H., *Proc. Soc. Exp. Biol. Med.*, **115**, 1005 (1964).
10. THORBECKE, G. J., HOCHWALD, G. M., VAN FURTH, R., MULLER-EBERHARD, H. J., AND JACOBSON, E. B., *Ciba Foundation Symposium on Complement*, J. and A. Churchill Ltd., London, 1965, p. 99.
11. SMITH, J. L., LAWTON, J. W. M., AND FORBES, I. J., *Aust. J. Exp. Biol. Med. Sci.*, **45**, 629 (1967).
12. MORGAN, E. H., *J. Physiol. (London)*, **171**, 26 (1964).
13. KUNKEL, H. G., AND WARD, S. M., *J. Biol. Chem.*, **182**, 597 (1950).
14. PETERS, T., JR., AND ANFINSEN, C. B., *J. Biol. Chem.*, **186**, 805 (1950).
15. KREBS, H. A., AND HENSELEIT, K., *Hoppe-Seyler's Z. Physiol.*

Chem., **210**, 33 (1932).
16. Ballard, F. J., and Oliver, I. T., *Biochem. J.*, **90**, 261 (1964).
17. Herberg, R. J., *Anal. Chem.*, **32**, 42 (1960).
18. Kingsley, G. R., *J. Lab. Clin. Med.*, **27**, 840 (1942).
19. Morgan, E. H., and Carter, G., *Australas. Ann. Med.*, **9**, 209 (1960).
20. Kaldor, I., *Aust. J. Exp. Biol. Med. Sci.*, **32**, 795 (1954).
21. Courtice, F. C., Harding, J., and Steinbeck, A. W., *Aust. J. Exp. Biol. Med. Sci.*, **31**, 215 (1953).
22. Hollingsworth, J. W., *Proc. Soc. Exp. Biol. Med.*, **87**, 493 (1964).
23. Campbell, P. N., and Stone, N. E., *Biochem. J.*, **66**, 19 (1957).
24. Wettstein, F. O., Noll, H., and Penman, S., *Biochim. Biophys. Acta*, **87**, 525 (1964).
25. Korner, A., *Biochem. J.*, **101**, 627 (1966).
26. Schimassek, H., and Gerok, W., *Biochem. A.*, **343**, 407 (1965).
27. Hanking, B. M., and Roberts, S., *Biochim. Biophys. Acta*, **104**, 427 (1965).
28. Sokoloff, L., and Kaufman, S., *J. Biol. Chem.*, **236**, 795 (1961).
29. Tata, J. R., Ernster, L., Lindberg, O., Arrhenius, E., Pedersen, S., and Hedman, R., *Biochem. J.*, **86**, 408 (1963).
30. Morgan, E. H., *Aust. J. Exp. Biol. Med. Sci.*, **39**, 361 (1961).
31. Morgan, E. H., *Amer. J. Physiol.*, **211**, 1486 (1966).
32. Picon-Reategui, E., Fryers, G. R., Berlin, N. I., and Lawrence, J. H., *Amer. J. Physiol.*, **172**, 33 (1953).
33. Hirsch, C. A., and Hiatt, H. H., *J. Biol. Chem.*, **241**, 5936 (1966).
34. Greengard, O., and Acs, G., *Biochim. Biophys. Acta*, **61**, 652 (1962).
35. Gleboin, H. V., and Blackburn, N. R., *Biochim. Biophys. Acta*, **72**, 657 (1963).
36. Drysdale, J. W., and Munro, H. N., *J. Biol. Chem.*, **241**, 3630 (1966).

AUTHOR INDEX

KEY-WORD TITLE INDEX